# Statistical Analysis of fMRI Data

# Statistical Analysis of fMRI Data

F. Gregory Ashby

The MIT Press
Cambridge, Massachusetts
London, England

For information about special quantity discounts, please email special_sales@mitpress.mit.edu

This book was set in Times New Roman and Syntax by Asco Typesetters, Hong Kong. Printed and bound in the United States of America.

Library of Congress Cataloging-in-Publication Data

Ashby, F. Gregory.
Statistical analysis of fMRI data / F. Gregory Ashby.
 p. ;  cm.
Includes bibliographical references and index.
ISBN 978-0-262-01504-2 (hardcover : alk. paper)
1. Magnetic resonance imaging. 2. Brain mapping. I. Title.
[DNLM: 1. Magnetic Resonance Imaging—statistics & numerical data. 2. Data Interpretation, Statistical. WN 185 A823s  2011]
QP376.6.A84  2011
616.07'548—dc22                                                                 2010018803

10  9  8  7  6  5  4  3  2  1

To Heidi, Duncan, Graham, and Coltrane

# Contents

Preface     xi

Acronyms     xv

**1    Introduction     1**

What Is fMRI?     2

The Scanning Session     4

Experimental Design     6

Data Analysis     7

Software Packages     8

**2    Data Formats     11**

Data Formats     11

    DICOM     11

    Analyze     13

    NIfTI     13

    MINC     14

Converting from One Format to Another     14

Reading fMRI Data into MATLAB     15

**3    Modeling the BOLD Response     17**

Linear Models of the BOLD Response     17

    Methods of Estimating the hrf     21

        Input an Impulse, and Observe the Response     21

        Deconvolution     22

        Open the Box; Study the Circuit     25

        Take a Guess     25

        Select a Flexible Mathematical Model of the hrf     28

Nonlinear Models of the BOLD Response     33

Conclusions     40

**4    Preprocessing     41**

Slice-Timing Correction     42

    Slice-Timing Correction during Preprocessing     43

Linear Interpolation    43
Spline Interpolation    44
Sinc Interpolation    45
Slice-Timing Correction during Task-Related Statistical Analysis    47
Head Motion Correction    51
Coregistering the Functional and Structural Data    58
Normalization    63
Spatial Smoothing    68
Temporal Filtering    73
Other Preprocessing Steps    77
Quality Assurance    78
Distortion Correction    78
Grand Mean Scaling    79
Conclusions    80

**5    The General Linear Model    81**
The FBR Method    81
Jittering    84
Microlinearity versus Macrolinearity    86
Using the General Linear Model to Implement the FBR Method    87
Modeling Baseline Activation and Systematic Non-Task-Related Variation in the BOLD Signal    88
Designs with Multiple Stimulus Events    90
The Correlation Approach    91
Block Designs    97
A Graphical Convention for Displaying the Design Matrix    99
The General Linear Model    100
Parameter Estimation    103
Parameter Estimation in the FBR and Correlation Models    104
Hypothesis Testing via the Construction of Statistical Parametric Maps    107
Nonparametric Approaches to Hypothesis Testing    118
Percent Signal Change    119
Comparing the Correlation and FBR Methods    123

**6    The Multiple Comparisons Problem    127**
The Sidak and Bonferroni Corrections    128
Gaussian Random Fields    130
False Discovery Rate    141
Cluster-Based Methods    147
Cluster-Based Methods Using a Spatial Extent Criterion    150
Cluster-Based Methods Using a Criterion That Depends on Cluster Height and Spatial Extent    153
Permutation-Based Solutions to the Multiple Comparisons Problem    156
Voodoo Correlations    157
Conclusions    158

**7    Group Analyses   159**
Individual Differences     159
Fixed versus Random Factors in the General Linear Model     162
A Fixed Effects Group Analysis     164
A Random Effects Group Analysis     170
Comparing Fixed and Random Effects Analyses     175
Multiple Factor Experiments     176
Power Analysis     178

**8    Coherence Analysis   185**
Autocorrelation and Cross-Correlation     186
Power Spectrum and Cross-Power Spectrum     193
Coherence     197
Partial Coherence     209
Using the Phase Spectrum to Determine Causality     211
Conclusions     219

**9    Granger Causality   221**
Quantitative Measures of Causality     226
Parameter Estimation     231
Inference     234
Conditional Granger Causality     235
Comparing Granger Causality to Coherence Analysis     242

**10    Principal Components Analysis   245**
Principal Components Analysis     246
PCA with fMRI Data     248
Using PCA to Eliminate Noise     251
Conclusions     256

**11    Independent Component Analysis   257**
The Cocktail-Party Problem     257
Applying ICA to fMRI Data     258
        Spatial ICA     260
        Assessing Statistical Independence     261
        The Importance of Non-normality in ICA     263
        Preparing Data for ICA     263
ICA Algorithms     266
        Minimizing Mutual Information     266
                Mathematical Definitions     267
                Conceptual Treatment     268
        Methods That Maximize Non-normality     269
        Maximum Likelihood Approaches     271
        Infomax     272
                Overview     272
                The Infomax Learning Algorithm     274

Interpreting ICA Results    277
    Determining the Relative Importance of Each Component    278
    Assigning Meaning to Components    279
The Noisy ICA Model    281
Other Issues    285
Comparing ICA and GLM Approaches    287
Conclusions    289

**12    Other Methods    291**
Pattern Classification Techniques    291
Partial Least Squares    292
Dynamic Causal Modeling    293
Bayesian Approaches    294

**Appendix A:  Matrix Algebra Tutorial    297**
Matrices and Their Basic Operations    297
Rank    304
Solving Linear Equations    306
Eigenvalues and Eigenvectors    310
    Definitions    310
    Properties    313

**Appendix B:  Multivariate Probability Distributions    315**
Multivariate Normal Distributions    316

References    321
Index    329

# Preface

My interests in functional magnetic resonance imaging (fMRI) began in the late 1990s. My lab (the Laboratory for Computational Cognitive Neuroscience) builds biologically detailed neural networks of a variety of cognitive behaviors (e.g., categorization, working memory, the development of automaticity, sequence learning). We had been testing these models against single-unit recording data at one extreme and behavioral data at the other. What was missing though were data at an intermediate level; that is, simultaneous measures of neural activation from a variety of brain regions as the subject performed the behavior under study. fMRI seemed the perfect methodology to fill this void. Our models made quantitative predictions about how neural activation changes in a set of interconnected, yet distributed brain regions as the subject performs some task. The goal was to use fMRI to test these predictions rigorously.

Using fMRI to test neural network models is not a standard application of fMRI. For example, the available fMRI software packages did not provide much help in achieving this goal. To proceed, I needed to understand fMRI data analysis at a deeper level than if my goals had been more conventional. After 4 or 5 years of study, I had learned enough to begin teaching a course, which I have offered regularly ever since. My course is a companion to one taught by Scott Grafton, who is the director of the University of California, Santa Barbara (UCSB) Brain Imaging Center. In a nutshell, Scott's course covers everything up through the end of data collection in a typical fMRI experiment, and my course covers everything after this. More specifically, I survey all topics a typical researcher needs to know to analyze a set of raw fMRI data. This text grew out of that teaching experience.

The goal of this book is for readers to understand the most important current methods for analyzing fMRI data. The aim is not to describe which buttons to push in the popular software packages. Rather, the goal for each method is for readers to understand the basic underlying logic, the assumptions, the strengths and weaknesses, and when the method is or is not appropriate to apply. In most cases, researchers who have read this book will still use a standard software package to analyze their data. However, they will now know what computations are being performed in each step of data analysis, and they will know the advantages and disadvantages of each of the various options they are offered.

The most important current topics in fMRI data analysis are all covered. Chapter 3 surveys models of how the fMRI blood oxygen level–dependent (BOLD) response is related to neural activation. Chapters 4–7 cover the basic analyses that are routinely done in virtually every fMRI article (preprocessing; using the general linear model to construct statistical parametric maps; solving the multiple comparisons problem; and group analyses). Chapters 8 and 9 cover the most popular methods for assessing functional connectivity (coherence analysis and Granger causality), and Chapters 10 and 11 cover the most popular multivariate approaches (principal components analysis and independent component analysis). Finally, chapter 12 briefly surveys a variety of other current fMRI methods.

The book also includes short examples of MATLAB code that implement many of the methods that are described. These were included to allow an interested reader to experiment with these methods on his or her own fMRI data. To facilitate this process, chapter 2 describes the most common fMRI data formats and includes a description of how to read data from any of these formats into MATLAB. In addition, appendix A includes a brief introduction to basic MATLAB matrix algebra commands.

The book assumes no prior background in fMRI. The only special background needed is basic statistical inference. As I was writing, I had in mind a student who had completed my two-quarter first-year statistics sequence, which surveys univariate statistical tests (e.g., t-tests) and analysis of variance. All relevant material not commonly taught in such courses is covered in this book. For example, appendix A is a brief tutorial on matrix algebra, and appendix B introduces multivariate probability distributions (including the multivariate normal distribution).

Many of the methods covered in the book are based on some fairly sophisticated mathematics. For example, a number of techniques for correcting for multiple comparisons depend on Gaussian random field theory, and coherence analysis depends on Fourier transforms of cross-correlation functions. In these cases, the necessary mathematics is explained at a conceptual level that will allow readers without an extensive mathematical background to understand the basic ideas. At the same time, enough mathematics is given so that mathematically sophisticated readers can gain more than a purely conceptual understanding.

I learned how to balance a conceptual presentation with one that is more mathematically rigorous during my 25-plus years of teaching graduate statistics. For example, in my first-year graduate statistics sequence that is required of all students pursuing a doctorate in psychology at UCSB, I once had a student with a graduate degree in mathematics sitting next to a student who had never had a course in calculus. Although this case was extreme, every course I taught included students with hugely diverse mathematical backgrounds. Struggling to simultaneously provide a fulfilling experience for all of these students taught me lessons that proved invaluable when writing this book.

Many people provided invaluable feedback on earlier drafts of the chapters in this book and for this I am deeply grateful. Included in this list are Kamal Agarwal, Michael Casale, Matthew Crossley, Christa Lynn Donovan, James Elliott, John Ennis, Amy Frithsen, Scott

Grafton, Sébastien Hélie, Arianne Johnson, Mari Jones, Ryan Kasper, Sangin Kim, Danielle King, Jennifer Kudo, Stephen Mack, Mario Mendoza, Jeffrey O'Brien, Erick Paul, Jessica Roeder, Dennis Rünger, Brian Spiering, Benjamin Turner, Jennifer Waldschmidt, Amber Westcott-Baker, Todd Wilkinson, and Julia Xin. Their comments and suggestions greatly improved the quality of every chapter in this book.

## Acronyms

| | |
|---|---|
| AFNI | Analysis of Functional NeuroImages (fMRI data analysis software package) |
| ANOVA | Analysis of variance |
| BOLD | Blood oxygen-level dependent |
| DTI | Diffusion tensor imaging |
| FBR | Finite BOLD response |
| FDR | False discovery rate |
| FIR | Finite impulse response |
| fMRI | Functional magnetic resonance imaging |
| FSL | FMRIB Software Library (fMRI data analysis software package) |
| FWHM | Full width at half maximum |
| GLM | General linear model |
| GRF | Gaussian random field |
| hrf | Hemodynamic response function |
| ICA | Independent component analysis |
| MVUE | Minimum variance unbiased estimator |
| PCA | Principal components analysis |
| pdf | Probability density function |
| ROI | Region of interest |
| SPM | Statistical Parametric Mapping (fMRI data analysis software package) |
| SSD | Sum of squared differences |
| SSE | Sum of squared errors |
| TR | Repetition time |

# 1 Introduction

Functional magnetic resonance imaging (fMRI) provides researchers the opportunity to observe neural activity noninvasively in the human brain, albeit indirectly, as it changes in near real time. This exciting technology has revolutionized the scientific study of the mind. The effects have probably been greatest within cognitive psychology and perception, but the influence of fMRI has spread to almost every area of the mind sciences. For example, there are now emerging new fields of social neuroscience, developmental neuroscience, and neuroeconomics, all largely because of fMRI. There is even a new field of neuromarketing.

fMRI has provided exciting new opportunities to study topics that had long seemed out of reach of rigorous scientific investigation. For example, the past few years have seen studies published in reputable journals in which researchers used fMRI to study the nature of consciousness (e.g., Lloyd, 2002), the effects of meditation on brain function (e.g., Cahn & Polich, 2006), and the neural basis of moral judgments (e.g., Greene, Sommerville, Nystrom, Darley, & Cohen, 2001). Researchers interested in using this new technology in their own research, however, have some notable challenges ahead when the time comes to analyze the data they collect. An fMRI experiment produces massive amounts of highly complex data. The statistical methods that most mind science researchers were trained on in graduate school, such as analysis of variance (ANOVA) and regression, provide a useful background for the most basic methods of fMRI analysis, but even the most straightforward fMRI analysis is considerably more complex than most classic treatments of ANOVA and regression. Furthermore, many other statistical methods that are now routinely used to analyze fMRI data are almost never covered in traditional statistics courses. Among many other topics, this includes, for example, Gaussian random field theory, false discovery rate, coherence analysis, Granger causality, and independent component analysis. Even worse (or better, depending on your perspective), complex new fMRI data analysis techniques are being proposed all the time. In fact, the statistical analysis of fMRI data is now a popular research area in statistics departments around the world.

This text introduces and surveys the most widely used current statistical methods of analyzing fMRI data. Every step is covered—from preprocessing to advanced methods for assessing functional connectivity. Because understanding the data analysis process is always a critical prerequisite to designing an efficient and powerful experiment, a naïve reader who works through this book will learn much about fMRI experimental design, though it should be understood by readers at the outset that this text focuses exclusively on data analysis. Just as a text on ANOVA and regression would not typically describe the computer equipment that may have been used to collect the data, this book does not include a description of the complex machinery and equipment one finds in a typical brain-imaging center or of how to run this equipment effectively (e.g., set the many parameters that control the scanner; spot and avoid artifacts that can corrupt the data). Neither is there any description of the physics of fMRI. The reader interested in learning more about these topics is urged to consult any of the several good books that concentrate on these issues (e.g., Buxton, 2002; Huettel, Song, & McCarthy, 2004).

This book assumes no previous background in fMRI. It does assume some statistical background, however, including basic univariate statistical inference (e.g., t-tests) and some exposure to ANOVA and regression. Anyone who has completed the basic first-year statistics sequence that is required, for example, in almost every doctoral psychology program in the United States should have more than enough statistical background to understand this book. Multivariate normal distributions will also be encountered in several chapters, but a brief overview of the necessary material on this topic is provided in appendix B. At the mathematics level, a few integrals will be encountered that require some calculus to understand. Nevertheless, motivated readers without calculus should be able to follow 95% of the material in the book. Basic matrix algebra is also used extensively, but a survey of everything a reader would need to know about this topic is included in appendix A.

## What Is fMRI?

Magnetic resonance imaging (MRI) provides a method to study the structure and function of the brain by measuring differences in the magnetic properties of certain molecules. The first human MRI scanner was built in 1977, and in 1985 the Food and Drug Administration approved MRI for clinical use. Within 10 years, thousands of MRI instruments were installed in hospitals throughout the United States, and today MRI is a routine medical procedure. Perhaps the most important reason for the dramatic rise in popularity in MRI for diagnostic and scientific purposes is that MRI is completely noninvasive and carries few health risks. In this sense, MRI was a significant improvement over other available neuroimaging techniques. For example, computed tomography (CT) scanning uses x-rays, and positron emission tomography (PET) scanning requires injecting the subject with a drug containing a radioactive label.

Currently, the most common clinical application of MRI is to assess brain structure (or the structure of other tissue) by measuring the density of water molecules (most typically).

Because the density of water is different in air, white matter, gray matter, blood vessels, and tumors, MRI becomes an effective method for visualizing brain structure. In most hospitals, structural MRI is a routine procedure, but few hospitals currently perform fMRI, though medical applications of fMRI are likely to rise in the future. For example, one useful clinical application of fMRI could be as a presurgical procedure to map out the functional architecture of a patient's brain. Such a map would be useful to a neurosurgeon who wants to avoid excising tissue associated with some critical skill (e.g., speech).

The goal of fMRI is to observe the brain as it is functioning in as close to real time as possible. The ideal fMRI methodology would measure neural activity with high spatial resolution in real time. This goal has not yet been realized, and in fact, the best available current methods fall far short of this goal. For example, currently the typical fMRI experiment records a sluggish, indirect measure of neural activity with a temporal resolution of 1–3 seconds and a spatial resolution of 3–5 $mm^3$. Nevertheless, as the thousands of fMRI publications attest, this highly imperfect technology has dramatically influenced the study of mind and brain.

The vast majority of fMRI experiments measure the blood oxygen level–dependent (BOLD) signal. The physics of this process is complex and far beyond the scope of this text. Interested readers should consult Hashemi, Bradley, and Lisanti (2004) for a mostly nontechnical description; for those readers with a background in physics, Haacke, Brown, Thompson, and Venkatesan (1999) provide a much more rigorous treatment. For our purposes, it suffices to know that the BOLD signal is a measure of the ratio of oxygenated to deoxygenated hemoglobin.

Hemoglobin is a molecule in the blood that carries oxygen from the lungs to all parts of the body. It has sites to bind up to six oxygen molecules. A key discovery that eventually led to BOLD fMRI was the observation that hemoglobin molecules fully loaded with oxygen have different magnetic properties than those of hemoglobin molecules with empty binding sites (Pauling & Coryell, 1936).

The theory, which is not yet fully worked out, is that active brain areas consume more oxygen than do inactive areas. When neural activity increases in an area, metabolic demands rise, and, as a result, the vascular system rushes oxygenated hemoglobin into the area. Immediately after the neural activity, there is (typically) an oxygen debt, so the ratio of oxygenated to deoxygenated hemoglobin often falls below baseline levels. The rush of oxygenated hemoglobin into the area causes the ratio (i.e., the BOLD signal) to rise quickly. As it happens, the vascular system overcompensates, in the sense that the ratio of oxygenated to deoxygenated hemoglobin actually rises well above baseline to a peak at around 6 seconds after the neural activity that elicited these responses. After this peak, the BOLD signal gradually decays back to baseline over a period of 20–25 seconds.

Current evidence suggests that the neural activity most closely related to changes in the BOLD signal is the local field potential (Logothetis, 2003; Logothetis, Pauls, Augath, Trinath, & Oeltermann, 2001). This is the summed total electrical activity in a small region around the recording site. Chapter 3 explores these issues in more detail and reviews mathematical models of the relationship between neural activation and the BOLD signal. These models are critical in fMRI data analysis because in most cases, we are interested in an unobservable, latent construct; namely, neural activity. For this reason, we can use fMRI data to make inferences about neural activity only if we have a rough understanding of how neural activity is related to the observable BOLD response.

**The Scanning Session**

An experimental session that collects fMRI data also commonly includes a variety of other types of scans. Typically, the first scan completed in each session is the *localizer*. This is a very quick structural scan (1–2 minutes) of low spatial resolution that is used only to locate the subject's brain in three-dimensional space. This knowledge is needed to optimize the location of the slices that will be taken through the brain in the high-resolution structural scan and in the functional scans that follow.

The ordering of the other scans that are commonly performed is not critical. Frequently, however, the *high-resolution structural scan* would follow the localizer. Depending on the resolution of this scan and on the exact nature of the pulse sequences that are used to control the scanner during acquisition, it may take 8–10 minutes to complete this protocol. This structural scan plays a key role in the analysis of the functional data. Because speed is a high priority in fMRI (i.e., to maximize temporal resolution), spatial resolution is sacrificed when collecting functional data. The high-resolution structural scan can compensate somewhat for this loss of spatial information. This is done during preprocessing when the functional data are aligned with the structural image (see chapter 4 for details). After this mapping is complete, the spatial coordinates of activation observed during fMRI can be determined by examining the aligned coordinates in the structural image.

The third step is often to collect the functional data. This can be done in one long run that might take 20–30 minutes to complete or can be broken down into two or three shorter runs, with brief rests in between. There are many parameter choices to make here, but two are especially important for the subsequent analysis of fMRI data. One choice is the time between successive whole-brain scans, which is called the *repetition time* and is abbreviated TR. If the whole brain is scanned, typical TRs range from 2 to 3 seconds, but TRs of 1 second or faster are possible on many machines, especially if some parts of the brain are excluded from the scanning.

Another important choice is voxel size, which determines the spatial resolution of the functional data. When a subject lies in the scanner, his or her brain occupies a certain volume. If we assign a coordinate system to the bore of the magnet, then we could identify any point in the subject's brain by a set of three coordinate values $(x, y, z)$. By convention, the $z$ direction runs down the length of the bore (from the feet to the head), and the $x$ and $y$ directions reference the plane that is created by taking a cut perpendicular to the $z$ axis. The brain, of course, is a continuous medium, in the sense that neurons exist at (almost) every set of coordinate values inside the brain. fMRI data, however, are discrete. The analog-to-digital conversion is performed by dividing the brain into a set of cubes (or, more accurately, rectangular right prisms). These cubes are called *voxels* because they are three-dimensional analogues of pixels; that is, they could be considered as volume pixels.

A typical voxel size might be 3 mm × 3 mm × 3.5 mm. In this case, in a typical human brain, 33 separate slices might be acquired, each containing a 64 × 64 array of voxels, for a whole-brain total of 135,168 voxels. In each fMRI run, a BOLD response is recorded every TR seconds in each voxel. Thus, for example, in a 30-minute run with a TR of 2 seconds, 135,168 BOLD responses could be recorded 900 separate times (i.e., 30 times per minute × 30 minutes), for a total of 121,651,200 BOLD values. This is an immense amount of data, and its sheer volume greatly contributes to the difficulties in data analysis.

Many studies stop when the functional data acquisition is complete, but two other types of scans are also common. One is to collect a *field map*. The ideal scanner has a completely uniform magnetic field across its entire bore. Even if this were true, placing a human subject inside of the bore will distort this field to some extent. After the subject is inside the scanner, all inhomogeneities in the magnetic field are corrected via a process known as *shimming*. If shimming is successful, the magnetic field will be uniform at the start of scanning. Sometimes, however, especially in less reliable machines, distortions in the magnetic field will reappear in the middle of the session. The field map, which takes only a minute or two to collect, measures the homogeneity of the magnetic field at the moment when the map is created. Thus, the field map can be used during later data analysis to correct for possible nonlinear distortions in the strength of the magnetic field that develop during the course of the scanning session.

A final common type of scan is *diffusion tensor imaging* (DTI). The goal here is to measure the major fiber tracts (e.g., bundles of axons) of the subject's brain. Although all human brains will theoretically contain the same major tracts, there is surprising variability across individuals in the robustness or thickness of these tracts. DTI can be useful for correlating performance in a task across subjects with the measured robustness of a theoretically relevant fiber tract.

DTI measures the distance and direction along which water molecules diffuse during a short but fixed amount of time. During any fixed time interval, water molecules outside of cells will tend to diffuse the same distance in every direction, but inside of a neuron, for example, water will diffuse farther up and down the length of an axon than it will diffuse in a direction perpendicular to the axon. Thus, the first step in analyzing DTI data is to find locations where diffusion in one direction is much greater than in any other direction. By linking together such directions from neighboring points, it may be possible to trace out fiber tracts. This linking process is called *tractography*. DTI is not covered in this book. Readers interested in learning about this important topic should consult any of several excellent reviews (e.g., Le Bihan et al., 2001; Mori, 2007).

**Experimental Design**

In clinical applications where the only goal is to collect a high-resolution structural scan, the subject lies passively inside the scanner during the entire procedure. In fMRI, however, subjects are typically given some task to perform. In the standard setup, a mirror is attached to the top of the bore and directed at the subject's eyes. A computer-controlled projector directs visual information onto this mirror, and the subject responds to this material, often by pressing a button on a hand-held device.

fMRI experiments use either a *block design* or an *event-related design*. In a block design, the functional run consists of a series of blocks, each of which may last for somewhere between 30 seconds to a couple of minutes. Within each block, subjects are instructed to perform the same cognitive, perceptual, or motor task continuously from the beginning of the block until the end. In almost all block design experiments, subjects will simply rest on some blocks. For example, a researcher interested in studying the neural network that mediates rhythmic finger tapping might use a block design in which blocks where the subject is resting alternate with blocks in which the subject taps his or her finger according to some certain rhythm.

Event-related designs are run more like standard psychological experiments, in the sense that the functional run is broken down into a set of discrete trials. Usually, each trial is one of several types, and each type is repeated at least 20 times over the course of the experiment (described more fully in chapter 5). As in a standard experiment, however, the presentation order of the trial types within each run is often random. When analyzing data from an event-related design, it is critical to know exactly when the presentation of each stimulus occurred relative to TR onset. A common practice is to synchronize stimulus presentation with TR onset. This is done in the following way. At the onset of each TR, the computer controlling the scanner sends a pulse to the computer that controls the experiment. The experiment is programmed in such a way that stimulus presentation is delayed until exactly the time when this pulse is received.

The first event-related designs included long rests between each pair of successive trials. In these *slow event-related designs*, rests of 30 seconds are typical. These are included so that the BOLD response in brain regions that participate in stimulus processing can decay back to baseline levels before the presentation of the next stimulus. This makes statistical sense, but it is expensive as it greatly reduces the number of trials a subject can complete in any given functional run. Another problem is that because subjects have so much time with nothing to do, they might think about something during these long rests, and any such uncontrolled cognition would generate an unwanted BOLD response that might contaminate the stimulus-induced BOLD response.

Most current event-related designs use much shorter delays. These *rapid event-related designs* became possible because statistical methods were developed for dealing with the overlapping BOLD responses that will occur anytime the BOLD response in a brain region has not decayed to baseline by the time another stimulus is presented. The most widely used of these methods are described in chapter 5. It is important to realize, however, that even in rapid event-related designs, the delay between trials is still significantly longer than in standard laboratory experiments. For example, a typical rapid event-related design might use random delays between successive trials that might cover a range between, say, 2 and 16 seconds. There are several reasons for this. First, because of the need to synchronize stimulus presentation with the TR, it is often necessary to delay stimulus presentation until the onset of the next TR. Second, to get unique estimates of the parameters of the standard statistical models that are used to analyze fMRI data, delays of random duration must be used (a process known as *jittering*). This topic is covered in detail in chapter 5.

### Data Analysis

A number of features of fMRI data make it especially challenging to analyze. First, as mentioned above, a typical scanning session generates a huge amount of data. Second, fMRI data are characterized by substantial spatial and temporal correlations. For example, the sluggish nature of the BOLD response means that a voxel in which the BOLD response is greater than average on some particular TR is also likely to be greater than average on the ensuing TR. Similarly, because brain tissue in neighboring voxels will be supplied by a similar vasculature, a large response in one voxel increases the likelihood that a large response will also be observed at neighboring voxels.

A third significant challenge to fMRI data analysis is the noisy nature of fMRI data. Typically, the signal that the data analysis techniques are trying to find is less than 2% or 3% of the total BOLD response. In other words, effect sizes are small. The noise has several sources. These can roughly be broken down into true noise and unaccounted-for signal.

One source of true noise is thermal motion of any electrons that are inside the bore of the magnet (i.e., including the brain) or in the equipment that is used to collect and process the raw data. A second true noise source is physiologic. For example, the same metabolic demand in the same brain region does not always elicit exactly the same BOLD response.

A number of other factors that contribute to observed noise in fMRI data might more accurately be described as unaccounted-for signal. These include head motion, scanner drift, and uncontrolled cognitive activity on the part of the subject. Relatively large head movements can be caused by the subject shifting his or her head position. Theoretically, these are corrected during preprocessing (as long as they are not too large; see chapter 4). Smaller movements occur as a result of heartbeat and respiration. One way to deal with these artifacts is to use biosensors to record heartbeat and respiration and then use these data as regressors during data analysis (see chapter 5). Scanner drift occurs when the strength of the magnetic field inside the bore slowly changes over the course of the scanning session. The possibility of such drift is often explicitly modeled during data analysis.

Finally, of course, anything the subject is thinking about that is unrelated to the task being studied will produce neural activation and changes in BOLD response. This is usually impossible to correct because such extraneous cognitive activity could presumably occur at any time and within almost any voxel. This seems especially likely in slow, event-related designs when the subject has long time periods without anything to do.

The analysis of fMRI BOLD data is broken down into two general stages: preprocessing and postprocessing. Preprocessing is covered in chapter 4, and the rest of this book is devoted to postprocessing. Preprocessing includes a number of steps that are required to prepare the data for statistical analysis. These include, for example, aligning the functional and structural scans, correcting for any possible head movements that might have occurred during the functional run, and various types of smoothing (to reduce noise).

Typically, the same preprocessing steps are always completed, regardless of the particular research questions that the study was designed to address. In contrast, postprocessing includes all analyses that are directed at these questions. This is a complex and rapidly changing field of statistics and is the main focus of this book.

**Software Packages**

A wide variety of software packages are available for fMRI data analysis. Many of these are free, and they each have their own advantages and disadvantages. The available software is frequently updated, so no attempt will be made here to thoroughly review each package.

The most widely used package is Statistical Parametric Mapping (SPM), which is written and maintained by the Wellcome Trust Centre for Neuroimaging at the University College London. SPM is freely available at <http://www.fil.ion.ucl.ac.uk/spm>. SPM is a collection of MATLAB functions and routines with some externally compiled C code that is included to increase processing speed. At the time of this writing, the most current version is SPM8, which was released in April 2009. A thorough description of the statistical foundations of SPM was provided by Friston, Ashburner, Kiebel, Nichols, and Penny (2007).

Another widely used fMRI data analysis software package is called FSL, which is an acronym for FMRIB Software Library. FSL is produced and maintained by the FMRIB Analysis Group at the University of Oxford in England. FSL is also freely available and can be downloaded at <http://www.fmrib.ox.ac.uk/fsl/index.html>. Descriptions of the statistical foundations of the FSL routines were provided by Smith et al. (2004) and by Woolrich et al. (2009).

BrainVoyager is a commercially available software package that contains routines written in C++ to optimize speed and that uses a sophisticated three-dimensional graphics environment. BrainVoyager is a product of the company Brain Innovation B.V. located in The Netherlands. A single license costs upward of $8000. More information about the package and its purchase are available at <http://www.brainvoyager.com/index.html>. A description of the underlying statistical foundations can be found in Goebel, Esposito, and Formisano (2006).

AFNI is a free software package created and maintained by neuroimaging researchers at the National Institute of Mental Health (NIMH) in Bethesda, Maryland. AFNI is an acronym for Analysis of Functional NeuroImages. AFNI is written in C and runs on Unix or Mac operating systems. It can be downloaded from <http://afni.nimh.nih.gov/afni>. The software is described by Cox (1996) and Cox and Hyde (1997).

# 2   Data Formats

The first challenge when analyzing fMRI data is to sort through the seemingly bewildering diversity of data formats. Unfortunately, different manufacturers of magnetic resonance (MR) systems and different data analysis software packages often use qualitatively different formats to store and process data. A further complication is that these different formats are highly complex, in the sense that they almost all include considerable qualitative and quantitative information other than the numerical values of the data collected during the experiment. The qualitative information might include the subject's name (usually in a coded format) and gender and a description of how particular spatial locations within the scanner are encoded in the data vector. The quantitative information could include numerical values of some of the scanner parameters used to collect the data and perhaps even the subject's age, height, and weight (again in a coded format).

This chapter describes some of the most commonly used fMRI data formats: DICOM, Analyze, NIfTI, and MINC. We will also consider methods for converting from one format to another. General purpose programming languages like MATLAB do not support any of these formats. Therefore, a researcher who writes his or her own MATLAB code for any data analysis step will have to convert from one of these standard formats to a format that is MATLAB compatible. Popular software packages such as SPM and FSL provide such code. The last section of this chapter describes several methods for taking fMRI data stored in a standard format and reading it into MATLAB. Later chapters will give short examples of MATLAB code that will implement the methods discussed in that chapter. By working through this chapter, readers will be able to load their own fMRI data into MATLAB and then use the MATLAB code presented in later chapters to experiment with most of the major data analysis methods described in this book.

## Data Formats

### DICOM

In the early 1980s, a number of different imaging technologies were available, including MRI, PET, and CT. Unfortunately, the images collected by these devices were stored in such idiosyncratic and nonintuitive ways that it was generally impossible for anyone other than the manufacturers to decode them. Thus, users were forced to rely solely on manufacturer-supplied software for data analysis. Because of this problem, in 1983 the American College of Radiology joined forces with the National Electrical Manufacturers Association with the goal of standardizing the formatting of medical imaging. This group established a series of data formatting standards that eventually became known as DICOM (*D*igital *I*maging and *Co*mmunications in *M*edicine). The DICOM standard has been continuously revised and expanded since 1983, and today a complete description of this standard runs to well over 1000 pages (available from <http://medical.nema.org>). Despite its complexity, DICOM is now the industry standard and has been adopted by the manufacturers of most MR systems. As a result, in most brain-imaging centers, the raw data collected in fMRI experiments come off the machine in DICOM format.

Every DICOM file includes two components: an *image* and a *header*. The image contains the data collected from the imaging device. In fMRI this could be the data from the high-resolution structural scan, the BOLD data collected during one particular TR, the localizer, diffusion tensor data, or a field map. The header includes a wide variety of information describing the subject and the scanning parameters. The DICOM committee wanted to ensure that imaging data would not become uninterpretable if it was somehow separated from any external documentation that described how and why it was originally collected. As a result, all of this information is routinely included as part of the header on each image file.

A typical header might include information related to the subject's name, age, height, and weight, the date and time when the data were collected, the type of data (e.g., MR vs. PET), and numerical values of many scanning parameters. Imaging centers routinely anonymize or de-identify the header to protect the subject's confidentiality according to Health Insurance Portability and Accountability Act (HIPPA) privacy rules (i.e., encoding all private information via a secure, unique key). In addition, the header also includes a description of exactly how each voxel location is encoded into the DICOM image file. This latter information is especially important for fMRI data analysis. For example, the high-resolution structural image is inherently three-dimensional; that is, for the purposes of data analysis, the location of each voxel is encoded as an ordered triple $(x, y, z)$, where, by convention, the $x$ axis runs through the subject's ears (from left to right), the $y$ axis runs from the back of the head through the forehead (posterior/anterior), and the $z$ axis is parallel to the scanner bore (and so runs from the feet through the head). The BOLD responses collected during one functional run are even more complex as these data are inherently four-dimensional. In addition to the three spatial dimensions, a fourth time dimension is needed to keep track of which TR the image is from.

In contrast, in all current MR image formats, including DICOM, the image file where these data are stored is inherently one-dimensional—essentially just a long string of numbers. Thus, to interpret this string, it is vital to know how a particular spatial location within the scanner [i.e., an (*x*, *y*, *z*) coordinate], and perhaps how a particular TR, maps to a particular position within the string. For more details about this problem, see Herrington, Sutton, and Miller (2007).

DICOM headers contain some standard information that is always the same (i.e., the public field) and other information that may be unique to the MR manufacturer (i.e., the private field). Because of this latter idiosyncratic information, DICOM is not exactly a standard format; rather, it is better described as a set of similar formats.

DICOM is not a useful format for fMRI data analysis. One problem is that a single fMRI session will typically generate several thousand DICOM files. Furthermore, each of these files will include its own header, even though all of these separate headers will be mostly identical. Thus, a single fMRI session creates an enormous number of large DICOM files that contain much redundant information. All of these files make data analysis difficult, so the raw DICOM files are often converted to some other more convenient format before data analysis begins.

## Analyze

The Analyze format was developed at the Mayo Clinic partly as an alternative to DICOM. For much of the past decade, Analyze was the most frequently used format in fMRI data analysis, and for a number of years it was the standard for both SPM and FSL. Analyze breaks the header and image components of the DICOM format into separate files. Header files end with a .hdr extension, whereas image files end with a .img extension. Analyze can also store three-dimensional and four-dimensional data in one file. As a result, the hundreds of separate DICOM files that are typically created from a single functional run can be collapsed into two Analyze files: one header file and one four-dimensional image file. This is much more convenient for data analysis.

The Analyze header file contains considerably less information than the DICOM header, and more importantly, it lacks certain details that are needed for unambiguous interpretation of Analyze data. Both SPM and FSL compensate for some of these omissions by adding extra data to nonessential fields in the Analyze header (e.g., coordinates that specify the location of the anterior commissure, which can be used during preprocessing). Nevertheless, some ambiguities remain. In particular, Analyze headers do not contain enough information about the orientation of data in the image file to know the exact spatial location within the scanner of each intensity value in the image file. At the minimum, therefore, it is often difficult to tell the left hemisphere from the right hemisphere when viewing Analyze data. Detailed information about Analyze software and formatting can be found at <http://www.wideman-one.com/gw/brain/analyze/formatdoc.htm>.

## NIfTI

A newer format, called NIfTI (<u>N</u>euroimaging <u>I</u>nformatics <u>T</u>echnology <u>I</u>nitiative), was created in an effort to preserve the major advantages of Analyze but to avoid some of the disadvantages. NIfTI retains the ability of Analyze to encode three- and four-dimensional data, but it uses a more extensive header and as a result avoids most of the ambiguities that arise with the Analyze format. NIfTI was created from the Analyze format by adding new standard information into the empty fields of the Analyze header. The most important addition was to include information that avoids the left–right ambiguity inherent to the Analyze format.

NIfTI data files carry a .nii extension, and like DICOM, the header and image fields are merged into the same file. Even so, by creating NIfTI as a modification of Analyze, it was hoped that the new NIfTI format would still be compatible with older software that was created for data in Analyze format. NIfTI has been a successful innovation, and it is rapidly replacing Analyze as the standard format for fMRI data analysis. For example, the newest version of SPM (i.e., SPM8) uses NIfTI as its default format, as do FSL and AFNI. For more details, see <http://nifti.nimh.nih.gov/nifti-1>.

### MINC

One other format that is widely used for fMRI data analysis is MINC, which is an acronym for *M*edical *I*maging *N*etCDF (Network Common Data Form). This is the format used, for example, by the Montreal Neurological Institute (MNI) software tools. MINC is a flexible format. For example, it can be used to encode data that have any number of dimensions (i.e., up to 100), and it includes a flexible header that can be used to store an arbitrary set of supporting information (both qualitative and quantitative). More detailed information is available at <http://en.wikibooks.org/wiki/MINC>.

### Converting from One Format to Another

As mentioned earlier, the data that come off the scanner with most MR systems are in DICOM format. So typically the first step in the data analysis process is to convert the data from DICOM to some other format. Fortunately, there are various software options for performing this task. In fact, free software is available for converting any of the formats described in this chapter into any of the other formats. During this conversion process, it is possible that some supporting information will be lost. For example, Analyze format tends to have smaller headers than those of DICOM or NIfTI. So when converting from either DICOM or NIfTI to Analyze, it is possible that some of the header information will be lost. Much more importantly, however, all of the intensity values collected from the scanner will be retained.

One of the most popular utilities for converting from DICOM to NIfTI was created by Chris Rorden of the University of South Carolina. This package, called dcm2nii, is available at <http://www.sph.sc.edu/comd/rorden/mricron/dcm2nii.html>. SPM has its own DICOM-to-NIfTI converter. FSL includes a toolbox called FSLUTILS, which contains a variety of utilities for manipulating data. One of these, called fslchfiletype, converts data back and forth between Analyze and NIfTI formats. A DICOM-to-MINC converter is available at <http://www.bic.mni.mcgill.ca/~jharlap/dicom>.

### Reading fMRI Data into MATLAB

There is a huge amount of software available for analyzing fMRI data. Even so, the time might come when one wants to manipulate the data in some way or to perform some unique analysis that is not easily accomplished with commercially available software packages. In such cases, the data must be formatted in a way that can be read by a standard computer language such as MATLAB.

MATLAB is a high-level programming language that is widely used in all areas of science. It can be used not only to analyze fMRI data but also to present the images to subjects in the MR scanner and to collect and record their responses. MATLAB is a matrix algebra–based language that can perform some extremely complex operations in a single line. For example, the eigenvalues and eigenvectors of a matrix can be computed in one line of code. Appendix A provides a tutorial on matrix algebra and along the way also provides a brief introduction to MATLAB commands.

All of the mathematical and statistical methods described in this book can be performed with MATLAB. For many of these, MATLAB code will be presented for implementing the method. Interested readers can therefore follow along with their own data. Running MATLAB code on one's own fMRI data, however, requires solving one additional problem—namely, that MATLAB does not read any of the data formats discussed so far. For example, MATLAB would not be able to interpret the header associated with any of the standard fMRI formats. Thus, one additional conversion is needed; namely, from a standard fMRI data format to a format that is MATLAB compatible.

A number of such converters have been written. One set of tools that can read either Analyze or NIfTI formats into MATLAB can be found at <http://www.mathworks.com/matlabcentral/fileexchange/8797> or at <http://www.rotman-baycrest.on.ca/~jimmy/NIfTI>. This software stores the information in the NIfTI file (for example) in a MATLAB cell array, which is a general purpose array in which each element can contain data of different qualitative types and sizes. For example, one cell can store descriptive information from the header and another cell can store the numerical data.

The numerical data file created by this package is denoted filename.img, where "filename" here substitutes for the actual filename. With functional data, filename.img will typically contain a four-dimensional array. The first two dimensions contain a matrix of all BOLD responses that were sampled in the same slice (e.g., dimensions $x$ and $y$). The third dimension typically denotes the slice number (e.g., dimension $z$), and the fourth dimension denotes the TR number.

The most widely used methods for analyzing fMRI data are run on the data from each voxel separately. Chapters 5–9 describe these methods. In these approaches, the first step is to load data from the to-be-analyzed voxel into a single vector that contains one entry for each TR of the experiment. The methods of chapters 5 and 6 can then be used to determine whether this voxel shows task-related activity. For example, consider an experiment with 284 TRs. The data from the voxel with $(x, y, z)$ coordinates equal to $(5, 7, 13)$ are loaded into the $284 \times 1$ vector B using the following MATLAB command:

B = filename.img(5, 7, 13, :).

The vector B would then be used in the subsequent data analysis, and this whole process would be repeated for every voxel in the brain or in the region of interest (ROI).

SPM and FSL have their own software for reading Analyze or NIfTI files into MAT-LAB. Although their implementation is slightly different, their results are essentially the same. For example, any software that reads NIfTI files into MATLAB should produce a data file with a similar name and structure as the filename.img file described above.

# 3   Modeling the BOLD Response

The goal of almost all fMRI experiments is to learn something about neural activity. Unfortunately, however, the BOLD response measured in most fMRI experiments provides only an indirect measure of neural activation (Ogawa, Lee, Kay, & Tank, 1990; Ogawa, Lee, Nayak, & Glynn, 1990). Although it is commonly assumed that the BOLD signal increases with neural activation, it is known that the BOLD response is much more sluggish than the neural activation that is presumed to drive it. As a result, for example, the peak of the BOLD signal lags considerably behind the peak neural activation (i.e., by about 6 seconds).

Logothetis and colleagues have presented evidence that the BOLD response is more closely related to local field potentials than to the spiking output of individual cells (Logothetis, 2003; Logothetis et al., 2001). Local field potentials integrate the field potentials produced by small populations of cells over a submillimeter range, and they vary continuously over time. Most applications of fMRI make no attempt to model neural activation at such a detailed biophysical level. Instead, neural activation is typically treated as a rather abstract latent (i.e., unobservable) variable. It is assumed to increase when a brain region is active and to decrease during periods of inactivity. As with any latent variable, however, to make inferences about neural activation from observable BOLD responses requires a model of how these two variables are related. This chapter reviews the most popular of these models.

## Linear Models of the BOLD Response

Almost all current applications of fMRI assume that the transformation from neural activation to BOLD response can be modeled as a linear, time-invariant system. Although it is becoming increasingly clear that the transformation is, in fact, nonlinear (e.g., Boynton, Engle, Glover, & Heeger, 1996; Buxton & Frank, 1998; Vazquez & Noll, 1998), it also appears that under appropriate conditions, these departures from linearity are not severe. For example, the approximation to linearity is improved if the intertrial interval exceeds

1 second and if brief exposure durations are avoided (Vazquez & Noll, 1998). These two conditions are commonly met in fMRI studies of high-level cognition.

In the linear systems approach, one can conceive of the vascular system that responds to a sudden oxygen debt as a black box. The input is neural activation, and the output is the BOLD response. Suppose we present a stimulus event $E_i$ to a subject at time 0. Let $N_i(t)$ denote the neural activation induced by this event at time $t$ and let $B_i(t)$ denote the corresponding BOLD response. Then from the systems theory perspective

$$N_i(t) \rightarrow \boxed{\phantom{xxx}} \rightarrow B_i(t),$$

where the gray box represents the set of all mathematical transformations that convert the neural activation $N_i(t)$ into the BOLD response $B_i(t)$. For convenience, we will express this mathematical relationship as

$$f[N_i(t)] = B_i(t),$$

where the operator $f$ symbolizes the workings of the gray box.

A system of this type is said to be linear if and only if it satisfies the *superposition principle,* which is stated as follows:

If $f[N_1(t)] = B_1(t)$ and $f[N_2(t)] = B_2(t)$, then it must be true that

$$f[a_1 N_1(t) + a_2 N_2(t)] = a_1 B_1(t) + a_2 B_2(t), \text{ for any constants } a_1 \text{ and } a_2.$$

In other words, if we know the BOLD responses to neural activations $N_1(t)$ and $N_2(t)$, then we can determine exactly what the BOLD response will be to any weighted sum of these two neural activations by computing the same weighted sum of the component BOLD responses.

If the superposition principle holds, then there is a straightforward way to determine the BOLD response to *any* neural activation from the results of one simple experiment. To understand this important result, we need to define a *delta function* $\delta(t - \tau)$,

$$\delta(t - \tau) = \begin{cases} 1 & \text{if } t = \tau \\ 0 & \text{if } t \neq \tau, \end{cases} \tag{3.1}$$

where $t$ is a variable and $\tau$ is a specific time point. The delta function, which is illustrated in figure 3.1, is a mathematical model of an impulse because it jumps from a value of 0 to 1 instantly (i.e., at time $\tau$) and then instantly drops back down to 0. This function is important because if we treat time as a discrete variable, then any neural activation can be written as a weighted sum of delta functions (which will allow us to apply the superposition principle). For example, consider the neural activation $N(t)$ illustrated in figure 3.2 that has numerical value $n_i$ at time (e.g., TR) $i$. Note that we can rewrite a discrete-time approximation of $N(t)$ as the following sum:

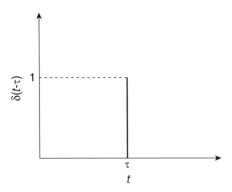

**Figure 3.1**
The delta function.

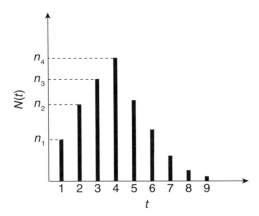

**Figure 3.2**
A hypothetical discrete-time neural activation function.

$$N(t) = n_1\delta(t - 1) + n_2\delta(t - 2) + \cdots + n_9\delta(t - 9).$$

When $t = 1$, all terms on the right drop out except the first term [because $\delta(1 - 1) = 1$ and $\delta(1 - i) = 0$ for $i = 2, 3, \ldots, 9$]. Thus, in this case, the right side reduces to $n_1$. Similarly, when $t = 2$, all terms on the right drop out except the second, and in this case the right side reduces to $n_2$. If we now define $n_0 = 0$, and $n_i = 0$ for all $i > 9$ then note that this sum can be rewritten as

$$N(t) = \sum_{\tau=0}^{\infty} n_\tau\delta(t - \tau). \tag{3.2}$$

For suitably chosen values of the $n_i$, every discrete-time function can be written in the form of equation 3.2.

Using the superposition principle, we can decompose the BOLD response to $N(t)$ into the separate BOLD responses to each of the delta functions in equation 3.2:

$$B(t) = f[N(t)]$$

$$= f\left[\sum_{\tau=0}^{\infty} n_\tau \delta(t-\tau)\right]$$

$$= \sum_{\tau=0}^{\infty} n_\tau f[\delta(t-\tau)]$$

$$= \sum_{\tau=0}^{t} n_\tau f[\delta(t-\tau)]. \tag{3.3}$$

The last equality holds because the BOLD response cannot begin before the neural activation. Thus, $f[N(t)] = 0$ for $t < 0$, and as a result, $f[\delta(t-\tau)] = 0$ for $\tau > t$.

In a time-invariant linear system, the response to an impulse is always the same, regardless of when the impulse occurs. Let $h(t-\tau) = f[\delta(t-\tau)]$ denote the response of the system to the delta function $\delta(t-\tau)$. Then equation 3.3 reduces to

$$B(t) = \sum_{\tau=0}^{t} n_\tau h(t-\tau). \tag{3.4}$$

If we now reduce the time between successive values of $\tau$ (i.e., take the limit as $\tau \to 0$), then the sum in equation 3.4 becomes an integral:

$$B(t) = \int_0^t N(\tau)h(t-\tau)\,d\tau. \tag{3.5}$$

Equation 3.5 is the well-known *convolution integral* that completely characterizes the behavior of any linear, time-invariant system (e.g., Chen, 1970). The function $h(t)$ is traditionally called the *impulse response function* because it describes the response of the system to an impulse. In the fMRI literature, however, $h(t)$ is known as the *hemodynamic response function*, often abbreviated as the hrf. Note that "hemodynamic response function" is not a synonym for "BOLD response." Rather, the hrf is the hypothetical BOLD response to an idealized impulse of neural activation. A common mathematical shorthand for the convolution integral is to write $B(t) = N(t) * h(t)$.

It is straightforward to evaluate the convolution integral numerically, but it is so common, for example, that MATLAB has its own convolution command. After defining the vectors N and h, one simply types

$$B = \text{conv}(N,h)$$

and the vector B is filled with values of the convolution integral (technically a sum because time is discrete).

Equation 3.5 tells us that if a system is linear and time invariant, we can perfectly predict how it will respond to any input, $N(t)$, no matter how complex, simply by observing its response to a single impulse and then by convolving this impulse response with the input $N(t)$. For example, electrical engineers frequently make use of this result because any electrical circuit constructed from resistors, inductors, and capacitors is linear and time invariant and so can be completely characterized by knowing how it will respond to an impulse. With fMRI, in cases where the transformation from neural activation to the BOLD response is linear and time invariant, equation 3.5 tells us how to predict the BOLD response to any neural activation perfectly from knowledge of the BOLD response to an impulse or single burst of neural activation. The superposition principle and the resulting convolution integral massively simplify the analysis of fMRI data, and as a result they form the basis for the most popular methods of fMRI data analysis.

## Methods of Estimating the hrf

Given that the hrf plays such a critical role in determining what sorts of BOLD responses we should look for in our data, the natural next question to ask is the following: How can we determine numerical values of the hrf? This section describes five different methods for estimating the hrf. These are not all commonly used in fMRI research, but they all are used widely in linear systems theory.

**Input an Impulse, and Observe the Response**    The most obvious method for determining the hrf, which is suggested by the name *impulse response function*, is simply to input an impulse to the system and record the output. If the system is linear and time invariant, then the output will exactly equal $h(t)$. With traditional fMRI experiments, of course, we cannot directly input a neural activation, so using this method to estimate the hrf is highly problematic.

Even so, this method has been used to estimate the hrf in primary visual cortex (i.e., area V1). For example, Richter and Richter (2003) presented subjects with a flashing checkerboard image for 500 milliseconds and recorded the BOLD response in area V1 for three different groups of subjects: children (ages 7–20 years), young adults (ages 21–27 years), and older adults (ages 30–61 years). The idea is that this brief visual stimulation should induce a brief neural activation that is approximately an impulse, and as a result, the BOLD response recorded in this experiment should approximate the hrf. Results are shown in figure 3.3. Note that, as expected, the peak occurs at around 5 or 6 seconds, and then there is a slow decay back to baseline. Note also that there are some age differences—primarily in decay back to baseline (i.e., decay rate decreases with age). Similar results were obtained by Huettel, Singerman, and McCarthy (2001).

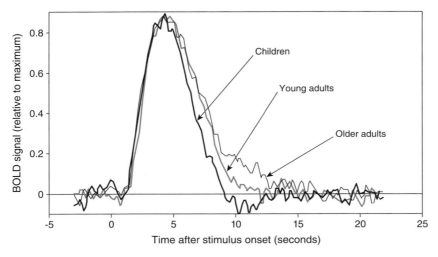

**Figure 3.3**
Empirical estimates of the hrf that were obtained using method 1. (Reprinted from Richter & Richter, "The shape of the fMRI BOLD response in children and adults changes systematically with age," *NeuroImage*, 2003, *20*, 1122–1131, with permission from Elsevier.)

Although this method may be plausible for estimating an hrf in early sensory areas, such as V1, it seems much more poorly suited to areas that are further removed from the stimulus. For example, what sort of stimulus is appropriate to produce an impulse of neural activation in prefrontal cortex or in the hippocampus? Another problem with the method is that, as we will see later, the brief, intense stimulus displays required to induce a neural impulse are also likely to cause violations of the superposition principle. If the superposition principle is violated, then the BOLD response to an impulse cannot be used to predict the BOLD response to other types of neural activation. Because of these two problems, this method does not provide a satisfactory solution to the general hrf estimation problem.

**Deconvolution** A second method of estimating the hrf is to solve equation 3.5 for $h(t)$, a technique known as deconvolution. In fMRI, the left side of equation 3.5 is just the observed BOLD response. But the right side includes two unobservable quantities: the hrf we are trying to estimate and the neural activation $N(t)$. Unless we can somehow specify $N(t)$, it will be mathematically impossible to determine $h(t)$ uniquely (i.e., because we would have only one equation, but two unknowns). It turns out that this is a common problem that plagues most of the popular methods for estimating the hrf. The only current solution is to substitute a hypothetical model of the neural activation for $N(t)$.

The field of computational neuroscience contains many examples of models that give plausible predictions of the neural activation one could expect in response to any particular stimulus presentation (e.g., Ashby & Valentin, 2007; Bower & Beeman, 1998; Johnston &

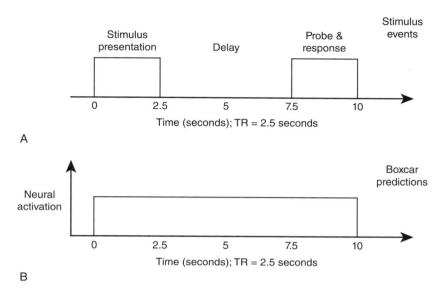

**Figure 3.4**
The boxcar model. Panel A shows the timing of stimulus events in a hypothetical experiment. Panel B shows the neural activation predicted by the boxcar model for any brain region that mediates performance in this experiment.

Wu, 1995; Koch, 1999). The fMRI literature, however, has almost uniformly adopted an exceedingly simple model that assumes neural activation turns instantly on when the stimulus is presented, it remains constant throughout the time assumed for processing of that stimulus, and it instantly returns to baseline when stimulus processing is complete. An example of this model is shown in figure 3.4 for a working memory task where a probe is presented for 2.5 seconds (the length of the TR in this example), which is followed by a blank screen for 5 seconds and then by a second stimulus for 2.5 seconds. The subject's task is to determine whether the second stimulus was the same or different from the first. The idea here is that brain areas mediating the representation and working memory of the first stimulus should remain active from the time of initial stimulus presentation until response. Applying the simple on–off model of neural activation produces the $N(t)$ function shown in the bottom panel of figure 3.4. Because of its characteristic rectangular shape, this model of neural activation is known as the *boxcar model*.

Suppose we know that a certain set of voxels in prefrontal cortex mediates the working memory required by the task illustrated in figure 3.4. In chapter 5, we will begin examining methods that might allow us to identify such voxels, but for now, assume that we have somehow already solved this problem. To estimate the hrf that characterizes these voxels, we could substitute the figure 3.4 boxcar model into the right side of equation 3.5. The left side is the observed BOLD response from this experiment, so only one unknown remains: $h(t)$.

Once $N(t)$ is specified, there are several numerical methods for solving equation 3.5 for $h(t)$. Perhaps the most straightforward is to use Fourier transforms. A brief overview of Fourier transforms is presented in chapter 8 when we discuss coherence analysis. For now, suffice it to say that almost any mathematical function can be written as a weighted linear combination of sinusoids. The Fourier transform of a function specifies the amplitude and phase of each sine-wave frequency required in this sum. Fourier transforms help solve the deconvolution problem because they convert convolution into multiplication. Let $\Im[B(t)]$ denote the Fourier transform of $B(t)$. Then,

$$\Im[B(t)] = \Im[N(t) * h(t)]$$
$$= \Im[N(t)] \times \Im[h(t)].$$

As a result,

$$\Im[h(t)] = \frac{\Im[B(t)]}{\Im[N(t)]}.$$

Thus, if we divide the Fourier transform of the observed BOLD response by the Fourier transform of the figure 3.4 boxcar function, the result will equal the Fourier transform of the hrf. Taking the inverse transform of this result produces an estimate of the hrf.

As with convolution, Fourier transforms are common enough that MATLAB has its own one-line Fourier transform (fft) and inverse Fourier transform (ifft) commands. For example, if the vectors N and B are defined, then the hrf could be estimated in MATLAB via the following command:

h = ifft(fft(B)/fft(N)).

Note that if the transformation from neural activation to BOLD response is truly a linear, time-invariant system, then the hrf estimated using this method should be identical for all possible experiments. In other words, if we change the stimulus—for example, by lengthening the delay period or perhaps even by fundamentally changing the task—then the boxcar function will change and so will the observed BOLD response. Even so, the BOLD response should change in a predictable way; that is, in a way such that deconvolving the observable BOLD with the new boxcar should produce exactly the same hrf as before.

The deconvolution method is effective as long as the system is linear and time invariant and the voxel from which the BOLD response is measured is mediating the performance of the task. If any of these conditions fail, then the assumption that the neural activation in that voxel is a boxcar will be wrong, and so our hrf estimate will be wrong. For this reason, the deconvolution method is appropriate for studying the nature of the hrf, but it is not an appropriate method for discovering which voxels are mediating performance in a task we are studying.

Deconvolution is not a widely used technique in fMRI data analysis. Even so, this method was used by Glover (1999) as a method to compensate for variability in the hrf across conditions and subjects.

**Open the Box; Study the Circuit**   A third method that is commonly used in linear systems theory to estimate the impulse response function is to open the black box, study the circuit, and then write equations that model the transformations that this circuit performs. For example, this is the method used by electrical engineers when confronted with a circuit constructed from resistors, inductors, and capacitors (i.e., resistors act as multipliers, inductors differentiate, and capacitors integrate). In fMRI, this was the method used to construct the balloon model (Buxton, Wong, & Frank, 1998), which we will encounter later in this chapter when we consider nonlinear models of the BOLD response. To my knowledge, however, this method has not been used to construct linear models.

**Take a Guess**   A fourth method is to select a specific mathematical function for the hrf based on our knowledge of what we think this function should look like. For example, we know the hrf should peak at roughly 6 seconds and then slowly decay back to baseline. Thus, we could select a mathematical function with these properties and then just assume that this is a good model of the hrf. In fact, this is, by far, the most popular method for determining the hrf in fMRI data analysis. It forms the basis, for example, of the standard correlation analysis (which is considered in detail in chapter 5).

Figure 3.5 shows one popular choice for the hrf. This particular hrf is a special case of a more general model described in the next section. In particular, figure 3.5 is an example of the gamma function hrf proposed by Boynton et al. (1996), with the parameters fixed at one typical set of values (i.e., $T_0 = 0$, $n = 4$, and $\lambda = 2$; see equation 3.6). Note that as we would

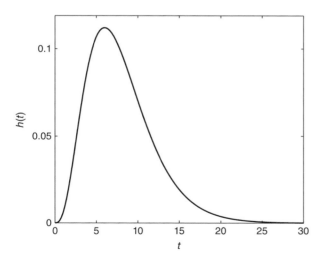

**Figure 3.5**
A typical hrf used in fMRI data analysis. This is the gamma function model of equation 3.6 that was proposed by Boynton et al. (1996) with $T_0 = 0$, $n = 4$, and $\lambda = 2$.

**MATLAB Box 3.1**
Create and plot an hrf (as in figure 3.5)

```
% Clear all workspaces
clear all; close all; clc;

% Set the parameter values of the hrf
T0=0; n=4; lamda=2;

% Define the time axis, i.e., from 0 to 30 sec in .01 sec increments
t=0:.01:30;

% Create the hrf
hrf=((t-T0).^(n-1)).*exp(-(t-T0)/lamda)/((lamda^n)*factorial(n-1));

% Plot the hrf
plot(t,hrf); axis([0 30 0 .12]);
```

expect, this model of the hrf peaks at around 6 seconds and then decays back to baseline after around 25 seconds. MATLAB box 3.1 gives the code used to produce this figure.

Figure 3.6 shows the results of convolving the hrf shown in figure 3.5 with boxcar models of hypothetical neural activation that persist for 5, 20, or 50 seconds. As the duration of the neural activation increases from 0 until around 20 seconds, the predicted BOLD response grows in magnitude. For durations longer than 20 seconds, the BOLD response saturates at its maximum value (i.e., 1.0). Once saturation is reached, the BOLD response remains at this high level as long as the neural activation persists. After the neural activation ceases, however, the BOLD response slowly decays back to its baseline level. MATLAB box 3.2 lists the code for these calculations.

This method has several obvious weaknesses. First, the function chosen may not be a particularly accurate model of the hrf. This weakness is similar to the problem that the boxcar function is not a particularly accurate model of neural activation. For example, neural activation will ramp up more slowly than the boxcar, it will slowly decay during the sustained activation period, and it will decay more slowly back to baseline than the boxcar. As we will see in chapter 5, inaccurate models of both the hrf and neural activation will reduce our ability to identify task-related voxels.

A more serious problem with this method of selecting an hrf, however, is that a single mathematical function has no flexibility that allows it to adjust for possible hrf differences across applications. This is a serious problem because research suggests that the hrf varies across brain regions (Schacter, Buckner, Koutstaal, Dale, & Rosen, 1997) and, as figure 3.3 shows, across subjects (Aguirre, Zarahn, & D'Esposito, 1998). Any inaccuracy in our model of the hrf will make it more difficult to identify task-related activity, and differences

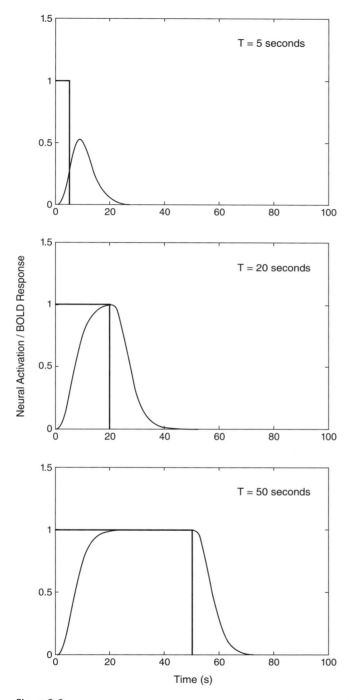

**Figure 3.6**
Results of convolving the hrf shown in figure 3.5 with boxcar neural activations of duration 5, 20, or 50 seconds. The rectangles denote the boxcar functions, and the curves denote the predicted BOLD response.

**MATLAB Box 3.2**
Convolve an hrf with a boxcar function to create a predicted BOLD response (as in figure 3.6)

```
clear all; close all; clc;    % Clear all workspaces
T0=0; n=4; lamda=2;          % Set the parameter values of the hrf

% Define the time axis and the 3 boxcar functions
t50=0:.01:50;
box5=[ones(1,500),zeros(1,4501)];
box20=[ones(1,2000),zeros(1,3001)];
box50=[ones(1,5000),0];

% Create the hrf
hrf=((t50-T0).^(n-1)).*exp(-(t50-T0)/lamda)/((lamda^n)*factorial(n-1));

% Compute the 3 convolutions. Divide by 100 to set time unit at .01 sec
BOLD5=conv(box5,hrf)/100;
BOLD20=conv(box20,hrf)/100;
BOLD50=conv(box50,hrf)/100;

% Plot the predicted BOLD responses
t=0:.01:100;
subplot(3,1,1); plot(t,BOLD5,t50,box5); axis([0 100 0 1.5]);
subplot(3,1,2); plot(t,BOLD20,t50,box20); axis([0 100 0 1.5]);
subplot(3,1,3); plot(t,BOLD50,t50,box50); axis([0 100 0 1.5]);
```

in the accuracy of the model across regions or subjects could introduce a systematic bias into these difficulties that could lead to inaccurate conclusions. For example, suppose current theories disagree as to whether performance in a particular task is primarily mediated by brain region A or brain region B. If the hrf model that we choose happens to be more accurate for region A, then our ability to identify voxels with task-related activity in region A will be greater than our corresponding ability in region B. As a result, it is likely that ambivalent data would be interpreted as evidence in favor of theories postulating a key role for region A.

**Select a Flexible Mathematical Model of the hrf**   The last method we will consider for estimating the hrf is a generalization of method 4. In this case, a canonical form is selected for the hrf, but this model is characterized by several free parameters that can be adjusted to account for differences in the hrf across brain regions or subjects. Many alternative models of this type have been proposed (Boynton et al., 1996; Clark, Maisog, & Haxby, 1998; Cohen, 1997; Dale & Buckner, 1997; Friston, Holmes, & Ashburner, 1999; Friston, Josephs, Ress, & Turner, 1998; Zarahn, Aquirre, & D'Esposito, 1997). For example, Boynton et al. (1996) proposed a gamma function of the type

$$h(t) = \begin{cases} \dfrac{(t-T_0)^{n-1}}{\lambda^n (n-1)!} & \text{for } t > T_0 \\ 0 & \text{for } t < T_0 \end{cases}, \tag{3.6}$$

where $\lambda$, $T_0$, and $n$ (an integer) are free parameters. The parameter $T_0$ is the lag between stimulus presentation and the initial rise in the BOLD response, whereas $\lambda$ and $n$ determine the shape of the hrf. For example, the peak of the hrf occurs at time $T_0 + (n-1)\lambda$. As mentioned earlier, figure 3.5 shows an example of this model with the parameters set to $T_0 = 0$, $n = 4$, and $\lambda = 2$.

The next question is the following: How do we determine the optimal values of the parameters $\lambda$, $T_0$, and $n$? This is typical of many parameter estimation problems, so standard methods can be used. In most of these, the following five steps are followed.

### Algorithm for Estimating the Parameters of a Canonical hrf

*Step 1*   Pick any reasonable initial values for $\lambda$, $T_0$, and $n$. For example, one might try $\lambda = 2$, $T_0 = 0.3$, and $n = 4$.

*Step 2*   Compute the predicted BOLD response, $B_P(t)$, by numerically evaluating the convolution integral

$$B_P(t) = \int_0^t N(\tau) h(t-\tau)\, d\tau, \tag{3.7}$$

where $h(t)$ is the equation 3.6 gamma function with the numerical parameter values from step 1, and $N(t)$ is the boxcar that describes the neural activation expected from the stimulus presentation.

*Step 3*   Compare the predicted and observed BOLD responses by computing the sum of squared errors across all $N$ TRs,

$$SSE = \sum_{TR=1}^{N} [B(TR) - B_P(TR)]^2,$$

where, as before, $B(TR)$ is the observed BOLD response when the TR equals $TR$.

*Step 4*   Try different values for $\lambda$, $T_0$, and $n$ and repeat steps 2 and 3.

*Step 5*   Repeat step 4 until you are convinced that no smaller value of $SSE$ is possible.

The optimal parameter estimates produced by this algorithm, called the least squares estimates, are those associated with the smallest possible value of $SSE$. Obviously, the time required to complete this process depends on how clever one is at selecting new values of the parameters to try. Fortunately, many sophisticated numerical algorithms are available to automate this process. In most cases, the user of such software would program steps 1, 2, and 3, and then the algorithm would complete the more labor-intensive steps 4 and 5. MATLAB has a whole toolbox containing a variety of such routines (i.e., the Optimization Toolbox), and even Excel has such a routine (i.e., Solver).

The slowest step in this process is step 2 because of the numerical integration it requires. If a separate hrf is estimated for each voxel in a whole-brain analysis, this entire procedure might be repeated more than 100,000 times. With this many repetitions of the analysis, the time needed for the numerical integrations of step 2 may be prohibitive.

One possible weakness of the equation 3.6 model of the hrf is that it has no negative dip. If the hrf is non-negative and neural activation is non-negative (as it is in the boxcar model), then a mathematical consequence of convolution is that the predicted BOLD response must also be non-negative. This contradicts considerable evidence that empirical BOLD responses often show a late negative dip (e.g., Fransson, Kruger, Merboldt, & Frahm, 1999; Glover, 1999). For example, such a dip is evident in the estimated hrf for children shown in figure 3.3. Because of results such as this, a number of models have been proposed in which the hypothesized hrf displays a late negative dip (e.g., Friston et al., 1998; Glover, 1999). For example, one popular choice is to model the hrf as a difference of two gamma functions: one that primarily models the early peak in the hrf, and one that primarily models the late dip (Glover, 1999). More specifically, according to this model the hrf is given by

$$h(t) = \frac{1}{C} \left[ \frac{t^{n_1 - 1}}{\lambda_1^{n_1} (n_1 - 1)!} e^{-t/\lambda_1} - a \frac{t^{n_2 - 1}}{\lambda_2^{n_2} (n_2 - 1)!} e^{-t/\lambda_2} \right], \tag{3.8}$$

where $a$ is a constant between 0 and 1, which measures the magnitude of the negative dip. The constant $C$, which equals the integral of the terms in the square brackets, guarantees that the area under this hrf is 1. An example of this model is shown in figure 3.7, with the following parameter values: $a = .3$, $n_1 = 4$, $\lambda_1 = 2$, $n_2 = 7$, and $\lambda_2 = 2$.

Friston et al. (1998) had a clever idea that eliminates most of the numerical integration required to estimate the parameters of hrfs like the one defined in equation 3.6. Their idea was to model the hrf as a weighted linear combination of basis functions,

$$h(t) = \theta_1 b_1(t) + \theta_2 b_2(t) + \theta_3 b_3(t), \tag{3.9}$$

where $b_i(t)$ is the i[th] basis function, and $\theta_i$ is its weight. Friston et al. (1998) suggested gamma probability density functions for the basis functions, with means and variances equal to 4, 8, and 16, respectively. Thus,

$$b_1(t) = \tfrac{1}{3!} t^3 e^{-t}, \tag{3.10}$$

$$b_2(t) = \tfrac{1}{7!} t^7 e^{-t}, \tag{3.11}$$

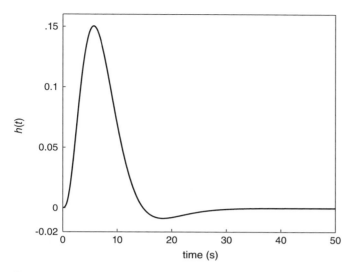

**Figure 3.7**
An example of the equation 3.8 model, in which an hrf is defined as the difference of two gamma functions. In this case, the equation 3.8 constants were set to $a = .3$, $n_1 = 4$, $\lambda_1 = 2$, $n_2 = 7$, and $\lambda_2 = 2$.

and

$$b_3(t) = \tfrac{1}{15!} t^{15} e^{-t}.$$  (3.12)

Note that none of these functions have any free parameters. Their specific forms were selected to model possible peaks during the early, intermediate, and late components of the anticipated BOLD response. The weighting parameters $\theta_1$, $\theta_2$, and $\theta_3$ can model differences in the hrf across participants and/or brain regions.

The advantage of defining the hrf in terms of basis functions can be seen when equation 3.9 is substituted into the convolution integral of equation 3.5:

$$B_P(t) = \int_0^t N(\tau)h(t-\tau)\, d\tau$$

$$= \int_0^t N(\tau)[\theta_1 b_1(t-\tau) + \theta_2 b_2(t-\tau) + \theta_3 b_3(t-\tau)]\, d\tau$$

$$= \theta_1 \int_0^t N(\tau)b_1(t-\tau)\, d\tau + \theta_2 \int_0^t N(\tau)b_2(t-\tau)\, d\tau + \theta_3 \int_0^t N(\tau)b_3(t-\tau)\, d\tau.$$  (3.13)

Note that none of these integrals include any free parameters. As a result, if we define

$$x_i(t) = \int_0^t N(\tau) b_i(t - \tau)\, d\tau, \qquad\qquad (3.14)$$

Then

$$B_P(t) = \theta_1 x_1(t) + \theta_2 x_2(t) + \theta_3 x_3(t), \qquad\qquad (3.15)$$

where the only free parameters are the $\theta_i$.

   With this reformulation of $B_P(t)$, the iterative and time-consuming parameter estimation process described by steps 1–5 can be avoided. Instead, optimal parameter estimates can be computed in one step. First, the three integrals specified by equation 3.14 are computed numerically. Each of these computations produces a vector of numerical values, $x_1(t)$, $x_2(t)$, and $x_3(t)$. The parameters $\theta_i$ can now be determined using standard linear regression techniques. In particular, if we treat $B(t)$ as the dependent variable and the $x_i(t)$ as the independent variables, then the $\theta_i$ can be interpreted as regression weights. As we will see in chapter 5, minimum variance unbiased estimators of the $\theta_i$ can therefore be computed directly from the normal equations of the general linear model.

   Various methods have been proposed that use basis functions that are different from those described by equations 3.10–3.12. One of these leads to what is known as the *finite impulse response (FIR) model* (Dale, 1999; Hinrichs et al., 2000). In this approach, the basis functions are a series of delta functions that each spike at a different TR. Recall from equation 3.1 that the delta function $\delta(t - \tau)$ equals 1 when $t = \tau$, and it equals 0 for all other $t$. In the FIR model, there are as many basis functions as there are TRs in the hrf. Thus, if the TR is 2.5 seconds and we assume the hemodynamic response to an impulse of neural activation would last for 20 seconds, then the FIR model uses the following nine basis functions:

$$b_1(t) = \delta(t),$$

$$b_2(t) = \delta(t - 2.5),$$

$$b_3(t) = \delta(t - 5),$$

$$\vdots$$

$$b_9(t) = \delta(t - 20).$$

Note that $b_1(t)$ has a numerical value of 1 at the moment the impulse is presented ($t = 0$) and it equals 0 at all other times; $b_2(t)$ has a numerical value of 1 exactly 2.5 seconds after the impulse is presented (i.e., after the first TR), and so forth. As in the Friston et al. (1998) model, the hrf is then defined by an equation like equation 3.9:

$$h(t) = \sum_{i=1}^{9} \theta_i b_i(t).$$

(3.16)

The FIR model has more free parameters than the Friston et al. (1998) model, but it makes fewer assumptions. If the hrf really does persist for no more than 20 seconds, then with a TR of 2.5 we will only have an opportunity to sample the hrf at nine time points. Thus, no matter what the form of the hrf, we can always find numerical values of the nine parameters (i.e., the $\theta_i$) that will perfectly fit these nine observed hrf values. This is not true of the Friston et al. (1998) model. Although it is mathematically flexible, because it only has three free parameters and makes the parametric assumption that the basis functions are all gamma probability density functions, it is possible that the model could provide a poor fit to some particular data set.

### Nonlinear Models of the BOLD Response

All of the methods that we have discussed so far in this chapter assume the superposition principle that characterizes all linear systems; in other words, that the response to a pair of stimuli presented simultaneously should equal the sum of the responses to each stimulus presented in isolation. As mentioned above, superposition is approximately satisfied if the intertrial interval exceeds 1 second and if brief stimulus exposure durations are avoided (Vazquez & Noll, 1998). However, if stimulus events quickly follow one another, or if brief stimulus exposure durations are used, then it is well documented that the BOLD response exhibits significant nonlinearities (i.e., violations of the superposition principle; Hinrinchs et al., 2000; Huettel & McCarthy, 2000; Ogawa et al., 2000; Pfeuffer, McCullough, Van de Moortele, Ugurbil, & Hu, 2003).

One of the earliest attempts to test the validity of the superposition principle in fMRI research was by Boynton et al. (1996). In this experiment, subjects viewed checkerboard patterns that were displayed for 3, 6, 12, or 24 seconds. A slow event-related design was used, and data analyses focused on primary visual cortex. One of these analyses directly tested the superposition principle. For example, a checkerboard pattern displayed at constant intensity for 6 seconds is equivalent to two successive displays of the same pattern displayed for 3 seconds. Therefore, if the superposition principle holds, then the BOLD response to the 6-second display should equal the sum of two BOLD responses to the 3-second display, with the second of these delayed for 3 seconds before the summing operation. Similarly, the BOLD response to the 12-second display should equal both the sum of two BOLD responses to the 6-second display, and the sum of four BOLD responses to

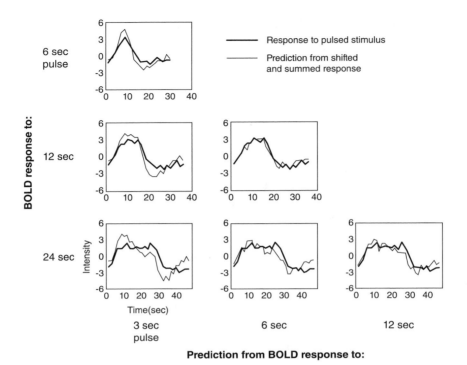

**Figure 3.8**
Observed BOLD response to a checkerboard pattern presented for a duration of 6, 12, or 24 seconds (thick lines) and the BOLD response predicted by the superposition principle from BOLD responses to the same stimulus presented for 3, 6, or 12 seconds (thin lines). (Reprinted from Boynton, Engel, Glover, & Heeger, "Linear systems analysis of functional magnetic resonance imaging in human V1," *Journal of Neuroscience*, 1996, *16*(13), 4207–4221, with permission from the Society for Neuroscience.)

the 3-second display. Figure 3.8 shows the results. The first column shows predictions for the 6-, 12-, and 24-second displays from the BOLD response that was recorded to the 3-second display. Column 2 shows predictions for the 12- and 24-second displays from the BOLD response to the 6-second display, and the last column shows predictions for the 24-second display that were generated from the BOLD response to the 12-second display. Superposition predicts that the thick and thin lines should be identical. Note that superposition is strongly supported for the data in columns 2 and 3. For column 1, however, there are systematic failures of superposition. In particular, the BOLD response to the 3-second display overpredicts the BOLD response to the 6-, 12-, and 24-second displays. Thus, these data suggest that linear systems approaches to modeling the BOLD response could be inaccurate when stimulus exposure durations are 3 seconds or less.

One reason these nonlinearities apparently occur is that even though blood flow increases with neural activity, the BOLD response has a nonlinear dependence on flow (e.g.,

Mechelli, Price, & Friston, 2001; Miller et al., 2001). For example, the BOLD signal might saturate at high levels of blood flow, in the sense that further increases in flow cause negligible increases in the concentration of deoxyhemoglobin. In this way, a moderately strong stimulus could evoke a near-maximal BOLD response, leaving little room for further increases in response (even to a stronger stimulus). This phenomenon could account for the violations of superposition seen in figure 3.8. In particular, note that in the Boynton et al. (1996) experiment, the BOLD responses to the longer-duration displays were smaller than what was predicted from the 3-second display.

There have been a number of attempts to model nonlinearities in the BOLD response. One of the earliest and best known nonlinear models is the balloon model of Buxton et al. (1998), which is based on the biomechanical properties of the brain's vasculature. The BOLD signal depends on blood flow, blood volume, and blood oxygenation, and the balloon model incorporates the conflicting effects of dynamic changes in both blood oxygenation and blood volume and assumes that the volume flow out of the system depends on a balloon-like pressure within the vasculature. For example, when the blood flow is high, the walls of the blood vessels are under greater tension, and as a result they push the blood out with greater force, which reduces the rate at which oxygen is extracted from the hemoglobin. The balloon model directly models this inherent nonlinearity using method 3 (see the earlier section "Open the Box; Study the Circuit"). On the other hand, the balloon model makes the simplifying assumption that there is no capillary contribution to the BOLD signal—an assumption that is challenged by more recent models (e.g., Zheng et al., 2002).

One practical drawback to the balloon model is its complexity. Implementing the model requires a major computational effort. Fortunately, computationally simpler alternatives exist. One especially attractive choice is to construct a Volterra series to model the nonlinearities in the BOLD signal. An important theorem in nonlinear systems theory states that the output of almost any time-invariant nonlinear system can be expressed as a Volterra series of its input (e.g., Schetzen, 1980). In the current case, this means that the BOLD response can be defined by the following function (i.e., the Volterra series) of the neural activation $N(t)$:

$$B(t) = \sum_{i=1}^{\infty} H_i[N(t)], \tag{3.17}$$

where

$$H_i[N(t)] = \int_{-\infty}^{\infty} \ldots \int_{-\infty}^{\infty} h_i(\tau_1, \ldots, \tau_i) N(t - \tau_1) \ldots N(t - \tau_i) \, d\tau_1 \ldots d\tau_i. \tag{3.18}$$

The function $h_i(t_1, \ldots, t_i)$ is called the $i^{th}$ Volterra kernel.

Note that

$$H_1[N(t)] = \int_{-\infty}^{\infty} h_1(\tau_1) N(t - \tau_1) \, d\tau_1$$

$$= \int_{-\infty}^{\infty} N(\tau_1) h_1(t - \tau_1) \, d\tau_1$$

$$= \int_{0}^{t} N(\tau_1) h_1(t - \tau_1) \, d\tau_1, \tag{3.19}$$

which is the familiar convolution integral of equation 3.5. As a result, $h_1(t)$ is just the hrf. In other words, $H_1[N(t)]$ models the linear response, and the higher-order terms model the nonlinearities in the response. Thus, the standard linear approach is to assume that $B(t) = H_1[N(t)]$. Friston et al. (1998) argued that many of the nonlinearities inherent to fMRI could be approximated by

$$B(t) = H_1[N(t)] + H_2[N(t)]. \tag{3.20}$$

Thus, we need only supplement the usual linear approach by adding a second-order correction for nonlinearity.

Now

$$H_2[N(t)] = \int_{-\infty}^{\infty} \int_{-\infty}^{\infty} h_2(\tau_1, \tau_2) N(t - \tau_1) N(t - \tau_2) \, d\tau_1 \, d\tau_2, \tag{3.21}$$

so to follow this approach we must specify the second-order Volterra kernel $h_2(\tau_1, \tau_2)$. Friston et al. (1998) suggested

$$h_2(\tau_1, \tau_2) = \sum_{i=1}^{3} \sum_{j=1}^{3} \beta_{ij} b_i(\tau_1) b_j(\tau_2), \tag{3.22}$$

where the $b_i(\tau)$ and the $b_j(\tau)$ are the gamma basis functions of equations 3.10–3.12, and the $\beta_{ij}$ are free parameters. The computational advantage of using basis functions to model the hrf extends to the second-order Volterra kernel because substituting equation 3.22 into equation 3.21 yields

$$H_2[N(t)] = \sum_{i=1}^{3}\sum_{j=1}^{3} \beta_{ij} \int_{-\infty}^{\infty} \int_{-\infty}^{\infty} b_i(\tau_1)b_j(\tau_2)N(t-\tau_1)N(t-\tau_2)\ d\tau_1\ d\tau_2$$

$$= \sum_{i=1}^{3}\sum_{j=1}^{3} \beta_{ij} \int_{-\infty}^{\infty} b_i(\tau_1)N(t-\tau_1)\ d\tau_1 \int_{-\infty}^{\infty} b_j(\tau_2)N(t-\tau_2)\ d\tau_2$$

$$= \sum_{i=1}^{3}\sum_{j=1}^{3} \beta_{ij} \int_{0}^{t} b_i(\tau_1)N(t-\tau_1)\ d\tau_1 \int_{0}^{t} b_j(\tau_2)N(t-\tau_2)\ d\tau_2$$

$$= \sum_{i=1}^{3}\sum_{j=1}^{3} \beta_{ij}[b_i(t)*N(t)][b_j(t)*N(t)]. \tag{3.23}$$

Thus, in this model, no double integrals are ever computed. Instead, we convolve each basis function with the predicted neural activation (a boxcar function), and to compute the second-order Volterra correction for nonlinearity, we compute a weighted sum of all possible products of these convolutions.

In summary, if as in equation 3.14, we define $x_i(t)$ as the function that results from convolving the $i^{th}$ basis function with the predicted neural activation, then the second-order Volterra series model of the BOLD response becomes

$$B(t) = \sum_{i=1}^{3} \alpha_i x_i(t) + \sum_{i=1}^{3}\sum_{j=1}^{3} \beta_{ij} x_i(t)x_j(t). \tag{3.24}$$

Note that, as with the linear basis function model, the parameters of equation 3.24 can be estimated using standard regression techniques.

Figure 3.9 shows the predicted BOLD response from this model to three successive 5-second-long boxcars that are each separated by 1 second. To generate this prediction, all nonlinear coefficients were set to zero except $\beta_{11}$, which was set to 0.25, and $\beta_{13}$, which was set to −0.25. The linear weights were all set to 0.2. Also shown is the linear version of this same model that was created by deleting all nonlinear (i.e., second-order) terms (with the linear weights normalized to $\alpha_1 = \alpha_2 = \alpha_3 = 0.33$). MATLAB box 3.3 provides the code that was used to generate this figure.

Note that the nonlinear BOLD response initially increases more quickly than the linear response and that it saturates after the second stimulus, whereas the linear response continues to rise at the same rate for all three stimulus presentations. The relatively reduced BOLD response to successive stimuli when the interstimulus interval is short is well documented (e.g., Wager, Vazquez, Hernandez, & Noll, 2005). Thus, when stimulus events closely follow one another, a second-order Volterra series might be a good choice to model the inevitable nonlinearities.

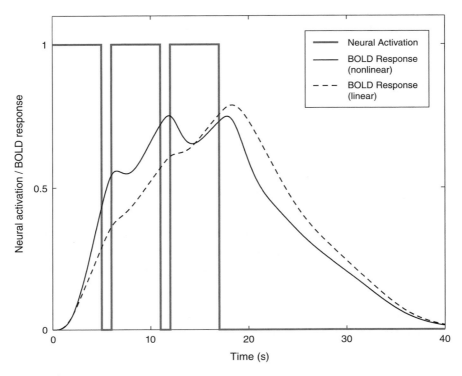

**Figure 3.9**
BOLD responses to the boxcar function shown in gray as predicted by the second-order Volterra series model
described in equations 3.17–3.22 (solid black curve) and by a model that assumes linearity (dashed curve). The
linear response was computed from the Volterra model with all nonlinear terms removed.

**MATLAB Box 3.3**
Generate BOLD predictions from the Volterra model (as in figure 3.9)

```
clear all; close all; clc;   % Clear all workspaces

% Define time, the 3 basis functions, and the boxcar
t50=0:.01:50;
b1=(t50.^3).*exp(-t50)/factorial(3);
b2=(t50.^7).*exp(-t50)/factorial(7);
b3=(t50.^15).*exp(-t50)/factorial(15);
box=[ones(1,500),zeros(1,100),ones(1,500),zeros(1,100),ones(1,500),zeros(1,3301)];

% Compute the 3 convolutions. Divide by 100 to set time unit at .01 sec
x1=conv(box,b1)/100; x2=conv(box,b2)/100; x3=conv(box,b3)/100;

% Compute the convolution products
% Only 2 given here. Others added in analogous fashion.
y11=x1.*x1; y13=x1.*x3;

% Set the weight parameters
a1=.2; a2=.2; a3=.2;
b11=.25; b13=-.25;

% Compute the predicted nonlinear BOLD response
H1=a1*x1+a2*x2+a3*x3;
H2=b11*y11+b13*y13;
B=H1+H2;

% Compute the predicted linear response (normalize weights so they sum to 1)
S=a1+a2+a3;
Lin=H1/S;

% Normalize area under nonlinear response to equal area under linear response
B=sum(Lin)*B/sum(B);

% Plot the boxcar and predicted nonlinear and linear responses
t=0:.01:100;
plot(t50,box,t,B,t,Lin); axis([0 40 0 1.1]);
```

**Conclusions**

The BOLD response measured in fMRI experiments provides only an indirect measure of neural activation. As cognitive neuroscientists, our primary interest is neural activation, not oxygen levels in the blood. Therefore, before we can hope to design fMRI experiments or to analyze fMRI data, it is vital that we understand how neural activation and the BOLD response are related. This chapter reviewed the most popular methods of modeling this relationship. These models form the basis, either directly or indirectly, for all other methods of analysis considered in this book.

# 4 Preprocessing

The most common goal of fMRI research is to identify brain areas activated by the task under study. The data that comes directly out of the scanner, however, are poorly suited to this goal. The *preprocessing* of fMRI data includes all transformations that are needed to prepare the data for the more interesting task-related analyses that are the focus of the rest of this book. Preprocessing steps typically are the same for all experiments, so any analyses that do not depend on the specific hypotheses that the experiment was designed to test are typically called preprocessing.

The variability in raw fMRI data is so great that it easily can swamp out the small changes in the BOLD response induced by most cognitive tasks. Some of this variability is unavoidable in the sense that it is due to factors that we cannot control or even measure (e.g., thermal and system noise). But other sources of variability are systematic. For example, when a subject moves his or her head, the BOLD response sampled from each spatial position within the scanner suddenly changes in a predictable manner. During the preprocessing phase of data analysis, as many of these systematic non-task-related sources of variability as possible are removed from the data.

In thermodynamics, noise is often interpreted as a fundamental uncertainty about the world that can never be reduced or eliminated. Within the field of statistics, however, noise is defined as any variability in the data that is not explained by our statistical model. Some of this variability might be quite systematic, as is the case, for example, with variability in fMRI data that is due to head movement. In many statistical models, including the model that is most commonly used to analyze fMRI data (i.e., the general linear model, which is the topic of chapter 5), all such sources of unexplained variability are modeled by a single error term, and the variance of this error term is a measure of the total unexplained variability. The magnitude of this variance is important because it is used to assess the statistical significance of any presumed task-related activation. Any analysis that reduces the error variance will increase the statistical power of our significance tests; that is, it will increase the probability that true task-related activations are discovered. Thus, the main goal of preprocessing is to reduce as much as possible the error variance of the statistical model used to detect task-related activation.

This chapter focuses on a number of common preprocessing steps. Six of these will be considered in detail, and at the end of the chapter several others will be considered more briefly. The first of the six, called slice-timing correction, corrects for variability in the BOLD responses that are due to the fact that data in different voxels are acquired at different times. The second step is to correct for variability due to head movement. The third step, called coregistration, is to align the structural and functional data. The fourth step, normalization, warps the subject's structural image to a standard brain atlas. Coregistration and normalization are not done so much to reduce variability but rather to help identify the anatomic location of a task-related activation that is discovered during data analysis. The fifth step spatially smoothes the data with the goal of reducing nonsystematic high-frequency spatial noise. Finally, in the sixth step, temporal filtering is done primarily to reduce the effects of slow fluctuations in the local magnetic field properties of the scanner.

### Slice-Timing Correction

Almost all fMRI data are collected in slices. Each slice includes an array of voxels. A scan of the whole brain might include 33 or more slices. The TR is the time between the onsets of consecutive whole-brain scans, so the TR is also the time it takes to collect all slices. This means that if the TR is 2.5 seconds, then the time between the acquisition of the first and last slice will be almost this long. This problem is compounded by the order in which slices are often collected. A common procedure is to use *interleaved* slice acquisition in which the odd-numbered slices are collected first (e.g., in ascending order) and then the even-numbered slices (in descending order). This means, for example, that slice 1 is taken first and slice 2 is taken last. As a result, with interleaved slice acquisition, the BOLD responses in neighboring voxels can be collected several seconds apart in time.

Slice-timing differences are not a critical problem in block designs. In these experiments, subjects often perform the same task for several minutes. As we will see in chapter 5, the statistical models for block designs assume that activation in task-sensitive brain regions will asymptote a few seconds after the task is initiated and then remain constant until the task block ends (after which activation should slowly decay back to baseline). In this case, differences in slice timing are not too important because the BOLD responses recorded at each TR should be the same regardless of the order in which the slices are acquired.

Slice-timing differences are much more problematic in event-related designs because in these experiments, subjects quickly alternate between task and rest. As a result, the BOLD responses in task-sensitive voxels are predicted to change frequently. If nothing is done about the slice-timing problem, then our statistical methods will be compromised. For example, suppose we present a stimulus on TR no. 10. Then our statistical models will assume that the BOLD response in brain areas responding to that stimulus will begin at the start of TR 10. But the last slice taken during TR 10 will lag behind the first slice taken by almost an entire TR (e.g., 2.5 seconds), so our statistical predictions will be off by this amount.

There are two possible ways to compensate for differences in the time of slice acquisition. Either the timing differences can be corrected during preprocessing or the statistical methods that are used for data analysis must somehow account for differences in acquisition time. Both solutions are common. We consider each in turn.

### Slice-Timing Correction during Preprocessing

Suppose the TR is $T$ seconds in duration. Then for any slice, the time between successive acquisitions is also $T$ seconds. Let $B(TR_i)$ denote the BOLD response collected during the $i$th TR from some voxel of interest. Note that the time when $B(TR_i)$ is acquired will be somewhere in the interval $[(i-1)T, iT]$. The slice-timing correction problem is to replace the observed BOLD response $B(TR_i)$ with the BOLD response we would expect if acquisition in this voxel had occurred exactly at time $t = (i-1)T$.

The most common preprocessing approach for correcting for differences in the timing of slice acquisition is to use some form of temporal *interpolation*. The idea here is to take the observed values we have, make a guess about how they might change over short time intervals, and then use this guess to predict what the BOLD response was at the beginning of the TR. The most common forms of interpolation are *linear*, *spline*, and *sinc*.

**Linear Interpolation**    Linear interpolation is the most widely known form of interpolation. This is the method that is routinely taught, for example, in beginning mathematics and statistics courses as a way to estimate missing values from numerical tables (e.g., Z tables). The idea behind linear interpolation is to run a straight line through every consecutive pair of points. Given the pair of points $(x_1, y_1)$ and $(x_2, y_2)$, the linear interpolation line is given by

$$y = y_1 + (x - x_1)\left(\frac{y_2 - y_1}{x_2 - x_1}\right).$$

An example is shown in figure 4.1. Figure 4.1A shows a hypothetical BOLD response. If the TR is 3 seconds, then the observed BOLD response at each TR is equal to the values denoted by the filled circles in figure 4.1A. Figure 4.1B shows the linear interpolation. Thus, if we were trying to estimate the BOLD response at some time point between TRs using linear interpolation, we would use the piecewise linear function shown in figure 4.1B. Note that this approximation is good, except during the first two TRs. Figure 4.1A shows why. The actual BOLD response in figure 4.1A is fairly linear between TRs, except at the beginning. Thus, linear interpolation is good as long as the unknown function we are trying to approximate does not change in a nonlinear way too much between our observed values. Fortunately, the sluggish nature of the BOLD response works to our advantage

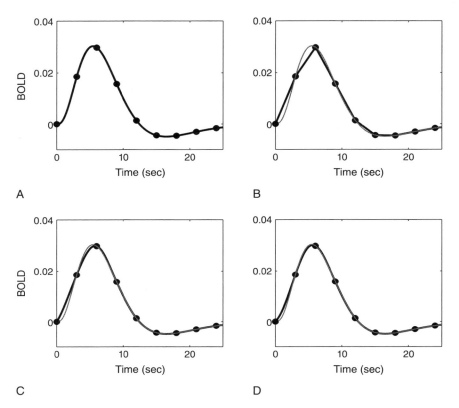

**Figure 4.1**
Different methods of interpolation. (A) A hypothetical BOLD response (solid curve) sampled at a TR of 3 seconds (circles). (B) The continuous BOLD response (gray) and a linear interpolation (black). (C) The continuous BOLD response (gray) and a sinc interpolation (black). (D) The continuous BOLD response (gray) and a cubic spline interpolation (black)

here. Because the BOLD response changes slowly, a linear interpolation cannot be too bad, and the errors caused by using this (or any other) method of interpolation will be smaller for shorter TRs.

**Spline Interpolation**   With spline interpolation, some function other than a line is used to connect the separate data points. In spline interpolation, the data points are often called knots, and the curves that connect each pair of successive knots are called splines. To produce a smooth curve, the coefficients of each spline are constrained to have the same (first) derivative at each knot. A common choice for the splines is a cubic polynomial. Figure 4.1D shows an example of cubic spline interpolation. Note that it is extremely accurate.

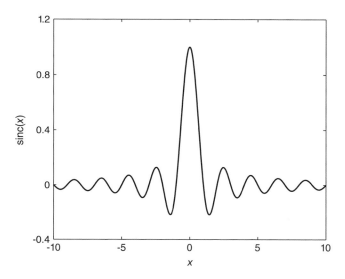

**Figure 4.2**
The sinc function.

**Sinc Interpolation**    One popular method for performing slice-timing correction, which has been used, for example, by SPM, is sinc interpolation. The sinc function, which is a damped sine wave, is defined as

$$\text{sinc}(t) = \frac{\sin(\pi t)}{\pi t},$$

for all $t$ in the interval $-\infty < t < \infty$. A graph of $\text{sinc}(t)$ is shown in figure 4.2.

To understand why sinc interpolation is used in slice-timing correction, consider first the hypothetical case of an infinitely long functional run. If the TR is T seconds, then the sinc interpolated value of the function at any arbitrary time point $t$ is given by

$$B(t) = \sum_{i=-\infty}^{\infty} B(TR_i) \, \text{sinc}\left(\frac{t - iT}{T}\right). \tag{4.1}$$

It can be shown that equation 4.1 will recover the $B(t)$ perfectly at all values of $t$ (i.e., with no error) if two conditions are met. The first is that $B(t)$ is *band-limited*. This means that $B(t)$ does not change too quickly in any small interval of time. Technically, band-limited means that the Fourier transform of $B(t)$ contains no frequencies above some finite upper value (see chapter 8 for a description of Fourier transforms). Task-related BOLD responses are almost certainly band-limited because of the slowly changing nature of the hrf. This point is explained in detail in chapter 8. The second condition required for equation 4.1 to recover $B(t)$ without error is that the observed samples $B(TR_i)$ are not too far apart in time (i.e., the TR is fairly small). The idea is that the samples need to be close enough together so that we can be certain that we did not miss anything important between samples. A famous result from information theory, called the Nyquist–Shannon sampling theorem, states that the highest frequency one could hope to recover from a set of discrete samples is one-half the sampling rate. Thus, if the TR is 2.5 seconds, which means the sampling rate is 0.4 of a TR per second, or 0.4 Hz, then the highest temporal frequency that can theoretically be measured in an fMRI experiment is 0.2 Hz. In other words, if a sine wave has a period of 5 seconds, then if we sample every 2.5 seconds we are guaranteed to see one peak and one trough, which is enough to fill in the missing values.

Note that equation 4.1 is in the same form as equation 3.4, and therefore equation 4.1 describes a convolution between the data vector $B$ and a sinc function. In the past chapter, we saw that the Fourier transform of a convolution of two functions equals the product of the Fourier transforms of the individual functions. The Fourier transform of a sinc function is a square wave that equals 1 for low frequencies and 0 for high frequencies. Thus, as long as the frequency where this square wave drops from 1 to 0 is higher than the highest frequency present in the data, then multiplying by a square wave, and therefore convolving with a sinc function, causes no loss of information. But because these operations produce a continuous function, they allow us to fill in the missing values (i.e., to interpolate). In other words, because the data are band-limited, they can be written as a finite sum of sine waves, and convolving with a sinc function essentially fills in the missing time points on all of the component sine waves.

Equation 4.1 is an infinite sum that assumes the data [i.e., the $B(TR_i)$] include an infinite number of nonzero values. Of course, with real data only some of the $B(TR_i)$ values will be nonzero. For example, consider an experiment with $n$ TRs. Then the only nonzero values of $B(TR_i)$ will be $B(TR_1)$, $B(TR_2)$, . . . , $B(TR_n)$. In this case, equation 4.1 reduces to

$$B(t) = \sum_{i=1}^{n} B(TR_i) \operatorname{sinc}\left(\frac{t - iT}{T}\right). \tag{4.2}$$

This form of sinc interpolation is much easier to use because there are only $n$ terms to compute, but it still requires computing all $n$ terms of the sum for every value of $t$. In practice, most of these terms will be negligible and can therefore be dropped. This is because $\operatorname{sinc}(t)$ converges to 0 as $t$ moves away from 0 (i.e., see figure 4.2). Thus, the contribution of the $B(TR_i)$ to the interpolation of $B(t)$ will be negligible for data points far in time from the value $t$. SPM eliminates these negligible terms from the computation by adding a multiplier to equation 4.2 that is nonzero only for values of $t$ near $t$. Many functions could be used, but SPM chooses the Hanning window:

$$H(t) = \begin{cases} \frac{1}{2}\left[1 + \cos\left(\frac{\pi t}{L}\right)\right] & -L \leq t \leq L \\ 0 & \text{otherwise} \end{cases}. \tag{4.3}$$

An example is shown in figure 4.3 where the width is $L = 5$. The bottom panel shows the results of multiplying a sinc function by this Hanning window.

When we put all this together, we arrive at the final form of sinc interpolation with a Hanning window:

$$B(t) = \sum_{i \in \{i | -L \le t - iT \le L\}} B(TR_i) \operatorname{sinc}\left(\frac{t - iT}{T}\right) H(t - iT). \tag{4.4}$$

MATLAB box 4.1 shows the code that implements equation 4.4 (i.e., on the difference-of-gammas hrf shown in figure 4.1).

To see how equation 4.4 would be used to correct for slice-timing differences, consider a voxel that is in a slice acquired 1 second after the beginning of each TR. Suppose the TR is 2 seconds, and we start the clock at the beginning of the first TR. Thus, the first TR starts at time $t = 0$, the second TR starts at time $t = 2$, and, for example, the fifth TR starts at time $t = 8$. Now because the BOLD response from this voxel is collected 1 second after the beginning of the TR, note that $B(TR_5)$ is collected at time $t = 9$. The slice-timing problem for this TR and voxel is to replace $B(TR_5)$ with $B(t = 8)$. So equation 4.4 is used with $t = 8$, and the BOLD response at this TR and voxel is replaced with the result.

### Slice-Timing Correction during Task-Related Statistical Analysis

If slice-timing differences are not corrected during preprocessing, then they should be accounted for during the statistical analysis that follows. The standard method of doing this is to choose a model of the hrf that has enough flexibility to account for moderate differences in timing. There are many ways to do this of course, but the most popular method, which was proposed by Friston et al. (1998), is to use an hrf that is a weighted sum of two terms. One is a standard hrf, such as a gamma or difference of gammas, and the other is the temporal derivative of that same hrf.

To see why this might be effective, consider the difference-of-gammas hrf. Recall from chapter 3 (equation 3.8) that according to this model, the hrf is given by

$$h_b(t) = \frac{1}{C}\left[\frac{t^{n_1-1}}{\lambda_1^{n_1}(n_1-1)!}e^{-t/\lambda_1} - a\frac{t^{n_2-1}}{\lambda_2^{n_2}(n_2-1)!}e^{-t/\lambda_2}\right]. \tag{4.5}$$

Its derivative equals

$$\dot{h}_b(t) = \frac{dh_b(t)}{dt}$$

$$= \frac{1}{C}\left[\frac{(n_1-1)t^{n_1-2}}{\lambda_1^{n_1}(n_1-1)!}e^{-t/\lambda_1} - \frac{t^{n_1-1}}{\lambda_1^{n_1+1}(n_1-1)!}e^{-t/\lambda_1} - a\frac{(n_2-1)t^{n_2-2}}{\lambda_2^{n_2}(n_2-1)!}e^{-t/\lambda_2} + a\frac{t^{n_2-1}}{\lambda_2^{n_2+1}(n_2-1)!}e^{-t/\lambda_2}\right]. \tag{4.6}$$

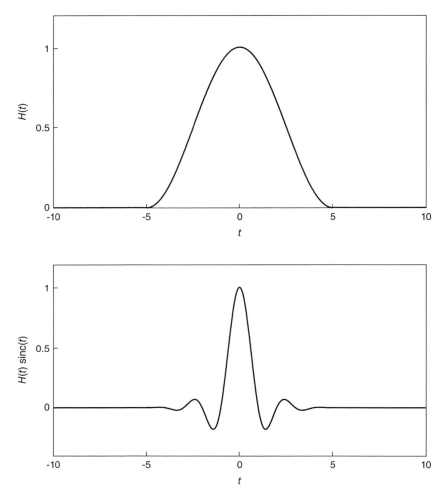

**Figure 4.3**
The top panel shows a Hanning window of width $L = 5$, and the bottom panel shows the results of multiplying a sinc function by this Hanning window. Compare figures 4.2 and 4.3.

**MATLAB Box 4.1**
The sinc interpolation of a difference-of-gammas hrf (as in figure 4.1C)

```
clear all; close all; clc;   % Clear all workspaces

% Create difference of gammas hrf and plot
t=0:.01:24;
n1=4; lamda1=2; n2=7; lamda2=2; a=.3; c1=1; c2=.5;
hx=(t.^(n1-1)).*exp(-t/lamda1)/((lamda1^n1)*factorial(n1-1));
hy=(t.^(n2-1)).*exp(-t/lamda2)/((lamda2^n2)*factorial(n2-1));
hrf=a*(c1*hx-c2*hy);
plot(t,hrf,'k'); axis([0 25 -.01 .04]); hold on;

% Sample hrf every TR=3 seconds. Plot these points as circles.
for i=1:9
    xx(i)=hrf(300*i-299);
    n(i)=300*i-299;
end;
tt=0:3:24;
plot(tt,xx,'o'); hold on;

% Sinc interpolate with Eq. 4.4. L = width of Hanning window.
L=10;
for i=1:2401;
    B_interp(i)=sum(xx.*sinc((i-n)/300).*(1+cos(pi*.01*(i-n)/L))/2);
end;

% Plot
plot(t,B_interp);
```

The top panel of figure 4.4 shows both of these functions. They are differentially weighted in this figure to have the same sum of squares because equation 4.6 produces numerical values that are much smaller than equation 4.5. Note that the derivative increases earlier than the difference of gammas, it reaches its peak earlier, and it has its negative component earlier.

The hrf model uses a weighted sum of these two functions. Specifically, a standard method to correct for slice-timing differences during postprocessing is to model the hrf as

$$h(t) = \theta_1 h_b(t) + \theta_2 \dot{h}_b(t). \tag{4.7}$$

By varying the values of $\theta_1$ and $\theta_2$, one can correct for small timing differences. To guarantee that both terms in equation 4.7 have an equal chance to contribute to the fit, it is common to normalize the derivative as we did in figure 4.4, so that $h_b(t)$ and $\dot{h}_b(t)$ have the same sum of squares.

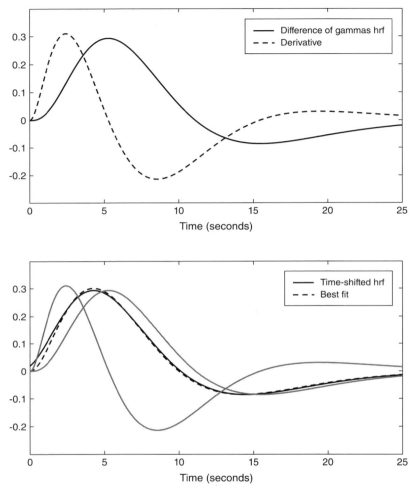

**Figure 4.4**
The top panel shows a standard difference-of-gammas hrf (solid line) along with its temporal derivative (broken line), which was normalized to have the same sum of squares. The bottom panel shows these same two functions (light gray) along with a hypothetical hrf (solid line) that peaks before the difference-of-gammas hrf shown in the top panel. Also shown is the best-fitting version of the equation 4.4 model.

As an illustration of the power of this model, consider a voxel from a brain region that responds strongly to a stimulus. Suppose we present the stimulus at the onset of the $i^{th}$ TR and, as before, denote the resulting BOLD response as $B(TR_i)$. Note that if we did not correct for slice-timing differences during preprocessing, then this notation only tells us that this response was collected sometime during TR $i$. It does not tell us when this response was collected within TR $i$. If the voxel is in a slice acquired late in the TR, then $B(TR_i)$ will tend to be greater than if the voxel belongs to a slice acquired earlier (i.e., because the BOLD response has more time to increase in later slices than in earlier slices). We can compensate for these different magnitudes by using an hrf that increases more quickly for voxels that are acquired later. In the equation 4.7 model, this is accomplished by increasing $\theta_2$, because the derivative rises more quickly than its hrf.

An example is shown in the bottom panel of figure 4.4. The solid curve shows the same hrf as the one displayed in the top panel except it is shifted earlier in time by 1 second. This simulates the case of a voxel in a slice that is acquired late in the TR (i.e., 1 second after TR onset). The broken line shows the best fit of the equation 4.7 model to this time-shifted hrf. For reference, the difference-of-gammas hrf and its derivative are shown in light gray. The parameters $\theta_1$ and $\theta_2$ were estimated using the methods of chapter 5. Note that the fit is nearly perfect.

The equation 4.7 model should be able to roughly fit any shift of the hrf that leaves its peak between the initial peaks of $h_b(t)$ and its derivative. In figure 4.4, the derivative peaks at around 2.5 seconds, and the difference-of-gammas hrf peaks at around 5 seconds. No weighted linear combination of these two functions can peak before 2.5 seconds or after 5 seconds. Note that variability in slice acquisition time should always shift the BOLD response to earlier rather than later time points (i.e., to the left), just as in the example shown in the bottom panel of figure 4.4. Thus, theoretically the equation 4.7 model should be able to correct for slice-timing errors of up to 2.5 seconds.

In summary, variability in fMRI data due to differences in the time that slices are acquired can be reduced either during preprocessing or during the statistical analysis of task-related activation. In the former case, some form of interpolation is used, whereas in the latter case temporal variability is accounted for with a flexible model of the hrf. Conservative researchers might choose to use both methods.

## Head Motion Correction

Correcting for head motion is probably the most important preprocessing step. Even small, almost imperceptible head movements can badly corrupt fMRI data. Huettel et al. (2004) give an example where a head movement of 5 mm increases activation values in a voxel by a factor of 5. For example, this can occur when a head movement causes a brain region that is richly supplied by blood to move to a location that was previously occupied by bone or air. A fivefold change in the BOLD response is much larger than we are likely to see from

any other source of variability considered in this chapter, and it is for this reason that accurately correcting for head movements is such a critical preprocessing step.

When a subject moves his or her head, brain regions will move to new spatial locations
within the scanner, and as a result, activation in those regions will be recorded in different
voxels than they were before the movement occurred. Without correcting for these movements, activation values in many voxels will therefore suddenly change in a way that is not
predicted by our statistical models. Even worse, larger movements could cause some brain
regions to move completely out of the scanning area (i.e., out of the field of view). This
creates an unrecoverable error that no head motion correction algorithm could ever overcome because there simply would be no data from these regions to correct. For this reason,
the best solution to the head motion problem is prevention rather than after-experiment
correction.

Mathematical methods for correcting for head movements depend heavily on the
assumption that when a subject moves his or her head, the brain does not change shape
or size. This is not exactly true because a sudden head movement can cause a slight change
in shape (e.g., a flattening), but for the small head movements that are common in fMRI
experiments, these shape changes are extremely small and can safely be ignored. If the
brain does not change size or shape, it can be treated as a rigid body. Head movement correction then becomes a problem of *rigid body registration* (e.g., Ashburner & Friston,
2007b).

Any movement of a rigid body can be described by six parameters. As illustrated in
figure 4.5, when a person lies inside a scanner, the center of any voxel in his or her head

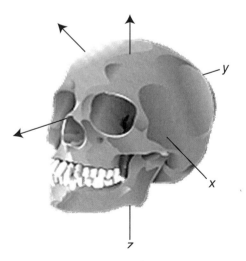

**Figure 4.5**
The standard (*x, y, z*) coordinate system used in fMRI analyses.

occupies a point in space that can be identified by a set of three coordinate values $(x, y, z)$. By convention, the $z$ axis runs parallel to the bore of the magnet and thus is a hypothetical pole that runs from the feet through the top of the head. The $x$ axis runs through the subject's ears (i.e., from left to right), and the $y$ axis is a pole that enters through the back of the head and exits the forehead. Using this coordinate system, note that the only possible rigid body movements are (1) a translation along the $x$ axis, (2) a translation along the $y$ axis, (3) a translation along the $z$ axis, (4) a rotation about the $x$ axis, (5) a rotation about the $y$ axis, and (6) a rotation about the $z$ axis. Each of these movements is characterized by a single parameter. Each translation is characterized by the distance moved along that axis, and each rotation is characterized by the angle of rotation.

Suppose we collect BOLD responses from the whole brain on two separate TRs. Suppose further that the BOLD responses on these two TRs are identical except that the subject moved his or her head between the TRs. Because of this head movement, the BOLD responses at the same physical $(x, y, z)$ coordinates within the scanner will be different on the two TRs. Because voxels are defined by their position within the scanner rather than by their position within the subject's brain, the activation values within at least some voxels will also be different on the two TRs. Thus, to correct for the head movement, we need to bring the two sets of data back into spatial alignment. If we could somehow do this, all differences between the two sets of (hypothetical) BOLD responses would disappear. Thus, one strategy for correcting for this head movement would be to take the data from the first TR as our standard and then perform rigid body movements on the data from the second TR until the BOLD responses from the two TRs agree as closely as possible at each $(x, y, z)$ coordinate point.

This process, called rigid body registration, is the standard method for correcting for head movements during preprocessing. The BOLD responses from one TR are taken as the standard, and then rigid body movements are performed separately on the data from every other TR until each of these data sets agrees as closely as possible with the data from the standard. Typically, the standard is defined as either the data from the first TR or from the middle TR. Note that this method assumes that the data at every TR are identical. Of course, if we believed this assumption were true, we never would have run the experiment. Regardless of whether a block or an event-related design was used, we expect task-related activation to differ from activation recorded during rest. Even so, the whole brain might include 100,000 or more voxels, and even our most optimistic expectation is that only a small fraction of these should show task-related activation. Thus, in almost all analyses, we expect activation in most voxels to remain roughly the same throughout the functional run. The efficacy of rigid body registration as a method for correcting for head movements critically depends on the assumption that activation in most voxels is invariant across TRs.

One method that compensates for task-related changes in activation in some voxels is to compute the variance across TRs in the BOLD responses in each voxel and then weight each voxel in the rigid body registration by the inverse of this variance. This method places less weight on voxels where activation changes across TRs and more weight on voxels where the BOLD response is relatively invariant across TRs.

There are a number of ways to formulate rigid body motion, but one conceptually straightforward method is as follows. Consider a point inside the scanner that has spatial coordinates

$$\underline{w} = \begin{bmatrix} w_x \\ w_y \\ w_z \end{bmatrix}.$$

Suppose we want to move point $\underline{w}$ to some new location with coordinates

$$\underline{u} = \begin{bmatrix} u_x \\ u_y \\ u_z \end{bmatrix}.$$

If a rigid body movement is performed, then

$$\underline{u} = R_x R_y R_z \underline{w} + \underline{b}, \tag{4.8}$$

where $R_x$, $R_y$, and $R_z$ are $3 \times 3$ matrices that rotate $\underline{w}$ around the $x$, $y$, and $z$ axes, respectively, and $\underline{b}$ is a vector of constants that performs the three possible translations.

To unpack equation 4.8, consider first the rotation matrix $R_x$. This matrix rotates the point $\underline{w}$ counterclockwise around the $x$ axis (i.e., when viewed from $x = -\infty$). Note that if we spin the $x$ axis, then any point on that axis retains its same position, but all other points move. Thus, a rotation about the $x$ axis primarily causes changes in the position of points in the $y - z$ plane. The form of $R_x$ that rotates $\underline{w}$ around the $x$ axis by $\theta_x$ degrees is

$$R_x = \begin{bmatrix} 1 & 0 & 0 \\ 0 & \cos(\theta_x) & \sin(\theta_x) \\ 0 & -\sin(\theta_x) & \cos(\theta_x) \end{bmatrix}. \tag{4.9}$$

Similarly, a rotation of the $y$ axis primarily causes changes in the position of points in the $x - z$ plane, and the rotation matrix that rotates the $y$ axis by $\theta_y$ degrees is

$$R_y = \begin{bmatrix} \cos(\theta_y) & 0 & -\sin(\theta_y) \\ 0 & 1 & 0 \\ \sin(\theta_y) & 0 & \cos(\theta_y) \end{bmatrix}. \tag{4.10}$$

Finally, a rotation of the $z$ axis primarily causes changes in the position of points in the $x - y$ plane, and the rotation matrix that rotates the $z$ axis by $\theta_z$ degrees is

$$R_z = \begin{bmatrix} \cos(\theta_z) & \sin(\theta_z) & 0 \\ -\sin(\theta_z) & \cos(\theta_z) & 0 \\ 0 & 0 & 1 \end{bmatrix}. \tag{4.11}$$

$R_x$, $R_y$, and $R_z$ can be changed to matrices that perform clockwise rotations (rather than counterclockwise) by reversing the sign on each sine term. Substituting equations 4.9–4.11 into equation 4.8 yields

$$\begin{bmatrix} u_x \\ u_y \\ u_z \end{bmatrix} = \begin{bmatrix} 1 & 0 & 0 \\ 0 & \cos(\theta_x) & \sin(\theta_x) \\ 0 & -\sin(\theta_x) & \cos(\theta_x) \end{bmatrix} \begin{bmatrix} \cos(\theta_y) & 0 & -\sin(\theta_y) \\ 0 & 1 & 0 \\ \sin(\theta_y) & 0 & \cos(\theta_y) \end{bmatrix} \begin{bmatrix} \cos(\theta_z) & \sin(\theta_z) & 0 \\ -\sin(\theta_z) & \cos(\theta_z) & 0 \\ 0 & 0 & 1 \end{bmatrix} \begin{bmatrix} w_x \\ w_y \\ w_z \end{bmatrix} + \begin{bmatrix} b_x \\ b_y \\ b_z \end{bmatrix}$$

$$\tag{4.12}$$

Thus, any (three-dimensional) rigid body movement can be described by six parameters: $\theta_x$, $\theta_y$, $\theta_z$, $b_x$, $b_y$, and $b_z$.

To see why these rotation matrices work, consider the point (1,0,0) that is shown in figure 4.6. To understand the effects of applying a rotation matrix to this point, it helps to think of it as a vector [i.e., beginning at (0,0,0) and ending at (1,0,0)]. Suppose we now rotate this vector counterclockwise around the $y$ axis by 45 degrees. The results of this rotation equal

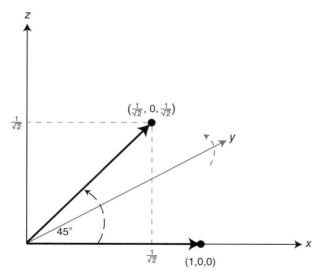

**Figure 4.6**
The effects of rotating the vector (1,0,0) counterclockwise around the $y$ axis by 45 degrees.

$$\begin{bmatrix} \cos(45°) & 0 & -\sin(45°) \\ 0 & 1 & 0 \\ \sin(45°) & 0 & \cos(45°) \end{bmatrix} \begin{bmatrix} 1 \\ 0 \\ 0 \end{bmatrix} = \begin{bmatrix} \cos(45°) \\ 0 \\ \sin(45°) \end{bmatrix} = \begin{bmatrix} \frac{1}{\sqrt{2}} \\ 0 \\ \frac{1}{\sqrt{2}} \end{bmatrix}.$$

Equation 4.12 rotates $\underline{w}$ around each of the three axes and then translates the result along these axes by amounts specified in the vector $\underline{b}$. When used as an fMRI preprocessing step, the rigid body registration described by equation 4.12 is applied simultaneously to all data from each TR. In other words, the same six parameter values are used to move every voxel from the TR that is being corrected in an effort to align it as closely as possible with the data from the TR that is taken as the standard. "As closely as possible" is formalized via an objective or loss function that increases with the mismatch between the two data sets. A variety of loss functions are possible, but one common choice is the sum of squared differences between the BOLD responses from the two TRs. These differences are computed at the spatial coordinates located at the center of each voxel in the standard TR.

The goal of rigid body registration is to find the values of the six parameters of equation 4.12 that minimize the loss function, or in other words that align the two data sets as closely as possible. This minimization is usually accomplished with some sort of optimization algorithm. MATLAB has an Optimization Toolbox that includes many such algorithms. As described in chapter 3, they all tend to work in a similar fashion. First, the user selects initial guesses about the values of each unknown parameter. For example, an obvious initial guess is that there were no movements between the TR currently being corrected and the standard TR. In this case, our initial guesses would be that all six parameters equal zero. The optimization routine would then compute the sum of squared differences (SSD; assuming this is the loss function we chose) for this choice of parameters. Next, the program automatically changes the parameters according to some rule that differs across optimization algorithms. The SSD associated with these new parameter values is then computed and compared with the SSD associated with our original guess. If the new SSD is smaller, then the program keeps changing the parameters in the same direction. If the new SSD is worse, it changes the parameters in some different direction. The program always keeps track of the smallest SSD it has found and keeps searching through all possible parameter values for a combination that produces a smaller SSD than the current best value. When it can no longer reduce the SSD it stops. Depending on the specific algorithm used, many hundreds of different parameter combinations might be tested. To correct a functional run for head movements, this minimization process must be repeated for every TR. The whole process can be very time consuming.

Figure 4.7 shows the results of applying this head motion correction algorithm to real fMRI data collected from a functional run that included more than 300 TRs. The figure shows estimates of the six parameters (on the ordinate) that minimized the SSD at each TR (on the abscissa). The top panel shows estimates of the three translation parameters, and the

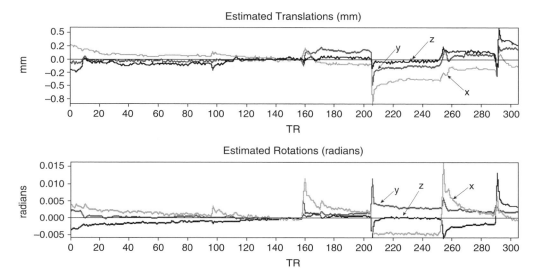

**Figure 4.7**
Parameter estimates from a head motion correction. The top panel shows the magnitude of the three translation parameters (in millimeters) on each of the 306 TRs of this experiment, and the bottom panel shows the magnitude of the three rotation parameters (in radians).

bottom panel shows estimates of the three rotation parameters. Head movements are readily identified by sudden discrete jumps in one or more parameters. Note that the subject had some small head movements early in the run, and then another small movement occurred at TR 95. Overall though, this subject remained very still throughout the first half of the session. During the second half of the session, however, at least four much larger head movements occurred, possibly because of fatigue. Even so, note that the largest translation during the entire session was less than 1 mm (on TR 207) and that the largest rotation was less than 1 degree (on TR 257). These are movements that should be correctable with standard head motion correction algorithms.

One difficult preprocessing decision is whether to correct for head movements before or after correcting for slice-timing differences. The separate effects of these two artifacts are often difficult to tease apart because they both affect the data in a similar way; that is, they both can cause the BOLD response in a particular voxel at a specific time to be different from the value our models predict.

Conventional thinking is that slice-timing correction should be performed first if the slices were acquired in an interleaved fashion, but head motion correction should be done first if the slices were acquired in an ascending fashion (e.g., Huettel et al., 2004). The logic is as follows. The first point to note is that head movements can corrupt fMRI data more than can slice-timing differences. For example, there is a relatively small fixed upper limit on the amount of error that slice-timing differences can cause (because the largest timing difference must be less than one TR), but there really is no such upper limit on the magnitude of the error that can be induced by a head movement. For this reason, the top priority should be to correct for head movements. Head movements and slice-timing differences interact because a small head movement will often move a particular point in the brain from one slice to another. When slices are acquired in ascending fashion, a shift to a neighboring slice causes only a very small delay in acquisition and, consequently, not much change in the observed BOLD response. On the other hand, a sudden head movement will often cause an abrupt change in the BOLD response at specific spatial locations within the subject's head. These discrete changes violate the assumptions of our slice-timing correction methods, and therefore they will cause slice-timing correction to fail. For this reason, with ascending slice acquisition, results are better if head movement corrections are made before slice-timing corrections.

With interleaved slice acquisition, a small head movement that moves a point in the brain into a neighboring slice will cause a significant change in acquisition time. As a result, timing differences will accentuate the effects of head movement, and the extra changes in the BOLD response induced by the change in acquisition time could defeat our head movement correction algorithms. To avoid this problem, slice-timing corrections are usually made before head movement corrections when interleaved slice acquisition is used.

### Coregistering the Functional and Structural Data

The next step in preprocessing also requires registration. In this case, however, the goal is to align the functional and structural images. This procedure is known as *coregistration*. Coregistering the functional and structural data is critical because the spatial resolution of the functional data is poor. This is mainly a simple matter of speed–accuracy trade-off. During a functional run, the whole brain might be scanned every 2 or 3 seconds, whereas a single structural scan might take 8 or 10 minutes to complete. Naturally, voxel size is much smaller in the structural data. With functional data, a voxel size of 3 mm × 3 mm × 3.5 mm is common. With structural images, however, the voxel size might be 0.86 mm × 0.86 mm × 0.89 mm, which is an improvement in resolution by a factor of almost 50.

After coregistration, the enhanced resolution of the structural data can be used to improve spatial localization of the functional data. For example, from the functional data alone it might be difficult to tell whether some significant task-related activation is localized in the supplementary motor area (SMA) or the pre-SMA, as these rather small cortical areas are adjacent. This difference is functionally important because the pre-SMA projects primarily to prefrontal cortex, whereas the SMA projects primarily to motor cortex and other premotor areas (Dum & Strick, 2005). However, it should be straightforward to resolve this ambiguity by mapping the functional activation onto the structural image.

At first, it might seem that the same methods used to correct for head movements could also be used for coregistration. In fact, it might seem that the coregistration problem is simpler than the head movement problem because only two images need to be aligned in coregistration, whereas many images must be aligned to correct for head movements. In coregistration, only the structural image and any one functional image must be aligned (as all functional images are already in alignment after our head movement corrections), but to correct for head movements we must successively align all functional images. Although this logic is valid, there are several new problems that arise with coregistration that we did not face when correcting for head movements.

The first problem is that the voxel sizes used in functional and structural imaging are different. As a result, there is no longer a 1-to-1 correspondence between voxels in the two images. This means that a simple SSD loss function will not work because there would be more numbers in one list of intensity values (i.e., values from the structural scan) than in the other list (BOLD responses from the functional scan). The second problem is that the structural and functional scans are run with different imaging parameters,[1] and as a result their contrasts are often different. An algorithm that tries to minimize SSD tries to minimize differences between the images, so this is a poor choice when trying to align images that have different intensity values even when alignment is perfect.

Early coregistration methods tried to solve these problems by first identifying key landmarks in the two images and then trying to align these landmarks. For example, the anterior commissure was often used for this purpose. Although this approach can lead to accurate solutions of the coregistration problem, it is rarely used today for a variety of reasons. Most of the problems occur because the process is difficult to automate; that is, it is difficult to write code that will accurately and reliably identify enough landmarks to ensure that coregistration will succeed. For this reason, landmark identification can only be guaranteed to work if it is done by hand. As a result, it is time consuming, and it depends on how skilled the researcher is in neuroanatomy. This latter factor introduces a degree of subjectivity into the landmark identification process. Different researchers will not always agree on the locations of the same landmarks in the same data.

As a result of these problems, methods were developed for coregistering functional and structural data using algorithms that did not require landmark identification, and therefore that could be easily automated. The most popular current technique is illustrated in figures 4.8 and 4.9. Two images are shown in each figure. Voxel sizes are the same in the images, but the contrasts are reversed. In figure 4.8 the images are in spatial alignment, but in figure 4.9 they are displaced (i.e., by a translation). The first step is to create a frequency histogram of the intensity values in each image. In figures 4.8 and 4.9, histograms with 50 bins

---

1. Structural scans are often collected with what is known as $T_1$-weighting, whereas functional scans often use $T_2^*$-weighting. See Hashemi et al. (2004), for example, for a description of these terms and a more thorough discussion of the differences between structural and functional scanning.

were used, but the technique does not depend on the number of bins. The second step is to replace the intensity value in each voxel with the bin number to which that intensity was assigned. Thus, note that each voxel has two associated bin numbers—one from each image. The final step is to plot these bin number pairs for every voxel. These scatterplots are shown in the bottom panels of figures 4.8 and 4.9. MATLAB box 4.2 shows the code that was used to generate figure 4.8.

Note that the bin values shown in the bottom panels of figures 4.8 and 4.9 are much more strongly correlated for the images in alignment. The correlation is negative because the contrasts in the two images are reversed. Thus, to solve the coregistration problem, we could find the alignment (e.g., via rigid body registration) that maximizes something like the squared correlation between the bin numbers of the two images.

This method works because when the images are aligned, regions where the intensity is roughly constant should fall on top of each other, even if the contrasts in the two images are different and even if the voxel sizes are different. Thus, if a group of neighboring voxels in image 1 are all in the same histogram bin, then when the images are aligned, the same voxels in image 2 should also be in the same bin, even if the bin numbers for the two images are different. As a result, the most popular intensity-based coregistration algorithms find the rigid body movement that maximizes the association between the histogram bins of the voxels in the two images (e.g., Ashburner & Friston, 2007b; Hill, Batchelor, Holden, & Hawkes, 2001; Woods, Mazziotta, & Cherry, 1993).

One complication is that there is not really any reason to expect that when the images are aligned the association between bins will be linear. Linearity is approximately satisfied in figure 4.8, but with natural images a nonlinear association is possible. The widely known Pearson correlation coefficient (commonly denoted by $r_{12}$) only measures the strength of a linear relationship between two variables. For example, if two variables are related via a U-shaped function, then they are strongly associated because knowledge of one allows perfect prediction of the other. Even so, the correlation between these two variables is zero because a U-shaped function is neither increasing nor decreasing.

To solve this problem, the most popular coregistration algorithms use an alternative measure of association that is sensitive to any linear or nonlinear form of association. The measure, called *mutual information*, comes from a branch of mathematics called information theory, which was developed by Claude Shannon at Bell Labs back in the 1940s (Shannon & Weaver, 1949). Information theory plays a key role in independent component analysis, which is the topic of chapter 11. That chapter includes a brief overview of information theory and mutual information. For now it suffices to know that the mutual information between two variables is zero if and only if there is no association of any kind between the variables, or in other words, if the variables are statistically independent. In addition, mutual information increases as the association between the variables increases. The most popular algorithm for solving the coregistration problem is therefore to find the

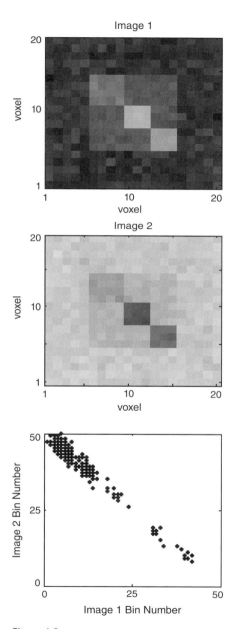

**Figure 4.8**
Two images and the scatterplot that is used for coregistration. Although the contrasts are reversed, note the obvious (negative) correlation in the scatterplot.

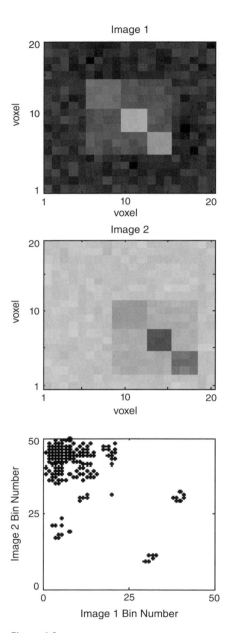

**Figure 4.9**
Two images and the scatterplot that is used for coregistration. Unlike in figure 4.8, the two images are now mis-aligned, and the scatterplot shows a much weaker correlation.

**MATLAB Box 4.2**
Coregistration using histogram bins (as in figure 4.8)

```
clear all; close all; clc;    % Clear all workspaces

% Read in the first image (i.e., X) and plot
X(1:20,1:20)=5; X(6:15,6:15)=12; X(6:9,6:9)=20;
X(10:12,10:12)=40; X(13:15,13:15)=32;
N=normrnd(0,1.5,[20,20]); X=X+N;
subplot(3,1,1); image(X); colormap(gray); brighten(.5);

% Read in the second image (i.e., Y) and plot
N=normrnd(0,1.5,[20,20]); Y=-X+N+50;
subplot(3,1,2); image(Y);

% Load the images into vectors
for i=1:20;
    XV(1+20*(i-1):20*i)=X(i,1:20);
    YV(1+20*(i-1):20*i)=Y(i,1:20);
end;

% Bin the entries in each vector (bin width = 1)
XBin=round(XV);
YBin=round(YV);

% Create a scatterplot
subplot(3,1,3); scatter(XBin,YBin,'k','.');
```

rigid body movement that maximizes the mutual information between the histogram bins of the voxels in the two images.

## Normalization

There are huge individual differences in the sizes and shapes of individual brains, and these differences extend to virtually every identifiable brain region. These differences make it difficult to assign a task-related activation observed in some cluster of voxels to a specific neuroanatomic brain structure. For example, suppose every subject in some experiment showed task-related activation in the same small cluster of voxels. How do we know what brain area this cluster is in? And how do we know that the cluster is in the same anatomic brain region in every subject?

A researcher particularly skilled in neuroanatomy could coregister the functional activation onto the structural image and then look for landmarks in the structural scan that would allow the neuroanatomic locus of the cluster to be identified. This process would then be repeated for every subject. As discussed in the preceding section, however, this process is time consuming and subjective, and it requires considerable neuroanatomic skill. An alternative is to register the structural scan of each subject separately to some standard brain where the coordinates of all major brain structures have already been identified and published in an atlas. Then we could determine the coordinates of a significant cluster within this standard brain, look these coordinates up in the atlas, and thereby determine which brain region the cluster is in. The process of registering a structural scan to the structural scan from some standard brain is called *normalization*.

Among the earliest and still most widely used brain atlases is the Talairach atlas (Talairach & Tournoux, 1988), which is based entirely on the detailed dissection of one hemisphere of the brain of a 60-year-old French woman. The coordinate system uses the same axes as in figure 4.5 with the origin [i.e., the point (0,0,0)] set to the midpoint of the anterior commissure. The atlas is essentially a look-up table containing major brain areas and their anatomic $(x, y, z)$ coordinates.

For many years, the Talairach atlas was almost universally used in neuroimaging, primarily because of the lack of any reasonable alternatives. But there has always been widespread dissatisfaction with this atlas because it is based on a single, rather unrepresentative brain. The brain it uses, for example, is smaller than the average brain by almost 10 mm in each direction. It is also flatter than the typical adult brain. This means that considerable morphing is usually required to register the structural scan of a typical subject to the Talairach atlas. More recently, an atlas produced by the Montreal Neurological Institute (MNI) has become popular. The MNI atlas was created by averaging the results of high-resolution structural scans that were taken from 152 different brains. The coordinate system was constructed to match the Talairach system, in the sense that it uses the same axes and origin.

Whichever atlas is used, it is important to note that the registration problem in normalization is considerably more complex than in head motion correction or coregistration. This is because normalization requires more than rigid body registration. Not only will there be rigid body differences between the standard brain and the brain of typical subjects, but there will also be size and shape differences. Size differences can be accommodated via a linear transformation, but a nonlinear transformation is almost always required to alter the shape of a subject's brain to match either the Talairach or MNI standards.

An added complication is that even when all these alignment differences have been optimally corrected, there will still be intensity differences between the subject's image and the reference image. We faced this same problem when solving coregistration, but with normalization the problem can be more severe. The functional and structural images that must be coregistered are collected using different scanning parameters, but at least they both come from the same subject and the same machine. For this reason, the intensity values in the aligned images should be highly correlated. In normalization, however, the two images we are trying to align were collected from different people on different machines. Thus, there is no way to predict the magnitude or the location of true differences beforehand. The goal of normalization is to correct for spatial differences between the test and reference images. Intensity differences are therefore only a nuisance factor that we must somehow deal with along the way (e.g., by using the histogram-binning procedure illustrated in figures 4.8 and 4.9).

There are many normalization algorithms (e.g., Ashburner & Friston, 2007a; Klein et al., 2009). In almost all, however, the first step is to find the linear transformation that aligns the subject's brain to the standard brain as closely as possible. The rigid body registration defined by equation 4.12 is a special case of a linear transformation that preserves size and shape. More general linear transformations will not only perform rigid body movements but also stretch or shrink the subject's brain along each axis to correct for size (and some shape) differences.

The most general linear transformation, called an *affine transformation* in mathematics, is given by

$$
\begin{bmatrix} u_x \\ u_y \\ u_z \end{bmatrix} = \begin{bmatrix} a_{xx} & a_{xy} & a_{xz} \\ a_{yx} & a_{yy} & a_{yz} \\ a_{zx} & a_{zy} & a_{zz} \end{bmatrix} \begin{bmatrix} w_x \\ w_y \\ w_z \end{bmatrix} + \begin{bmatrix} b_x \\ b_y \\ b_z \end{bmatrix}. \tag{4.13}
$$

Note that this transformation has 12 parameters: 9 $a_{ij}$ and 3 $b_i$. These typically would be estimated using the same procedures we used to solve the coregistration problem. For example, we could use an optimization algorithm to find the values of each of these parameters that maximize the mutual information between the histogram bin numbers of the two images.

Thus, the first step in the normalization process is to align the images as closely as possible using an affine transformation. This procedure will guarantee that the two images have roughly the same location, orientation, and size on each dimension. The differences that remain will typically require local stretching and shrinking to reduce. For example, the subject might have a larger prefrontal cortex than that of the standard brain but a smaller hippocampus. To align these two brains, therefore, we would have to stretch the hippocampus and shrink the prefrontal cortex. Linear transformations are incapable of such subtlety. Any operation performed by a linear transformation, such as stretching or shrinking, is applied equally everywhere. Therefore, to continue, a nonlinear transformation is required.

Whereas any (three-dimensional) linear transformation is defined by equation 4.13, a nonlinear transformation, by definition, is any transformation not defined by equation 4.13. Thus, nonlinear transformations are characterized by a definition of exclusion. This means, of course, that there are an infinite number of nonlinear transformations that can take wildly different forms.

In all forms of nonlinear registration, however, transformations are performed that differentially move separate parts of one image in an effort to align it with another image.

These movements change the spatial coordinates of the centroids of each voxel in the image that is moved. After the movements therefore, it is necessary to redefine the voxels. Without this redefinition, the voxels would no longer be rectangular volumes of equal size. The redefinition creates a slight problem though; namely, the new voxel centroids will tend to be positioned between the centroids of the voxels that were created during data collection. As a result, some form of interpolation is required to set the intensity values in the newly defined voxels. As we saw in the slice-timing correction section of this chapter, interpolation is straightforward and quite accurate when the to-be-interpolated function is fairly smooth. But this smoothness requirement places constraints on the nonlinear transformation that is used. In other words, the nonlinear transformation that is used must be locally smooth. This will guarantee that nearby image positions have similar intensity values. This same problem occurs with the linear registration methods that are used to correct for head movements and to coregister the functional and structural images, but as linear functions are always locally smooth, the resulting interpolations are not a concern.

Despite this smoothness constraint, many different nonlinear registration methods have been proposed. Some use a form of flexible curve fitting, and some use a form of local averaging. A different approach is to treat the to-be-moved image as an elastic body or a viscous fluid that is pushed and pulled by some external force. In all nonlinear approaches, the methods perform different transformations in each small brain region, and therefore they have many free parameters. Most nonlinear registration algorithms have thousands of parameters, and many have millions.

As an example of the way that a nonlinear registration method might align two small images, consider the two-dimensional hypothetical data denoted by the solid gray curve in the top panel of figure 4.10. For illustrative purposes, these data are continuous, but suppose they represent voxels that are each 2.5 mm wide. Specifically, suppose that the centers of these voxels are at the locations identified by the black dots. Suppose further that the best affine transformation has already been found, so that the data from the whole brain have been linearly aligned as well as possible. Finally, suppose that the black broken-line curve in figure 4.10 represents analogous spatial positions in the standard brain atlas. The problem here is to drag the dots on the gray curve to the dots on the black curve in such a way that all the points on the gray curve get dragged along (i.e., to guarantee local smoothness). In this simple example, we will only move each data point vertically, so the only issues to consider are how far to move each point and how to drag the other points on the data curve along in a way that guarantees smoothness. The algorithm could be generalized to allow both vertical and horizontal movements, but this would complicate the mathematics without much added pedagogical value.

There are many ways to warp the gray curve onto the black curve, but a simple way is to use a form of local averaging that is implemented via radial basis functions (e.g., Buhmann, 2003). In the current case, the algorithm would proceed as follows. Let $d(x)$ denote the vertical position at horizontal value $x$ on the data curve. Denote the vertical position

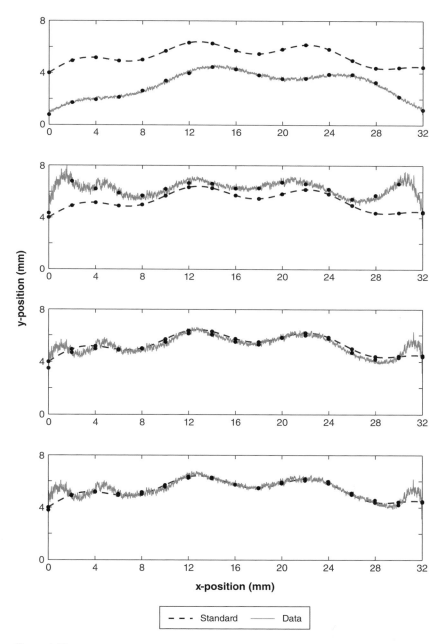

**Figure 4.10**
An example of a nonlinear warping step that might be used during the normalization process. The black broken-line curve represents the standard, and the solid gray curve represents our hypothetical data. The dots represent the voxel centroids. The warping process gradually aligns the data to the standard at each voxel centroid in a way that pulls along the points that are between the centroids.

of the $i^{th}$ reference voxel by $r_i$ and the vertical position of the $i^{th}$ data voxel by $d_i$. To determine the magnitude of the movement at the $i^{th}$ voxel, we compute

$$A_i = \frac{r_i - d_i}{d_i}.$$

Next we compute the correction factor at point $x$

$$C_i(x) = A_i d(x) b_i(x),$$

where

$$b_i(x) = e^{-\frac{(x-d_i)^2}{\theta}}.$$

Note that $b_i(x)$ is a Gaussian function centered at $d_i$ (where it has height 1) and with a width that increases with $\theta$. Finally, the warped version of $d(x)$ becomes

$$d_W(x) = d(x) + C_i(x).$$

This process is then repeated for all voxels (i.e., at all $d_i$).

The second panel in figure 4.10 shows the results. Note that the alignment with the referent is much better, but there is still considerable error. The error can be further reduced by simply repeating the process again. The bottom two panels of figure 4.10 show the effects of repeating this process one and two more times. Note that the final result is quite accurate, except for some small errors at the edges.

Klein et al. (2009) reported the results of comparing the accuracy of 14 different fully automated nonlinear normalization algorithms. Each algorithm was used several thousand times on 80 different manually labeled brain images, and the accuracy of these registrations was evaluated using eight different error measures. The top-rated algorithms were SyN (*Sy*mmetric Image *N*ormalization; Avants, Epstein, Grossman, & Gee, 2008) and ART (*A*utomatic *R*egistration *T*oolbox; Ardekani et al., 2005). Not far behind were IRTK (*I*mage *R*egistration *T*oolkit; Rueckert et al., 1999) and SPM's DARTEL (*D*iffeomorphic *A*natomical *R*egistration Using *E*xponentiated *L*ie Algebra; Ashburner, 2007). FSL uses FNIRT (*F*MRIB's *N*onlinear *I*mage *R*egistration *T*ool; Andersson, Smith, & Jenkinson, 2008), which was in the third tier of algorithms.

## Spatial Smoothing

The next preprocessing step is spatial smoothing. In this step, the BOLD value in each voxel is replaced by a weighted average of the BOLD responses in neighboring voxels. The weight is greatest at the voxel being smoothed and decreases with distance. Thus, voxels far from the to-be-smoothed voxel contribute almost nothing and nearby voxels contribute a lot. The rate at which the weights decrease with distance determines the amount of smoothing. Spatial smoothing essentially blurs the data at each TR by smoothing off peaks and filling in valleys.

There are a number of advantages to spatially smoothing fMRI data. Most of these are due to the effects of the smoothing process on noise in the data. First, because smoothing replaces each BOLD response with a weighted sum of BOLD responses, the central limit theorem tells us that smoothing will make the distribution of the BOLD responses more normal. As we will see in the next chapter, the statistical models that dominate fMRI data analysis assume normally distributed noise. Thus, smoothing transforms the data in a way that makes it more likely to satisfy the assumptions of our statistical models.

A second benefit of smoothing is that it is required by a number of popular methods for solving the multiple comparisons problem. In the standard fMRI analysis, a separate decision is made about whether each voxel displays task-related activation. The multiple comparisons problem, which is the topic of chapter 6, is to protect all these decisions against the possibility of too many false positives. Several of the most popular methods for solving this problem are derived from Gaussian random field theory, and the significance thresholds recommended by all of these methods assume spatial smoothing with a Gaussian kernel. Thus, if smoothing is not done, then Gaussian random field theory should not be used as a solution to the multiple comparisons problem.

A third benefit of smoothing, which is the most important of all, is that it can reduce noise and therefore increase signal-to-noise ratio. As mentioned before, fMRI data are noisy, and changes in the BOLD response that are task related are small. Thus, any preprocessing step that can increase signal-to-noise ratio can greatly increase the chances of success in an fMRI experiment. Later in this section, we will consider the technical reasons that smoothing can increase signal-to-noise ratio. First, however, we describe the mathematical details of the smoothing operation.

Spatial smoothing is implemented by applying a three-dimensional filter or kernel to the BOLD responses. Let $B(x_i, y_j, z_k)$ denote the BOLD response at the voxel with spatial coordinates $(x_i, y_j, z_k)$. Then the smoothing step replaces $B(x_i, y_j, z_k)$ with the value

$$B_S(x_i, y_j, z_k) = \frac{\sum_q \sum_r \sum_s f_x(x_q - x_i) f_y(y_r - y_j) f_z(z_s - z_k) B(x_q, y_r, z_s)}{\sum_q \sum_r \sum_s f_x(x_q - x_i) f_y(y_r - y_j) f_z(z_s - z_k)}. \qquad (4.14)$$

This equation is applied successively at every voxel $(x_i, y_j, z_k)$ in the brain. The functions $f_x, f_y,$ and $f_z$ are the smoothing kernels along directions $x$, $y$, and $z$, respectively. The product of these, $f_x(x_q - x_i) \times f_y(y_r - y_j) \times f_z(z_s - z_k)$, equals the weight given to the BOLD response at voxel $(x_q, y_r, z_s)$ when smoothing the BOLD response at voxel $(x_i, y_j, z_k)$. The denominator of equation 4.14 simply guarantees that the sum of all weights applied when smoothing

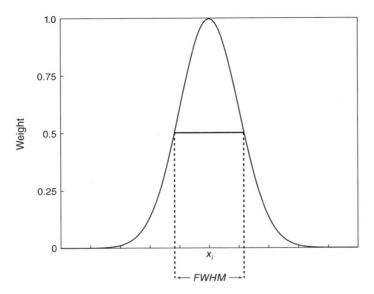

**Figure 4.11**
A Gaussian smoothing kernel and an illustration of its width parameter FWHM (full width at half maximum).

$B(x_i, y_j, z_k)$ equals 1. This is critical to ensure that the smoothing operation does not change the mean BOLD response across the whole brain at any TR.

The standard choice for the smoothing kernel is a Gaussian function that is centered at the to-be-smoothed voxel. For example, with a Gaussian kernel

$$f_x(x - x_i) = e^{-\frac{(x-x_i)^2}{2\sigma_x^2}},$$
                                                                                    (4.15)

which is proportional to the probability density function of a normal distribution with mean $x_i$ and variance $\sigma_x^2$. Analogous definitions hold for $f_y(y - y_j)$ and $f_z(z - z_k)$. The amount of smoothing that occurs depends on the numerical values of the three variances $\sigma_x^2$, $\sigma_y^2$, and $\sigma_z^2$. The larger these values, the more smoothing because voxels far from $(x_i, y_j, z_k)$ will be given a greater weight when the variance is large. So $\sigma_i^2$ measures the width of the kernel in direction $i$. In fMRI, a more common measure of width is the so-called *full width at half maximum* (FWHM), which is illustrated in figure 4.11. The FWHM along direction $i$, denoted $FWHM_i$, is equal to the width of the interval between the points at which the height of the smoothing kernel along direction $i$ is exactly half its peak height. In figure 4.11, the peak height of the kernel is 1, so half this height is 0.5. The width of the kernel at height 0.5 therefore equals its FWHM. With a Gaussian kernel, $FWHM_i$ is equal to

$$FWHM_i = \sqrt{8 \ln 2} \, \sigma_i.$$
                                                                                    (4.16)

The $FWHM_i$ values measure the width of the kernel and therefore the amount of smoothing that occurs in each direction. Rewriting the Gaussian kernel in equation 4.15 in terms of this measure of width produces

$$f_x(x - x_i) = e^{-\frac{4\ln 2(x-x_i)^2}{FWHM_x^2}}. \tag{4.17}$$

At the beginning of this section, it was noted that spatial smoothing can increase signal-to-noise ratio. The key result here is the matched filter theorem of signal processing (e.g., Allen & Mills, 2004), which states that the filter that maximizes signal-to-noise ratio is the one with the same size and shape as the signal. The theorem is illustrated in figure 4.12. The top panel shows a Gaussian signal. The middle panel shows the same signal embedded in noise. Note that the signal is now barely visible. The bottom panel shows the results of smoothing the middle panel with a kernel that exactly matches the signal. This was done with a one-dimensional version of equation 4.14; that is, where there is an $f_x$ (i.e., equal to the signal) but no $f_y$ or $f_z$, and $B_S(x, y, z)$ and $B(x, y, z)$ are replaced with $B_S(x)$ and $B(x)$, respectively. Note that the smoothing almost perfectly recovers the signal. The MATLAB code used to produce this figure is shown in MATLAB box 4.3.

Figure 4.12 shows that spatial smoothing can dramatically improve signal-to-noise ratio, provided we have some good idea about the nature of the signal we are trying to recover. The ability of smoothing to increase signal-to-noise ratio is reduced if the filter or smoothing kernel is either narrower or wider than the signal. The effects of these two errors though are different. If the kernel is too narrow, then the data will not be smoothed enough, and there may still be too much noise present to detect the signal. Smoothing too much with a kernel that is wider than the signal may cause even more serious problems. First, when the kernel is centered over the signal, other regions that contain only noise will be averaged in, thereby reducing the estimated signal intensity. If too much noise is included in the averaging process, the signal may disappear.

A second problem that can result from too much averaging is that separate signals can be fused together (e.g., Fransson, Merbolt, Petersson, Ingvar, & Frahm, 2002). This problem is illustrated in figure 4.13. The top panel shows two separate signals: a stronger and slightly wider signal centered at 15, and a weaker and narrower signal centered at 22 (the solid black curve). The middle panel shows these same two signals embedded in noise. The bottom panel shows the results of smoothing the noisy data in the middle panel with the smoothing kernel shown in the top panel (the broken gray curve). Note that this kernel is slightly wider than either signal. The bottom panel shows that smoothing with this kernel causes the two signals to fuse together. The best that any statistical analysis could do with such a result is to identify a single signal. The identity of the two separate signals was lost even though the smoothing kernel is only slightly wider than the wider of the two signals.

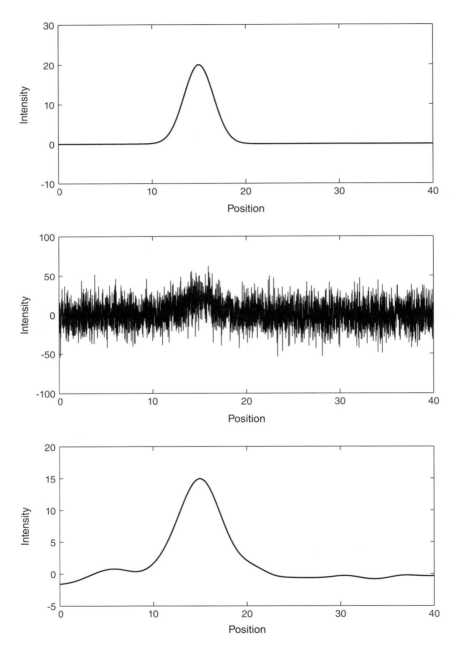

**Figure 4.12**
An illustration of the matched filter theorem. The top panel shows a signal. The middle panel shows the same signal embedded in noise. The bottom panel shows the results of smoothing the middle panel with a filter that exactly matches the signal.

**MATLAB Box 4.3**
The matched filter theorem (as in figure 4.12)

```
clear all; close all; clc;    % Clear all workspaces

% Define time and the signal. Plot.
t=[0:.01:40]; ystand=20*exp(-(t-15).^2/5);
subplot(3,1,1); plot(t,ystand); axis([0 40 -10 30]);

% Read in (or create) the data. Plot.
ydat=ystand+normrnd(0,35,1,length(t));
subplot(3,1,2); plot(t,ydat); axis([0 40 -200 200]);

% correlate the matched filter with the data & plot the results.
for j=1:4001;
    r=exp(-(t-j*.01).^2/5);
    Corect=r.*ydat;
    ypred(j)=sum(Corect)/sum(r);
end;
subplot(3,1,3); plot(t,ypred); axis([0 40 -5 20]);
```

For these reasons, it is important to choose a kernel width that is not wider than the smallest signal that one hopes to identify. In practice, a common choice for kernel width (i.e., the FWHM) is somewhere between 1 and 3 voxel widths. For example, if the voxel size is 3 mm × 3 mm × 3.5 mm, then a standard choice might be $FWHM_x = FWHM_y = 6$ mm and $FWHM_z = 7$ mm.

## Temporal Filtering

The last preprocessing step we consider in detail is temporal filtering. Spatial filtering smoothes the data at each TR across neighboring voxels. In contrast, temporal filtering smoothes the data at each voxel across neighboring TRs. Thus, in spatial filtering, the data to be smoothed are three-dimensional spatial maps. In temporal filtering, the data are one-dimensional time series.

The goal of both types of filtering is to reduce noise and thereby make it easier to identify the signal. The two procedures focus on very different types of noise, however. Spatial smoothing primarily reduces high-frequency noise; that is, noise that changes quickly across small regions of the brain. The blurring caused by the local averaging that defines spatial smoothing reduces or eliminates intensity (e.g., BOLD) changes that happen over smaller distances than we expect from task-related activation.

The time series that are the focus of temporal filtering contain no high-frequency noise. The Nyquist–Shannon sampling theorem mentioned earlier states that to determine the

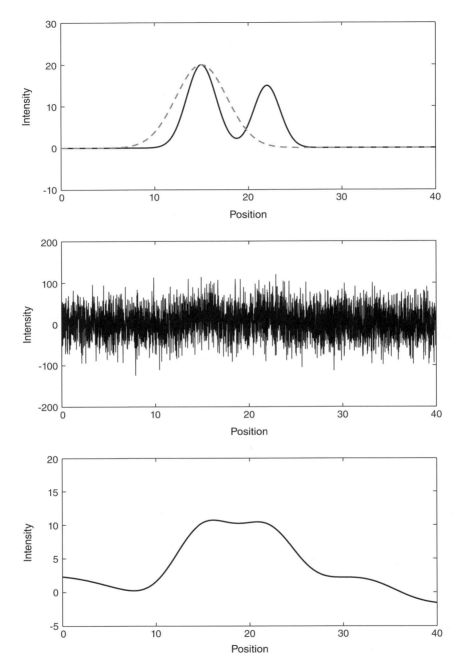

**Figure 4.13**
Results of smoothing with a kernel that is wider than the signal. The solid black curve in the top panel is an example of two spatially separated signals. The dotted-line gray curve is the smoothing kernel. The middle panel shows the same signals embedded in noise. The bottom panel shows the results of smoothing the middle panel with the dotted-line gray curve of the top panel.

frequency of a sine wave, we must record at least two samples per period. In an fMRI time series, we record one value of the BOLD response (in each voxel) every TR seconds. Thus, if the TR is 2 seconds, the highest temporal frequency we can collect information about has a period of 4 seconds. This means that in 1 second, it has completed one-quarter of a cycle and therefore has a frequency of 0.25 Hz (i.e., cycles per second). Frequencies higher than 0.25 Hz are lost in the discrete-time sampling process. In other words, the poor temporal resolution of fMRI effectively filters out all high temporal frequency noise.

For this reason, temporal filtering only makes sense as a method to reduce temporal low-frequency noise; that is, unexplained and very slow changes in the BOLD response across time. In chapter 3, we saw that the hrf changes slowly over time—rising to a peak after about 6 seconds and decaying back to baseline after about 25 seconds. Clearly, we do not want to interfere with our ability to observe this response, so any low temporal frequencies we try to eliminate must be considerably slower than this. In practice, it is common only to eliminate frequencies less than about 0.0083 Hz, which corresponds with a period of 2 minutes or longer. In event-related designs, such slow changes are almost surely not due to any task-related factor. A likely cause is slow fluctuations in the local magnetic field properties of the scanner (Smith et al., 1999). Such fluctuations can be especially problematic with older machines. In many newer scanners, measurable drift is negligible. At any rate, temporal filtering can reduce or eliminate the effects of such drift from the data.

With block designs, temporal filtering can be dangerous. For example, if we alternate blocks of rest and task every 2 minutes, then we can expect periodic changes in task-related activation that repeat every 4 minutes, or at a frequency of $\frac{1}{240} = 0.0042$ Hz. Filtering out frequencies below 0.0083 Hz would therefore reduce or eliminate most of the effect we were trying to discover. For this reason, with most block-design data, we would have to set our frequency cutoff considerably lower than with event-related data. A common choice is twice the period at which the task-related activation is expected to repeat. In our example with 2-minute blocks, this rule produces a cutoff period of 8 minutes and therefore a cutoff frequency of $\frac{1}{480} = 0.0021$ Hz.

As with the other preprocessing steps discussed in this chapter, temporal filtering can be implemented in a variety of different ways. In SPM, temporal filtering is done by adding a set of discrete cosine transform basis functions to the design matrix of the general linear model (the topic of chapter 5). Essentially, this correlates the BOLD response with cosine functions of different low frequencies. Because the correlations are specifically modeled in this way, low-frequency fluctuations do not affect the analysis of task-related activation.

FSL uses a different approach, which is illustrated in figure 4.14. The solid curve in the top panel shows a hypothetical BOLD response from a block design that is corrupted by low-frequency scanner drift. The design alternates blocks of task and rest that are each 25 seconds in duration. Thus, the task-related activation has a period of 50 seconds. The scanner drift, which is modeled here as a simple low-frequency sine wave, has a period of roughly 630 seconds. This causes the task-related activation to fluctuate slowly over time.

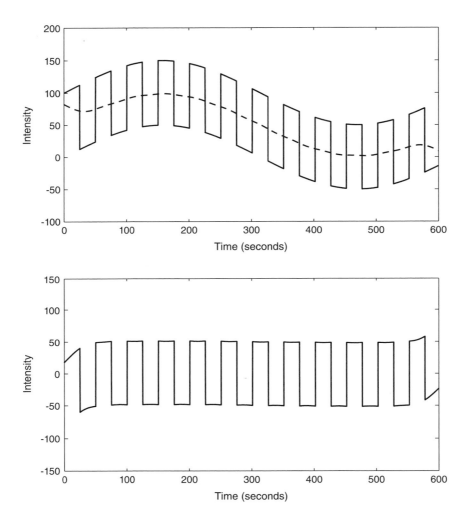

**Figure 4.14**
The high-pass temporal filtering algorithm used by FSL. The solid curve in the top panel shows a hypothetical BOLD response from a block design that is corrupted by low-frequency scanner drift. The broken-line curve shows the results of low-pass filtering these data. The bottom panel shows the results of subtracting the low-pass filtered data from the raw data.

**MATLAB Box 4.4**
High-pass temporal filtering (as in figure 4.14)

```
clear all; close all; clc;   % Clear all workspaces

% Create and plot the data
t=[0:.1:600];
y=50+50*sin(.01*t)+50*square(.25*t);
subplot(2,1,1); plot(t,y); axis([0 600 -100 200]); hold on;

% Low-pass filter by smoothing with a Gaussian kernel & plot
W=250;                    % W = kernel width
for j=1:6001;
   r=exp(-(t-j*.1).^2/W);
   Corect=r.*y;
   ylow(j)=sum(Corect)/sum(r);
end;
plot(t,ylow,'k');

% Subtract low-pass filtered data from raw data & plot
ypred=y-ylow;
subplot(2,1,2); plot(t,ypred); axis([0 600 -100 100]);
```

The first step in the FSL approach is to low-pass filter the data using a Gaussian kernel with a large FWHM. The broken line curve in the top panel of figure 4.14 shows the results of this smoothing. Mathematically, this step is identical to the procedures we used to construct figures 4.12 and 4.13, except a large FWHM is used. In figure 4.14, the FWHM is approximately equal to 59. Note that this value is large enough to smooth away the task-related activation but not large enough to reduce the variation due to scanner drift. Thus, after this filtering step, the higher frequencies have been removed from the data, and all that is left is the low-frequency noise.

The second and final step, which is illustrated in the bottom panel of figure 4.14, is to subtract the low-pass filtered data from the raw data. Both data sets contain roughly the same low frequencies, but only the raw data contains any high frequencies. All that is left after the subtraction, therefore, is the high-frequency components of the raw data. Figure 4.14 shows that this procedure effectively removes the influence of scanner drift from our data. MATLAB box 4.4 shows the code that implements this high-pass filtering algorithm.

## Other Preprocessing Steps

The six steps discussed in this chapter are common preprocessing procedures. In addition, however, several other steps are also often included as part of the preprocessing analysis.

## Quality Assurance

Anyone collecting any kind of data on human subjects knows the importance of inspecting the data to ensure that it is not corrupted because of some unexpected problem. fMRI data are no different. In fact, because of the complexity of the data acquisition process, quality assurance is especially important with fMRI data.

A psychologist who collects human behavioral data in his or her own laboratory is responsible for all aspects of quality assurance. fMRI data, however, are typically collected in a brain-imaging center that is a shared research facility with its own dedicated professional staff. Although the final responsibility for the quality of the data rests with the investigator who designed and ran the experiment, quality assurance very much depends on the skill and dedication of the imaging center personnel and on the quality of the scanner and other brain-imaging center equipment.

A strong imaging center will run frequent quality assurance tests to check on the reliability and accuracy of the scanner (e.g., Firbank, Harrison, Williams, & Coulthard, 2000). As just one example, it is common for imaging centers to regularly scan *phantoms*, which are artificial objects, such as fluid-filled spheres, that are used to test MR systems. A skilled MR professional can identify and then correct many potential problems by examining the results of such tests. An excellent brain-imaging center can therefore greatly reduce (but not eliminate) the need for aggressive quality assurance by the investigator.

Even so, every investigator should do some quality assurance. At the very least, the raw images from each individual subject should be visually examined. Unfortunately, this is a process that is difficult to automate. There are many potential problems that could occur during the data collection process, and at least with modern MR systems, most of these have low probability. Many of these problems leave a telltale signature in the raw data that can quickly be identified by an experienced MR researcher. But the ability to troubleshoot MR data acquisition by looking at raw images is a skill that only comes slowly with much hard work.

## Distortion Correction

As briefly discussed in chapter 1, an ideal scanner produces a perfectly uniform magnetic field throughout its bore (i.e., before the gradients are applied). No scanner is perfect, however, and even if it were, placing a person inside the scanner will distort that field. Modern scanners have *shimming coils* that are adjusted after the subject is inside the scanner in an effort to correct for inhomogeneities in the magnetic field. There are at least two reasons though why adjusting these coils might not produce a completely uniform magnetic field that is maintained throughout the experimental session. First, scanner drift might cause inhomogeneities to reappear sometime during the session, even if initial shimming was successful. This is more of a problem with older machines. Second, the sinus cavities can cause local inhomogeneities that are not easily corrected via shimming. This can be an especially serious problem if there is research interest in brain regions that lie near the sinuses, such as the orbitofrontal cortex. In particular, inhomogeneities near the sinuses can distort data collected in nearby brain regions.

For these reasons, it is common to collect one or more field maps during the scanning session (see chapter 1). A field map, which takes only a minute or two to collect, measures the homogeneity of the magnetic field. It can be used to correct for inhomogeneities via a process that is similar to normalization (Jezzard & Balaban, 1995). The basic idea is to find the transformation that corrects the inhomogeneities in the field map and then apply this same transformation to the functional and structural images. If scanner drift is a problem, several field maps can be collected during the scanning session. For example, a field map might be collected before the start of each functional run. During preprocessing, the data for each run could then be corrected for the inhomogeneities that existed at the start of the run.

### Grand Mean Scaling

Grand mean scaling normalizes the mean of the BOLD responses from each functional run to the same numerical value. This step is routinely carried out by both SPM and FSL. The goal is to eliminate any global differences across sessions or subjects that might be due to extraneous effects. For example, the magnitude of the overall BOLD response could change from one session to another because of differences in magnetic field strength or because of differences in the subject's respiration and heart rate (e.g., Petersson, Nichols, Poline, & Holmes, 1999). Some of these effects will be removed during preprocessing by temporal filtering and during statistical analysis by the general linear model (see chapter 5). Even so, neither of these methods will correct for slow changes in magnetic field strength that occur over the course of hours or days or in cerebral blood oxygenation differences between subjects. Normalizing the overall mean BOLD response in each session to the same numerical value corrects for these session-to-session differences.

Grand mean scaling originated with PET scanning. Because of variability in the time course and efficacy of the radioactive label, the global mean in PET scanning changes significantly over time and across subjects. Grand mean scaling can correct for differences across subjects but not for differences across time. As a result, other more complex methods were also developed. The collection of all these is often called *global normalization*. One approach, called proportional scaling, essentially constrains all voxels to have the same mean at every TR. When applied to fMRI, many of these more complex methods have been shown to bias the experimental results (e.g., Gavrilescu et al., 2002; Murphy, Birn, Handwerker, Jones, & Bandettini, 2009). Because the problems that global normalization methods were designed to address are not nearly as severe with fMRI data as they are with PET scanning data, a conservative approach is to avoid proportional scaling or any other method of global normalization except grand mean scaling.

Grand mean scaling is automatically performed by both SPM and FSL. First, a single mean BOLD response is computed for each functional run (i.e., across all TRs and all voxels). Next, each single BOLD response from that run (i.e., on each TR in every voxel) is divided by this mean. The overall mean is now 1. Finally, each single BOLD response is multiplied by a constant (e.g., 100 or 10,000), which becomes the new global mean.

## Conclusions

As this chapter should make clear, there are many preprocessing steps and many choices to make about how to preprocess fMRI data. Researchers must decide how much quality assurance to do, whether to motion correct before or after slice-timing correction, whether to slice-timing correct and temporal filter during preprocessing or during statistical analysis, how much spatial smoothing to do, and which normalization algorithm to use. Some of these decisions will depend on methodology and parameter choices made by the brain-imaging center where the data are collected. For example, we saw that the convention is to slice-timing correct before motion correction with interleaved slice acquisition, but to use the opposite order with ascending slice acquisition. Other choices may depend on a personal decision about how to resolve the trade-off between statistical power and computing time.

One significant challenge that must be overcome when beginning an fMRI research program is to make all these choices. Because some are facility dependent, the imaging center director and other researchers using the same facility should be consulted. Once a set of procedures is selected, the procedures are usually used without significant modification for every experiment run on the same scanner. Because of the repetitive nature of these preprocessing steps, the particular set of preprocessing procedures used by a research laboratory is often referred to as the *preprocessing pipeline*.

After data collection has been completed in an fMRI experiment, the first step in data analysis then is to run all the data through the preprocessing pipeline. Once this process is complete, the more interesting search can begin for task-related activation. This latter problem is the topic of the rest of this book.

# 5    The General Linear Model

This chapter surveys the most popular current methods for identifying brain regions that show task-related activity. Number one on this list is a correlation-based technique that is the foundation of most fMRI software packages (Friston, Frith, Liddle, & Frackowiak, 1991; Friston et al., 1995b). More recently, a method that generalizes the FIR model of the hrf (see chapter 3) to the BOLD response (Ollinger, Corbetta, & Shulman, 2001a; Ollinger, Shulman, & Corbetta, 2001b) has also become popular. The FIR model considers the hrf as a discrete sequence of impulses (i.e., delta functions). As we saw in chapter 3 the hrf is the impulse response of the black box that converts neural activation to a BOLD response, hence FIR is named "finite impulse response." The method proposed by Ollinger et al. (2001a, 2001b) models the BOLD response (rather than the hrf) as a discrete sequence of impulses, so in this book the method will be called the finite BOLD response (FBR) model. Although the correlation and FBR methods are based on philosophically different approaches, they are analyzed using the same statistical model (i.e., the general linear model, or GLM), and for this reason, both methods are covered in this chapter.

The correlation and FBR methods both apply to data from a single voxel at a time. Thus, if an experiment collects data from the whole brain, both of these analyses would have to be repeated as many as 100,000 times to analyze all of the data collected in the experiment. Because both methods analyze one voxel at a time, they are examples of *univariate* statistical techniques. Chapters 10 and 11 consider *multivariate* methods that analyze data from all voxels simultaneously.

The correlation method preceded the FBR method by a decade or so, and the older method is also the more popular. Nevertheless, the FBR method is conceptually simpler, and it makes fewer assumptions. For this reason, we begin by considering the FBR method, and then later in this chapter we turn to the correlation method. Our main focus is on event-related designs, but later in the chapter we will also consider block designs.

## The FBR Method

Consider a rapid event-related design with only one stimulus type. Suppose the TR equals 3 seconds, and for convenience suppose that the BOLD response to each stimulus onset persists for a total of only 14 seconds. Suppose also that we present a stimulus every 6 seconds. Then the sequence of events on consecutive TRs will be

TR:     1   2   3   4    5    6    7  . . .
Time:   0   3   6   9   12   15   18
Events: E       E        E         E

where E denotes a stimulus presentation. On TRs 1 and 2, note that the observed BOLD response in this experiment will exactly equal the BOLD response to the stimulus event. However, on TR 4, the observed BOLD response will be affected by the event that occurred on TR 1 and the event that occurred on TR 3. If we want to estimate the complete BOLD response to the stimulus, then at TR 4 we must somehow separate the contributions of the events that occurred at TRs 1 and 3. This is exactly the problem that the FBR method (Ollinger et al., 2001a, 2001b) was designed to solve.

To proceed, we must have a model that specifies how the separate BOLD responses from events 1 and 2 combine. Chapter 3 introduced the superposition principle, which assumes that the BOLD response to two separate neural activations is the sum of the BOLD response to each activation separately. If the superposition principle holds in the current experiment, our problem is solved because then the observed BOLD response at TR 4 will be the sum of the residual BOLD response to the event that occurred at TR 1 plus the BOLD response to the event that occurred at TR 3.

If the TR is 3 seconds, and if the BOLD response to a stimulus onset lasts for 14 seconds, then the BOLD response to any stimulus presentation will last[1] for five TRs. In this case, the FBR method defines five different parameters that describe the BOLD response to the stimulus presentation at each of the ensuing five TRs. Call these five parameters $\beta_1$, $\beta_2$, $\beta_3$, $\beta_4$, and $\beta_5$. Figure 5.1 illustrates this notation. If we assume instead that the BOLD response to a stimulus onset lasts for 25 seconds, then nine different $\beta_i$ would be needed, rather than five. Note that figure 5.1 models the BOLD response at each TR as a delta function and that $\beta_i$ denotes the height or magnitude of the $i$th of these delta functions. Thus, the figure 5.1 model is mathematically identical to the FIR model of chapter 3 where $\beta_i$ plays the same role as $\theta_i$ in equation 3.16. The only difference between the models is that FIR models the hrf in this way and FBR models the BOLD response. Remember that the hrf is the BOLD response to an idealized impulse of neural activation, whereas the BOLD response in figure 5.1 could be generated by any neural activation.

---

1. Technically the word "finite" in both the FIR and FBR names comes from the assumption that the hrf and BOLD responses are nonzero for only a finite number of TRs. Thus, for example, the FBR model needs only a finite number of $\beta_i$ parameters. Note that mathematically this contradicts most of the other hrf models we considered in Chapter 3. For example, the gamma function model of the hrf (equation 3.6) assumes the hrf > 0 for all TRs after event presentation. In practice this is not a serious problem though because the gamma function assumes that the magnitude of this positive hrf is negligible for large values of time.

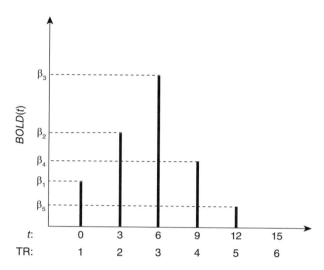

**Figure 5.1**
Illustration of how the FBR method defines the $\beta_i$ parameters.

If we also assume that every time the same stimulus is presented the exact same BOLD response occurs, then the stimulus events and their BOLD responses at each TR will be:

| TR: | 1 | 2 | 3 | 4 | 5 | 6 | 7 | 8 | ... |
|---|---|---|---|---|---|---|---|---|---|
| Time: | 0 | 3 | 6 | 9 | 12 | 15 | 18 | 21 | |
| Events: | E | | E | | E | | E | | |
| BOLD response to 1st event: | $\beta_1$ | $\beta_2$ | $\beta_3$ | $\beta_4$ | $\beta_5$ | | | | |
| BOLD response to 2nd event: | | | $\beta_1$ | $\beta_2$ | $\beta_3$ | $\beta_4$ | $\beta_5$ | | |
| BOLD response to 3rd event: | | | | | $\beta_1$ | $\beta_2$ | $\beta_3$ | $\beta_4$ | |
| BOLD response to 4th event: | | | | | | | $\beta_1$ | $\beta_2$ | |

Therefore, if the superposition principle holds, then the observed BOLD response at each TR will equal:

| TR | BOLD |
|---|---|
| 1 | $\beta_1$ |
| 2 | $\beta_2$ |
| 3 | $\beta_1 + \beta_3$ |
| 4 | $\beta_2 + \beta_4$ |
| 5 | $\beta_1 + \beta_3 + \beta_5$ |
| 6 | $\beta_2 + \beta_4$ |
| 7 | $\beta_1 + \beta_3 + \beta_5$ |
| 8 | $\beta_2 + \beta_4$ |

**Jittering**

The FBR method uses these equations and the observed BOLD responses from this experiment to estimate the unknown values of all $\beta_i$. If this experimental design was extended to include many TRs, then note that a new stimulus would be presented on every odd TR, and on every even TR the subject would rest. In this case, it is straightforward to see that except for the first and last three TRs, the predicted BOLD response on every even TR is $\beta_2 + \beta_4$, and the predicted BOLD response on every odd TR is $\beta_1 + \beta_3 + \beta_5$. In other words, the FBR method predicts that in this experiment, the observed BOLD response on virtually every odd-numbered TR would equal one value, whereas on almost all even-numbered TRs it would equal another value. If this were true, then note that we could get a good estimate of the sum $\beta_2 + \beta_4$, but we could not separately estimate the components $\beta_2$ and $\beta_4$. Similarly, we could get a good estimate of the sum $\beta_1 + \beta_3 + \beta_5$, but we could not uniquely estimate the components $\beta_1$, $\beta_3$, and $\beta_5$. Thus, our design is flawed because $\beta_2$ (almost) always appears with $\beta_4$, and $\beta_1$, $\beta_3$, and $\beta_5$ almost always appear together.

To avoid this identification problem, we need to vary the amount of time between events. For example, consider the following design:

| | TR: | 1 | 2 | 3 | 4 | 5 | 6 | 7 | 8 | ... |
|---|---|---|---|---|---|---|---|---|---|---|
| | Time: | 0 | 3 | 6 | 9 | 12 | 15 | 18 | 21 | |
| | Events: | E | | E | E | | | E | | |
| BOLD response to 1st event: | | $\beta_1$ | $\beta_2$ | $\beta_3$ | $\beta_4$ | $\beta_5$ | | | | |
| BOLD response to 2nd event: | | | | $\beta_1$ | $\beta_2$ | $\beta_3$ | $\beta_4$ | $\beta_5$ | | |
| BOLD response to 3rd event: | | | | | $\beta_1$ | $\beta_2$ | $\beta_3$ | $\beta_4$ | $\beta_5$ | |
| BOLD response to 4th event: | | | | | | | | $\beta_1$ | $\beta_2$ | |

In this case, the observed BOLD response at each TR will equal:

| TR | BOLD |
|---|---|
| 1 | $\beta_1$ |
| 2 | $\beta_2$ |
| 3 | $\beta_1 + \beta_3$ |
| 4 | $\beta_1 + \beta_2 + \beta_4$ |
| 5 | $\beta_2 + \beta_3 + \beta_5$ |
| 6 | $\beta_3 + \beta_4$ |
| 7 | $\beta_1 + \beta_4 + \beta_5$ |
| 8 | $\beta_2 + \beta_5$ |

$$(5.1)$$

Note that now every equation is different, so we have a much better chance of obtaining unique and accurate estimates of each $\beta_i$.

In the fMRI literature, the process of varying the amount of time between events is called *jittering*. Jittering is a necessary design feature in any rapid, event-related design.

Without jittering, it would be impossible to separate BOLD responses from successive events or to obtain unique estimates of model parameters. A variety of jittering algorithms could prove effective, but one approach, which is both effective and popular, is to determine the time between events by sampling randomly from a truncated geometric distribution.

If a geometric distribution was used to determine the interevent intervals, then the probability that the delay between events would equal $n$ TRs would be given by

$$P(\text{Delay} = n) = p(1 - p)^n, \tag{5.2}$$

where $p$ is a parameter between 0 and 1. A common choice is $p = .5$. The geometric distribution, which is the discrete analogue of the exponential distribution, is an attractive choice for an intertrial interval because it provides the subject no information about when the next stimulus presentation will occur. For example, with a uniform distribution there would be a fixed upper limit on the delay length, so an ideal observer would know that every blank TR increases the probability that the stimulus will appear on the next TR. At the extreme, on trials when the longest possible delay occurs, the ideal observer knows with certainty that the stimulus will appear on the next TR. The geometric is the only discrete distribution (and the exponential is the only continuous distribution) that provides an ideal observer no opportunity to anticipate the stimulus presentation. If $M$ blank TRs have elapsed, the probability that the stimulus will appear on the next TR is $p$, regardless of the value of $M$. For this reason, the geometric and exponential distributions are widely used to define intertrial intervals in experiments where such anticipations could bias the results, such as simple reaction time experiments (e.g., Luce, 1986).

One problem with the geometric distribution, though, is that it ensures that some extremely long delays are possible. This is not usually a problem in experiments run in a psychological laboratory, but in fMRI experiments long delays are expensive. A common solution is to truncate the distribution, or in other words to place an upper limit on the length of the longest possible delay. This allows an ideal observer some opportunity to anticipate the stimulus presentation, but it guarantees no long and expensive delays.

Suppose the longest delay we allow is $N_{max}$ TRs. If we use the first $N_{max}$ terms in equation 5.2 to calculate the probabilities of the various delays, then the sum of probabilities will be less than 1. Therefore, we must condition equation 5.2 by dividing by the sum of the first $N_{max}$ terms in equation 5.2. In other words,

$$P(\text{Delay} = n) = \frac{p(1-p)^n}{\displaystyle\sum_{i=0}^{N_{max}} p(1-p)^i}. \tag{5.3}$$

For example, setting $p = .5$ and disallowing any delay longer than four TRs produces the following probability distribution:

| No. of TRs in Delay | $P$(Delay) |
|---|---|
| 0 | 16/31 |
| 1 | 8/31 |
| 2 | 4/31 |
| 3 | 2/31 |
| 4 | 1/31 |

Note that, as required, the probabilities sum to 1. This same sampling scheme would be used regardless of the number of event types; that is, samples from the equation 5.3 distribution would be used to define the delays between all consecutive events, whether or not they are the same type.

To sample values from this distribution, the following algorithm can be used. Draw a random sample from a uniform (0, 1) distribution. If the sampled value is in the interval (0, .516], the next delay is zero TRs (i.e., .516 = 16/31). If the value is in the interval (.516, .774], the delay is one TR. If the value is in the interval (.774, .903], then the delay is two TRs. If the value is in the interval (.903, .968], the delay is three TRs. Finally, if a value greater than .968 is obtained, then the delay is four TRs. Later in this chapter, we will consider one method for evaluating the effectiveness of any particular jittering strategy.

### Microlinearity versus Macrolinearity

The FBR method uses the superposition principle to predict how BOLD responses from separate events will combine at each TR. This is the same assumption that we used in chapter 3 to predict BOLD responses to arbitrary neural activations from the hrf. Even so, it is important to note that the timescales of these two applications of the superposition principle are different. In particular, the FBR method assumes that superposition can be used to predict how BOLD responses to events that are well separated in time will combine, whereas the hrf approach assumes that superposition can be used to predict the BOLD response to individual neural activations, no matter how brief. As a result, we refer to the hrf use of superposition as *microlinearity* and the FBR use as *macrolinearity*.

As discussed in chapter 3, Boynton et al. (1996) showed that microlinearity holds for long-duration neural events but not for shorter durations. Dale and Buckner (1997) tested macrolinearity directly. They found strong support for this version of the superposition principle across three experiments that included conditions in which consecutive stimuli were separated by as little as 2 seconds. Thus, macrolinearity should be considered a weaker assumption than microlinearity. It is logically possible that convolving the neural activation with the hrf poorly predicts the BOLD response to each stimulus event, but that the BOLD responses to separate events nevertheless add. In this case, microlinearity is violated but macrolinearity holds. Note that such a result would not invalidate the FBR method. In other words, the FBR method assumes macrolinearity, but it does not assume microlinearity. In contrast, note that the FIR model from chapter 3 assumes both microlinearity and macrolinearity.[2]

## Using the General Linear Model to Implement the FBR Method

The parameters of the FBR method (i.e., the $\beta_i$) are most easily estimated within the context of the general linear model. To see this, note that equations 5.1 can be rewritten into matrix form as:

$$
\begin{bmatrix} B(TR_1) \\ B(TR_2) \\ B(TR_3) \\ B(TR_4) \\ B(TR_5) \\ B(TR_6) \\ B(TR_7) \\ B(TR_8) \end{bmatrix} = \begin{bmatrix} 1 & 0 & 0 & 0 & 0 \\ 0 & 1 & 0 & 0 & 0 \\ 1 & 0 & 1 & 0 & 0 \\ 1 & 1 & 0 & 1 & 0 \\ 0 & 1 & 1 & 0 & 1 \\ 0 & 0 & 1 & 1 & 0 \\ 1 & 0 & 0 & 1 & 1 \\ 0 & 1 & 0 & 0 & 1 \end{bmatrix} \begin{bmatrix} \beta_1 \\ \beta_2 \\ \beta_3 \\ \beta_4 \\ \beta_5 \end{bmatrix},
$$

where $B(TR_i)$ is the BOLD response on TR $i$. Of course, in real data, these equations would never hold exactly because of noise—even if all assumptions of the method were met. A standard method for modeling noise is to assume that the noise is normally distributed with mean 0 across TRs and that its effects add to the BOLD responses. Let $\varepsilon_i$ denote the noise on TR $i$. Then the FBR model becomes

$$
\begin{bmatrix} B(TR_1) \\ B(TR_2) \\ B(TR_3) \\ B(TR_4) \\ B(TR_5) \\ B(TR_6) \\ B(TR_7) \\ B(TR_8) \end{bmatrix} = \begin{bmatrix} 1 & 0 & 0 & 0 & 0 \\ 0 & 1 & 0 & 0 & 0 \\ 1 & 0 & 1 & 0 & 0 \\ 1 & 1 & 0 & 1 & 0 \\ 0 & 1 & 1 & 0 & 1 \\ 0 & 0 & 1 & 1 & 0 \\ 1 & 0 & 0 & 1 & 1 \\ 0 & 1 & 0 & 0 & 1 \end{bmatrix} \begin{bmatrix} \beta_1 \\ \beta_2 \\ \beta_3 \\ \beta_4 \\ \beta_5 \end{bmatrix} + \begin{bmatrix} \varepsilon_1 \\ \varepsilon_2 \\ \varepsilon_3 \\ \varepsilon_4 \\ \varepsilon_5 \\ \varepsilon_6 \\ \varepsilon_7 \\ \varepsilon_8 \end{bmatrix}. \tag{5.4}
$$

If we define

2. The FIR model assumes microlinearity because it only provides a model of the hrf. The predicted BOLD response in the FIR model is still computed by convolving the hrf with a model of the neural activation (e.g., a boxcar model). The FIR and FBR models have other differences. For example, the FIR model can assume different boxcar durations and therefore different BOLD responses for every event presentation, whereas the FBR model is constrained to always predict the same BOLD response to the same stimulus event.

$$
\underline{B} =
\begin{bmatrix}
B(TR_1) \\
B(TR_2) \\
B(TR_3) \\
B(TR_4) \\
B(TR_5) \\
B(TR_6) \\
B(TR_7) \\
B(TR_8)
\end{bmatrix}, \quad
X =
\begin{bmatrix}
1 & 0 & 0 & 0 & 0 \\
0 & 1 & 0 & 0 & 0 \\
1 & 0 & 1 & 0 & 0 \\
1 & 1 & 0 & 1 & 0 \\
0 & 1 & 1 & 0 & 1 \\
0 & 0 & 1 & 1 & 0 \\
1 & 0 & 0 & 1 & 1 \\
0 & 1 & 0 & 0 & 1
\end{bmatrix}, \quad
\underline{\beta} =
\begin{bmatrix}
\beta_1 \\
\beta_2 \\
\beta_3 \\
\beta_4 \\
\beta_5
\end{bmatrix}, \quad \text{and} \quad
\underline{\varepsilon} =
\begin{bmatrix}
\varepsilon_1 \\
\varepsilon_2 \\
\varepsilon_3 \\
\varepsilon_4 \\
\varepsilon_5 \\
\varepsilon_6 \\
\varepsilon_7 \\
\varepsilon_8
\end{bmatrix},
$$

then in matrix shorthand the model can be written as

$$\underline{B} = X\underline{\beta} + \underline{\varepsilon}, \tag{5.5}$$

where $\underline{\varepsilon}$ is a multivariate normal random vector with mean $E(\underline{\varepsilon}) = \underline{0}$ (i.e., a vector of all zeros) and variance-covariance matrix $\Sigma_{\underline{\varepsilon}}$. Appendix B provides a brief overview of random vectors and the multivariate normal distribution.

Equation 5.5 is the well-known general linear model (GLM). Note that the matrix X has a row for every TR and a column for every parameter in the $\underline{\beta}$ vector. X is called the design matrix because it describes the design of the experiment. For example, because $\beta_1$ always appears at stimulus onset, by noting which rows of column 1 (i.e., the column that corresponds with $\beta_1$) have ones, we can identify every TR when a stimulus was presented. The GLM is a widely used and well-understood statistical model. As we will see in later sections, using it to analyze fMRI data solves many statistical problems.

### Modeling Baseline Activation and Systematic Non-Task-Related Variation in the BOLD Signal

There are several shortcomings of the model as formulated in equation 5.4. First, in its current form, the resting or baseline activation would be incorporated into the $\beta_i$ estimates. In other words, all the $\beta_i$ estimates would be greater than zero even in a voxel from a brain area that did not respond to the stimulus. This problem can be corrected by adding a baseline activation term to the model.

Second, as we saw in chapter 4, fMRI data frequently have a slow, or low-frequency, drift in intensity over the course of an experimental session that is mostly due to slight changes in the local magnetic field properties of the scanner (Smith et al., 1999). If there is scanner drift, then the average resting values of the BOLD response will vary slightly throughout the session. Temporal filtering during preprocessing will correct for periodic changes in magnetic field strength (see chapter 4). A simple method of correcting for monotonic (i.e., either increasing or decreasing) changes in field strength is to augment the model with a linear regression term.

Adding the baseline and linear regression terms to the model produces:

$$
\begin{bmatrix} B(TR_1) \\ B(TR_2) \\ B(TR_3) \\ B(TR_4) \\ B(TR_5) \\ B(TR_6) \\ B(TR_7) \\ B(TR_8) \end{bmatrix} =
\begin{bmatrix}
1 & 0 & 0 & 0 & 0 & 1 & 1 \\
0 & 1 & 0 & 0 & 0 & 1 & 2 \\
1 & 0 & 1 & 0 & 0 & 1 & 3 \\
1 & 1 & 0 & 1 & 0 & 1 & 4 \\
0 & 1 & 1 & 0 & 1 & 1 & 5 \\
0 & 0 & 1 & 1 & 0 & 1 & 6 \\
1 & 0 & 0 & 1 & 1 & 1 & 7 \\
0 & 1 & 0 & 0 & 1 & 1 & 8
\end{bmatrix}
\begin{bmatrix} \beta_1 \\ \beta_2 \\ \beta_3 \\ \beta_4 \\ \beta_5 \\ B_0 \\ \Delta \end{bmatrix} +
\begin{bmatrix} \varepsilon_1 \\ \varepsilon_2 \\ \varepsilon_3 \\ \varepsilon_4 \\ \varepsilon_5 \\ \varepsilon_6 \\ \varepsilon_7 \\ \varepsilon_8 \end{bmatrix}.
\tag{5.6}
$$

The parameter $B_0$, which is assumed to have the same constant value at all TRs, is a measure of the baseline activation. With this parameter added to the model, the $\beta_i$ should be nonzero only in task-related voxels. The $\Delta$ parameter measures the amount of linear signal drift that occurs at each TR. More complex models of signal drift could be constructed (e.g., quadratic rather than linear), but as complexity increases, we would have to worry more and more about whether parameters of the drift model are tracking changes in the psychological state of the subject rather than changes in the magnetic field properties of the machine. For example, a quadratic drift model could account for a gradual increase in average BOLD response during the first half of the experimental session and a gradual decrease in the second half. But one could also imagine that the subject's attention could follow a similar pattern. For example, during the first half of the session, the subject could become increasingly engaged in the task, but in the second half, as fatigue sets in, the subject's attention might wane. With a quadratic (or even more complex) drift model, slow fluctuations in attention like this could be misinterpreted as drifts in the MR signal. For this reason, many researchers are satisfied with a simple linear model of drift (as in equation 5.6). In fact, with many newer machines, drift is often negligible over the course of any single functional run, so it is becoming more common to omit even a linear model of drift from the GLM.

Drift in the magnetic field strength adds systematic variation to the observed BOLD response that is unrelated to task processing. If the drift is not explicitly modeled (or is not removed during preprocessing) it will be absorbed into the error term as unexplained variation. This will increase the estimated error variance and therefore reduce the power of our subsequent statistical tests. For this same reason, it is often also advantageous to include regressors in the model that account for other non-task-related sources of systematic variability. For example, the BOLD response can be affected by both respiration and heart rate. Thus, some researchers might use external monitors to record the subject's respiration and heart rate throughout the functional run. After the experiment, these data could be used to construct two new vectors: one containing the heart rate measure at each TR and the other containing the respiration measure at each TR. Next, these two vectors would be added as new columns to the design matrix, and two new regression weights would be added to the analogous positions in the $\underline{\beta}$ vector (e.g., call them $\Delta_{heart}$ and $\Delta_{respiration}$). In this way, systematic variation in the BOLD response due to changes in heart rate or respiration would be removed from the error term, thereby reducing error variance and increasing statistical power.

**Designs with Multiple Stimulus Events**

Many experiments include more than one type of stimulus event. For example, in many experiments, a feedback signal is provided after the subject's response. Typically, one would assume that the brain regions that mediate processing of the stimulus and selection of a response are different from the regions that would process the feedback signal. And even if some regions were common to both tasks, we would expect the BOLD response to the stimulus to differ from the BOLD response to the feedback. The FBR method handles multiple event types by assigning a new set of $\beta$ parameters to each new event. Let $E_i$ denote the onset of an event of type $i$, and let $\beta_{ij}$ denote the BOLD response to event type $i$ on the $j^{th}$ TR after event onset. Now consider the following design that includes two separate event types $E_1$ and $E_2$ (e.g., $E_1$ might denote stimulus presentation and $E_2$ might signal the presentation of feedback):

| TR: | 1 | 2 | 3 | 4 | 5 | 6 | 7 | 8 |
|---|---|---|---|---|---|---|---|---|
| Time: | 0 | 3 | 6 | 9 | 12 | 15 | 18 | 21 |
| Events: | $E_1$ | $E_2$ | $E_1$ | | | $E_2$ | | $E_1$ |

The FBR method assumes the following BOLD responses will be generated:

| TR: | 1 | 2 | 3 | 4 | 5 | 6 | 7 | 8 |
|---|---|---|---|---|---|---|---|---|
| Time: | 0 | 3 | 6 | 9 | 12 | 15 | 18 | 21 |
| Events: | $E_1$ | $E_2$ | $E_1$ | | | $E_2$ | | $E_1$ |
| BOLD to 1st $E_1$: | $\beta_{11}$ | $\beta_{12}$ | $\beta_{13}$ | $\beta_{14}$ | $\beta_{15}$ | | | |
| BOLD to 1st $E_2$: | | $\beta_{21}$ | $\beta_{22}$ | $\beta_{23}$ | $\beta_{24}$ | $\beta_{25}$ | | |
| BOLD to 2nd $E_1$: | | | $\beta_{11}$ | $\beta_{12}$ | $\beta_{13}$ | $\beta_{14}$ | $\beta_{15}$ | |
| BOLD to 2nd $E_2$: | | | | | | $\beta_{21}$ | $\beta_{22}$ | $\beta_{23}$ |
| BOLD to 3rd $E_1$: | | | | | | | | $\beta_{11}$ |

As a result, the model becomes

$$
\begin{bmatrix} B(TR_1) \\ B(TR_2) \\ B(TR_3) \\ B(TR_4) \\ B(TR_5) \\ B(TR_6) \\ B(TR_7) \\ B(TR_8) \end{bmatrix}
=
\begin{bmatrix}
1 & 0 & 0 & 0 & 0 & 0 & 0 & 0 & 0 & 0 & 1 & 1 \\
0 & 1 & 0 & 0 & 0 & 1 & 0 & 0 & 0 & 0 & 1 & 2 \\
1 & 0 & 1 & 0 & 0 & 0 & 1 & 0 & 0 & 0 & 1 & 3 \\
0 & 1 & 0 & 1 & 0 & 0 & 0 & 1 & 0 & 0 & 1 & 4 \\
0 & 0 & 1 & 0 & 1 & 0 & 0 & 0 & 1 & 0 & 1 & 5 \\
0 & 0 & 0 & 1 & 0 & 1 & 0 & 0 & 0 & 1 & 1 & 6 \\
0 & 0 & 0 & 0 & 1 & 0 & 1 & 0 & 0 & 0 & 1 & 7 \\
1 & 0 & 0 & 0 & 0 & 0 & 0 & 1 & 0 & 0 & 1 & 8
\end{bmatrix}
\begin{bmatrix} \beta_{11} \\ \beta_{12} \\ \beta_{13} \\ \beta_{14} \\ \beta_{15} \\ \beta_{21} \\ \beta_{22} \\ \beta_{23} \\ \beta_{24} \\ \beta_{25} \\ B_0 \\ \Delta \end{bmatrix}
+
\begin{bmatrix} \varepsilon_1 \\ \varepsilon_2 \\ \varepsilon_3 \\ \varepsilon_4 \\ \varepsilon_5 \\ \varepsilon_6 \\ \varepsilon_7 \\ \varepsilon_8 \end{bmatrix}.
\tag{5.7}
$$

Note that the time between different events has also been jittered. As before, this is necessary to guarantee unique estimates of the various $\beta_{ij}$ parameters. Another, conceptually similar method for guaranteeing unique parameter estimates is to use a *partial-trials design* (Ollinger et al., 2001a, 2001b; Serences, 2004). This approach excludes one event type on some proportion of trials (usually 20% to 40% of trials). For example, if $E_1$ is stimulus presentation and $E_2$ is feedback about the accuracy of the subject's response, then in a partial-trials design the feedback would be omitted on say, 30% of all trials. Jittering is still required between successive $E_1$ presentations, but using this approach there is no need to jitter between $E_1$ and $E_2$ presentations. The idea is that the BOLD response to $E_1$ can be estimated uniquely because there are many trials where $E_1$ occurs alone. This unique estimate of the $E_1$ BOLD response can then be used to uniquely estimate the BOLD response to $E_2$ from those trials where $E_1$ and $E_2$ occur together. A partial-trials design is a highly effective way to produce unique and stable estimates of the model parameters. Jittering is most effective when the jitter distribution (equation 5.3) is truncated at some large value of $N_{max}$. A partial-trials design can be about as effective as this optimal form of jittering (Serences, 2004).

We will consider parameter estimation and hypothesis testing within the FBR model later in this chapter. First, we turn to an alternative correlation approach that is currently more popular than the FBR method.

## The Correlation Approach

The idea behind the correlation approach is to first predict as accurately as possible what the BOLD response should look like in task-sensitive voxels. Next, the observed BOLD response in each voxel is correlated with this predicted signal. Voxels where this correlation is high are identified as task related.

To see exactly how the method works, we begin by considering a rapid event-related design with only one stimulus type. Suppose the TR again equals 3 seconds and that we have already added jitter to the stimulus onsets. To take a concrete example, suppose the sequence of events on the first eight TRs is

| TR:    | 1 | 2 | 3 | 4 | 5  | 6  | 7  | 8  | . . . |
|--------|---|---|---|---|----|----|----|----|-------|
| Time:  | 0 | 3 | 6 | 9 | 12 | 15 | 18 | 21 |       |
| Events:|   | E |   | E | E  |    |    | E  |       |

where, as before, E denotes a stimulus presentation. Suppose further that the duration of each event is one TR (i.e., 3 seconds).

To predict the BOLD response to each of these stimulus events, we must first make an assumption about how long the neural activation will last in brain regions that process this stimulus. Because the stimulus exposure duration is 3 seconds, we will assume for this example that the neural activation induced by the stimulus onset will also last 3 seconds. The FBR method did not require any assumptions about neural activation. However, it did require an assumption about how long the BOLD response would last after stimulus onset.

Once the duration of the neural activation that is induced by each stimulus event is determined, the correlation approach models that activation via a boxcar function (see chapter 3). The boxcar function for this example is shown in the top panel of figure 5.2. Note that it equals 1 when the stimulus is present and equals 0 when the stimulus is absent.

To generate the BOLD response that would be predicted by this boxcar model, micro-linearity is typically assumed, in which case a model of the hrf is needed. As mentioned in chapter 3, the most popular choice is to select a specific mathematical function for the hrf that has no free parameters (see method 4 of chapter 3). Next, the relevant boxcar is convolved with the hrf (see equation 3.5). The middle panel of figure 5.2 shows the result of convolving a gamma function hrf (i.e., the hrf shown in figure 3.5) with the boxcar function shown in the top panel.

Let $x(t)$ denote the result of this integration:

$$x(t) = N(t) * h(t) = \int_0^t N(\tau)h(t - \tau)\, d\tau.$$

Because there are no free parameters in either the boxcar function $N(t)$ or the hrf $h(t)$, this integral can be evaluated numerically, and the numerical values that result can be used to compute the values of $x(t)$ at the time of each TR [i.e., each $x(\text{TR}_i)$]. The bottom panel of figure 5.2 shows the values of $x(t)$ at each of the first 13 TRs. These values are used in the correlation approach to identify voxels that show task-related activation. MATLAB box 5.1 shows the code that was used to generate all three panels of figure 5.2.

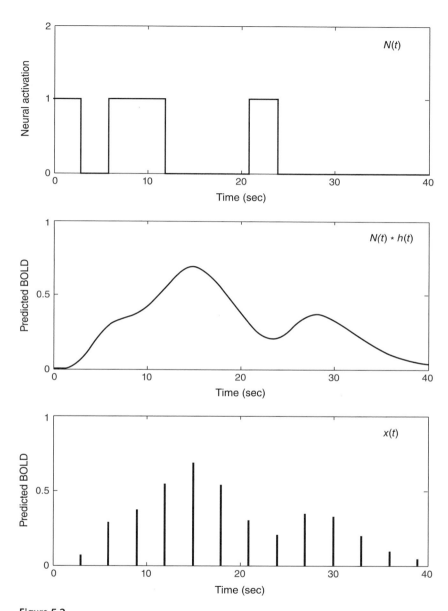

**Figure 5.2**
The top panel shows a boxcar model for an experiment with a TR of 3 seconds and stimulus presentations on TRs 1, 3, 4, and 7. The middle panel shows the convolution of this boxcar with a canonical hrf (gamma function), and the bottom panel depicts the entries in the vector $x(t)$ (i.e., the value of the convolution at the beginning of each TR).

**MATLAB Box 5.1**
Generate a predicted BOLD vector for GLM analysis (as in figure 5.2)

```
clear all; close all; clc;   % Clear all workspaces

% Define the time axis and the hrf
t25=0:.01:25; T0=0; n=4; lamda=2;
hrf=((t25-T0).^(n-1)).*exp(-(t25-T0)/lamda)/((lamda^n)*factorial(n-1));

% Define and plot the boxcar
box=[ones(1,300),zeros(1,300),ones(1,600),zeros(1,900),ones(1,300),zeros(1,101)];
subplot(3,1,1); plot(t25,box); axis([0 40 0 2]);

% Convolve the hrf and boxcar and then plot
B=conv(hrf,box)/100;
t=0:.01:50; subplot(3,1,2); plot(t,B); axis([0 40 0 1]);

% Discretize the predicted BOLD response (i.e., in the vector N) & plot
Nplot=zeros(1,5001);
for i=1:13
   N(i)=B(i*300);
   Nplot(i*300)=N(i);
end;
subplot(3,1,3); plot(t,Nplot); axis([0 40 0 1]);
```

The correlation approach correlates these predicted values with the observed BOLD response in each voxel. It does this by multiplying each predicted value by a parameter $\theta$ and then finding the value of $\theta$ that provides the best fit of the predicted BOLD response to the observed BOLD response. If the observed BOLD response exactly equals the predicted response, then $\theta$ will equal 1. If the observed BOLD response is from a voxel that did not participate in the task, then the predicted and observed BOLD responses will be uncorrelated, and $\theta$ will be nearly zero. This whole strategy is implemented via the following version of the GLM:

$$
\begin{bmatrix} B(TR_1) \\ B(TR_2) \\ B(TR_3) \\ B(TR_4) \\ B(TR_5) \\ B(TR_6) \\ B(TR_7) \\ B(TR_8) \end{bmatrix} = \begin{bmatrix} x(TR_1) & 1 & 1 \\ x(TR_2) & 1 & 2 \\ x(TR_3) & 1 & 3 \\ x(TR_4) & 1 & 4 \\ x(TR_5) & 1 & 5 \\ x(TR_6) & 1 & 6 \\ x(TR_7) & 1 & 7 \\ x(TR_8) & 1 & 8 \end{bmatrix} \begin{bmatrix} \theta \\ B_0 \\ \Delta \end{bmatrix} + \begin{bmatrix} \varepsilon_1 \\ \varepsilon_2 \\ \varepsilon_3 \\ \varepsilon_4 \\ \varepsilon_5 \\ \varepsilon_6 \\ \varepsilon_7 \\ \varepsilon_8 \end{bmatrix}.
$$

Note that, as with the FBR method, we have modeled baseline activation and allowed for linear drift in the magnetic field properties of the scanner.

This correlation method makes strong assumptions about the nature of the neural activation (i.e., boxcar), the shape of the hrf (e.g., gamma), and the relationship between neural activation and BOLD response (e.g., micro-linearity and macrolinearity). In contrast, the FBR method only assumes macrolinearity. This imbalance is somewhat offset, however, by an increased flexibility in the manner via which the correlation method treats stimulus onsets and offsets.

The FBR method assumes that each time the same event occurs, it initiates an identical BOLD response. This is a continuous function of time that might persist for, say, 25 seconds. If the TR is 2 seconds, then we will sample this waveform 13 times before it disappears. In the FBR method, we create 13 parameters to measure the magnitude of this BOLD response at each of our 13 sampling points. To estimate these parameters, we must average the observed BOLD responses over many repetitions of this same event. Because of this averaging process, it is critical that each event repetition elicits the exact same BOLD response. For example, suppose that on some TRs we delay event onset by 1 second. Then it is reasonable to assume that the same BOLD response will ensue, but it will be delayed from TR onset by 1 second. However, this means that at each of the next 13 TRs, we will sample the BOLD response at a different relative time point compared with that of TRs when the event is not delayed. This is problematic for the FBR method because it means we would need to create 13 new parameters to measure these 13 new BOLD responses that we were sampling.

However, in the correlation method, we assume we already know exactly the entire 25-second-long waveform. Thus, delaying stimulus onset causes no problems at all. In fact, we could randomize the time of event onset on every event TR so that the relative time of event onset is always unique (to create within-TR jittering). We could also assume that each event onset initiates a neural activation (i.e., a boxcar) of unique duration. For example, suppose the event is the presentation of some stimulus that requires a response from the subject. One reasonable assumption is that the duration of the neural activation equals the subject's response time on that trial. Thus, we could create a boxcar function that begins at stimulus onset (whenever that is relative to TR onset) and ends when the subject makes a response. This would be repeated for every such stimulus presentation during the course of the scanning session. Next, we would convolve this long chain of boxcar functions with an hrf to generate a predicted BOLD response for the entire experiment. The last step would be to read off the numerical value of this convolution integral at each TR (onset) in the experiment and load these values into column 1 of the design matrix.

Thus far, we have assumed that the correlation method uses a fixed hrf with no free parameters. Suppose instead that we decide to use one of the basis function models of the hrf introduced in chapter 3. For example, recall that the Friston et al. (1998) model assumes

$$h(t) = \theta_1 b_1(t) + \theta_2 b_2(t) + \theta_3 b_3(t),$$

where the $\theta_i$ are free parameters and the $b_i(t)$ are fixed basis (e.g., gamma) functions with no free parameters (i.e., see equations 3.9–3.15). In this case, the first step is to compute the following three convolution integrals:

$$x_1(t) = N(t) * b_1(t), \quad x_2(t) = N(t) * b_2(t), \quad \text{and} \quad x_3(t) = N(t) * b_3(t).$$

As before, none of these integrals involve any free parameters, so they each can be evaluated numerically. After this procedure, $x_1(t)$, $x_2(t)$, and $x_3(t)$ will contain known numerical values. Next, we construct the following model:

$$
\begin{bmatrix}
B(TR_1) \\
B(TR_2) \\
B(TR_3) \\
B(TR_4) \\
B(TR_5) \\
B(TR_6) \\
B(TR_7) \\
B(TR_8)
\end{bmatrix}
=
\begin{bmatrix}
x_1(TR_1) & x_2(TR_1) & x_3(TR_1) & 1 & 1 \\
x_1(TR_2) & x_2(TR_2) & x_3(TR_2) & 1 & 2 \\
x_1(TR_3) & x_2(TR_3) & x_3(TR_3) & 1 & 3 \\
x_1(TR_4) & x_2(TR_4) & x_3(TR_4) & 1 & 4 \\
x_1(TR_5) & x_2(TR_5) & x_3(TR_5) & 1 & 5 \\
x_1(TR_6) & x_2(TR_6) & x_3(TR_6) & 1 & 6 \\
x_1(TR_7) & x_2(TR_7) & x_3(TR_7) & 1 & 7 \\
x_1(TR_8) & x_2(TR_8) & x_3(TR_8) & 1 & 8
\end{bmatrix}
\begin{bmatrix}
\theta_1 \\
\theta_2 \\
\theta_3 \\
B_0 \\
\Delta
\end{bmatrix}
+
\begin{bmatrix}
\varepsilon_1 \\
\varepsilon_2 \\
\varepsilon_3 \\
\varepsilon_4 \\
\varepsilon_5 \\
\varepsilon_6 \\
\varepsilon_7 \\
\varepsilon_8
\end{bmatrix}.
$$

In this case, we would conclude that the voxel showed task-related activity if any of the $\theta_i$ are greater than zero. For example, the null hypothesis that the voxel does not participate in the task could be formalized as

$$H_0 : \sum_{i=1}^{3} \theta_i^2 = 0.$$

We would conclude that the voxel did display task-related activity if this null hypothesis was rejected in favor of the alternative

$$H_1 : \sum_{i=1}^{3} \theta_i^2 > 0.$$

Later in this chapter, we will construct the statistics needed to test this hypothesis.

Next, consider the following experiment with two event types, $E_1$ and $E_2$:

| TR:     | 1     | 2     | 3     | 4 | 5     | 6  | 7  | 8  |
|---------|-------|-------|-------|---|-------|----|----|----|
| Time:   | 0     | 3     | 6     | 9 | 12    | 15 | 18 | 21 |
| Events: | $E_1$ | $E_2$ | $E_1$ |   | $E_2$ |    |    |    |

Suppose we are again using a model with no free hrf parameters. In this case, we create one vector $\underline{x}_1$ containing the numerical convolution of the hrf and the presumed neural activation produced by event $E_1$ (i.e., a boxcar) and a second vector $\underline{x}_2$ containing the numerical convolution of the hrf and the presumed neural activation produced by event $E_2$ (another boxcar). Thus,

$$x_1(t) = N_1(t) * h(t) \quad \text{and} \quad x_2(t) = N_2(t) * h(t).$$

Note that because the hrfs are the same in these two operations, if the neural activations for events $E_1$ and $E_2$ are assumed to persist for the same amount of time, then the predicted BOLD responses to events $E_1$ and $E_2$ will be identical, except for their onsets. After these calculations are complete, the model can be constructed:

$$\begin{bmatrix} B(TR_1) \\ B(TR_2) \\ B(TR_3) \\ B(TR_4) \\ B(TR_5) \\ B(TR_6) \\ B(TR_7) \\ B(TR_8) \end{bmatrix} = \begin{bmatrix} x_1(TR_1) & x_2(TR_1) & 1 & 1 \\ x_1(TR_2) & x_2(TR_2) & 1 & 2 \\ x_1(TR_3) & x_2(TR_3) & 1 & 3 \\ x_1(TR_4) & x_2(TR_4) & 1 & 4 \\ x_1(TR_5) & x_2(TR_5) & 1 & 5 \\ x_1(TR_6) & x_2(TR_6) & 1 & 6 \\ x_1(TR_7) & x_2(TR_7) & 1 & 7 \\ x_1(TR_8) & x_2(TR_8) & 1 & 8 \end{bmatrix} \begin{bmatrix} \theta_1 \\ \theta_2 \\ B_0 \\ \Delta \end{bmatrix} + \begin{bmatrix} \varepsilon_1 \\ \varepsilon_2 \\ \varepsilon_3 \\ \varepsilon_4 \\ \varepsilon_5 \\ \varepsilon_6 \\ \varepsilon_7 \\ \varepsilon_8 \end{bmatrix}.$$

If there are more than two event types, then these are handled in an analogous way; that is, a new column is added to the design matrix for each new event (the predicted BOLD response for this event), and new $\theta_i$ are added to the $\underline{\beta}$ vector.

## Block Designs

For the sake of data analysis, a block design can be considered a special case of an event-related design in which there are fewer events that are each of a much longer duration. For example, if the TR is 2.5 seconds and the design includes alternating on–off blocks of 20 seconds, then the correlation method would use the simple boxcar model shown in figure 5.3 (dotted line) that assumes task-related neural activation is constant during the length of the block and zero during the rest period.

As with event-related designs, the correlation method generates a predicted BOLD response from this experiment by convolving the figure 5.3 boxcar with a fixed model of the hrf. The predicted BOLD response that results from this convolution is also shown in figure 5.3 (solid line curve). Figure 3.6 shows how the duration of the block affects the shape of the predicted BOLD response. If the subject performs the same task during each active block (e.g., finger tapping), then the correlation model has only a single $\theta$ parameter. In the

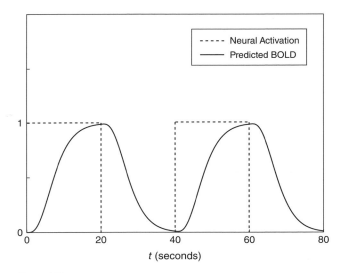

**Figure 5.3**
Boxcar model of the neural activation expected from a block design with two 20-second on/off periods (dotted line) and the predicted BOLD response in this experiment (solid line curve).

simple experiment illustrated in figure 5.3, in which there are only two active blocks, or on-blocks, and two rest blocks, or off-blocks, and the TR is 2.5 seconds, the correlation model is

$$
\begin{bmatrix} B(TR_1) \\ B(TR_2) \\ \vdots \\ B(TR_{33}) \end{bmatrix} = \begin{bmatrix} x(TR_1) & 1 & 1 \\ x(TR_2) & 1 & 2 \\ \vdots & \vdots & \vdots \\ x(TR_{33}) & 1 & 33 \end{bmatrix} \begin{bmatrix} \theta \\ B_0 \\ \Delta \end{bmatrix} + \begin{bmatrix} \varepsilon_1 \\ \varepsilon_2 \\ \vdots \\ \varepsilon_{33} \end{bmatrix}.
\tag{5.8}
$$

We assume here that the clock is started at the beginning of the first TR. Therefore, $B(TR_1)$ is the observed BOLD response at time 0, $B(TR_5)$ is the observed response at time $t = 10$ seconds, and $B(TR_{33})$ is the observed response at the last TR (i.e., at time $t = 80$ seconds).

The FBR method is rarely applied to block designs. First, the main benefit of the method is to separate out the contributions of separate neural activations to the current BOLD response. This is not an issue in block designs because the rest blocks are long enough that the residual activation from the task block decays to baseline well before the rest block ends. Second, as the bottom panel in figure 3.6 shows, the predicted BOLD response in a block design is constant for much of each block (in the case of task blocks because of saturation, and in the case of rest blocks because of decay). This is true regardless of what model is chosen for the hrf, so if an application of the correlation method chooses the wrong hrf, it will have little effect on the predicted BOLD response. Thus, a second sig-

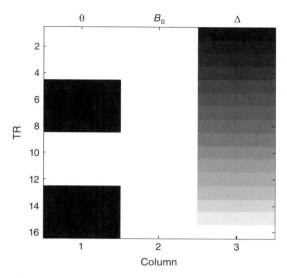

**Figure 5.4**
Graphical representation of the design matrix for a block design experiment with two on-blocks and two off-blocks that each persist for 4 TRs. Maximum values in each column are presented in white and minimum values in black.

nificant advantage of the FBR method over the correlation method is reduced in block designs; namely, that the FBR method makes weaker assumptions about the shape of the BOLD response.

## A Graphical Convention for Displaying the Design Matrix

The design matrix gives a complete picture of an experimental session because it describes exactly what neural activations are expected to be present at every TR. On the other hand, the design matrix in fMRI experiments is often a very large matrix, and this makes it difficult to present. For this reason, a common convention is to display a design matrix with grayscale values substituted for the numerical entries. Typically, minimum values are represented by black and maximum values by white.

The design matrix for a block design is presented in this way in figure 5.4. This functional run begins with an active block and alternates between two active and two rest blocks each of which has a duration of four TRs. The design matrix is of order $16 \times 3$. Note that the first column shows values of the boxcar function rather than the predicted BOLD response. This is conventional because the boxcar function, rather than the predicted BOLD response, would be input into most fMRI data analysis software packages (e.g., SPM). Strictly speaking, of course, this means that the figure 5.4 matrix is not a design

**MATLAB Box 5.2**
Present a design matrix visually (as in figure 5.4)

```
clear all; close all; clc;   % Clear all workspaces

% Define number of TRs (nTRs) & scale factor for plotting
nTRs=16; scalefac=4;

% Create the boxcar
box=[ones(1,4),zeros(1,4),ones(1,4),zeros(1,4)];

% Create the design matrix
X(:,1)=box';
X(:,2)=ones(nTRs,1);
X(:,3)=linspace(1, nTRs, nTRs)';

% Scale columns 1 and 2 so all columns have same maximum
X(:,1)=max(max(X))*X(:,1); X(:,2)=max(max(X))*X(:,2);

% Scale and plot the matrix
X=scalefac*X;
colormap(gray); image(X);
```

matrix in the traditional GLM sense. No harm is done, however, as SPM, for example, would use this matrix to construct the actual design matrix (like the one shown in equation 5.8). The figure 5.4 matrix can be converted into a true design matrix by numerically convolving the boxcar function shown in the first column of the figure 5.4 matrix with a canonical model of the hrf, and then replacing column 1 with predicted BOLD responses.[3] MATLAB box 5.2 shows the code that was used to generate this figure.

### The General Linear Model

As we have seen, the result of applying either the FBR or correlation methods is the well-known GLM, which is the mathematical foundation of both analysis of variance (ANOVA) and linear regression. This provides a huge computational and statistical advantage to these methods because both parameter estimation and statistical inference are straightforward in the GLM. This section introduces and provides a brief review of the GLM. Readers already familiar with the GLM should skip to the next major section (i.e., "Parameter Estimation in the FBR and Correlation Models").

---

3. Note that the coefficients for $\Delta$ run from 0 to 1, whereas in equation 5.6 they run from 1 to $n$. The conversion to a 0 to 1 scale is done only to facilitate visual presentation.

Within ANOVA, the standard structural model for a factorial (ANOVA) design with two experimental factors A and B is (e.g., Winer, Brown, & Michels, 1991)

$$y_{ijk} = \mu + \alpha_i + \beta_j + \alpha\beta_{ij} + \varepsilon_{ijk},$$

where $y_{ijk}$ is the observed score of subject $k$ who received level $i$ of factor A and level $j$ of factor B, $\mu$ is the grand mean, $\alpha_i$ is the treatment effect for level $i$ of factor A, $\beta_j$ is the treatment effect for level $j$ of factor B, $\alpha\beta_{ij}$ is the interaction effect between level $i$ of factor A and level $j$ of factor B, and $\varepsilon_{ijk}$ is the normally distributed error (with zero mean) associated with the score $y_{ijk}$. With 2 levels of each factor and two subjects per condition, the eight structural equations (i.e., one for each subject) can be written in matrix form as

$$
\begin{bmatrix}
y_{111} \\
y_{112} \\
y_{211} \\
y_{212} \\
y_{121} \\
y_{122} \\
y_{221} \\
y_{222}
\end{bmatrix}
=
\begin{bmatrix}
1 & 1 & 0 & 1 & 0 & 1 & 0 & 0 & 0 \\
1 & 1 & 0 & 1 & 0 & 1 & 0 & 0 & 0 \\
1 & 0 & 1 & 1 & 0 & 0 & 1 & 0 & 0 \\
1 & 0 & 1 & 1 & 0 & 0 & 1 & 0 & 0 \\
1 & 1 & 0 & 0 & 1 & 0 & 0 & 1 & 0 \\
1 & 1 & 0 & 0 & 1 & 0 & 0 & 1 & 0 \\
1 & 0 & 1 & 0 & 1 & 0 & 0 & 0 & 1 \\
1 & 0 & 1 & 0 & 1 & 0 & 0 & 0 & 1
\end{bmatrix}
\begin{bmatrix}
\mu \\
\alpha_1 \\
\alpha_2 \\
\beta_1 \\
\beta_2 \\
\alpha\beta_{11} \\
\alpha\beta_{21} \\
\alpha\beta_{12} \\
\alpha\beta_{22}
\end{bmatrix}
+
\begin{bmatrix}
\varepsilon_{111} \\
\varepsilon_{112} \\
\varepsilon_{211} \\
\varepsilon_{212} \\
\varepsilon_{121} \\
\varepsilon_{122} \\
\varepsilon_{221} \\
\varepsilon_{222}
\end{bmatrix}.
\tag{5.9}
$$

If we define

$$
\underline{y} =
\begin{bmatrix}
y_{111} \\
y_{112} \\
y_{211} \\
y_{212} \\
y_{121} \\
y_{122} \\
y_{221} \\
y_{222}
\end{bmatrix},
\quad
X =
\begin{bmatrix}
1 & 1 & 0 & 1 & 0 & 1 & 0 & 0 & 0 \\
1 & 1 & 0 & 1 & 0 & 1 & 0 & 0 & 0 \\
1 & 0 & 1 & 1 & 0 & 0 & 1 & 0 & 0 \\
1 & 0 & 1 & 1 & 0 & 0 & 1 & 0 & 0 \\
1 & 1 & 0 & 0 & 1 & 0 & 0 & 1 & 0 \\
1 & 1 & 0 & 0 & 1 & 0 & 0 & 1 & 0 \\
1 & 0 & 1 & 0 & 1 & 0 & 0 & 0 & 1 \\
1 & 0 & 1 & 0 & 1 & 0 & 0 & 0 & 1
\end{bmatrix},
\quad
\underline{\beta} =
\begin{bmatrix}
\mu \\
\alpha_1 \\
\alpha_2 \\
\beta_1 \\
\beta_2 \\
\alpha\beta_{11} \\
\alpha\beta_{21} \\
\alpha\beta_{12} \\
\alpha\beta_{22}
\end{bmatrix},
\quad \text{and} \quad
\underline{\varepsilon} =
\begin{bmatrix}
\varepsilon_{111} \\
\varepsilon_{112} \\
\varepsilon_{211} \\
\varepsilon_{212} \\
\varepsilon_{121} \\
\varepsilon_{122} \\
\varepsilon_{221} \\
\varepsilon_{222}
\end{bmatrix},
$$

then equation 5.9 can be rewritten as

$$\underline{y} = X\underline{\beta} + \underline{\varepsilon}, \tag{5.10}$$

where the random vector $\underline{\varepsilon}$ has a multivariate normal distribution with mean vector $\underline{0}$ and variance-covariance matrix $\Sigma_{\underline{\varepsilon}}$ (for a review of multivariate normal distributions, see appendix B).

Equation 5.10 defines the GLM. As mentioned earlier, the matrix X is known as the *design matrix*. In this application, it contains a row for every subject and a column for every parameter. It is called the design matrix because it identifies which experimental treatments each subject received. For example, row 3 tells us that the third subject (whose score was $y_{211}$) did not receive level 1 of factor A (because of the 0 in column 2), did receive level 2 of factor A (because of the 1 in column 3), did receive level 1 of factor B (because of the 1 in column 4), and did not receive level 2 of factor B (because of the 0 in column 5).

Next, consider a regression design with two independent variables and one dependent variable. The standard structural model in this case is

$$y_i = \alpha + \beta_1 x_{1i} + \beta_2 x_{2i} + \varepsilon_i,$$

where $y_i$ is the observed score of subject $i$, $\alpha$ is the baseline score, $x_{1i}$ and $x_{2i}$ are the amounts or magnitudes of the first and second independent variables, respectively, which were associated with or given to subject $i$, $\beta_1$ and $\beta_2$ are the effects of one unit of the two independent variables, and $\varepsilon_i$ is the normally distributed error (with zero mean) associated with the score $y_i$.

With four subjects in this experiment, the structural equations in matrix form would be

$$\begin{bmatrix} y_1 \\ y_2 \\ y_3 \\ y_4 \end{bmatrix} = \begin{bmatrix} 1 & x_{11} & x_{21} \\ 1 & x_{12} & x_{22} \\ 1 & x_{13} & x_{23} \\ 1 & x_{14} & x_{24} \end{bmatrix} \begin{bmatrix} \alpha \\ \beta_1 \\ \beta_2 \end{bmatrix} + \begin{bmatrix} \varepsilon_1 \\ \varepsilon_2 \\ \varepsilon_3 \\ \varepsilon_4 \end{bmatrix},$$

and again, if we define

$$\underline{y} = \begin{bmatrix} y_1 \\ y_2 \\ y_3 \\ y_4 \end{bmatrix}, \quad X = \begin{bmatrix} 1 & x_{11} & x_{21} \\ 1 & x_{12} & x_{22} \\ 1 & x_{13} & x_{23} \\ 1 & x_{14} & x_{24} \end{bmatrix}, \quad \underline{\beta} = \begin{bmatrix} \alpha \\ \beta_1 \\ \beta_2 \end{bmatrix}, \quad \text{and} \quad \underline{\varepsilon} = \begin{bmatrix} \varepsilon_1 \\ \varepsilon_2 \\ \varepsilon_3 \\ \varepsilon_4 \end{bmatrix},$$

then the linear regression model becomes

$$\underline{y} = X\underline{\beta} + \underline{\varepsilon}.$$

Thus, both ANOVA and linear regression are special cases of the GLM.

Note that the design matrix X in ANOVA contains only zeroes and ones, whereas the design matrix in regression could contain any values (i.e., as the $x_{ji}$ could conceivably take on any value). For this reason, one could view ANOVA as a special case of regression. In ANOVA designs, subjects receive either a whole treatment or no treatment, whereas in regression, fractional treatments are possible. Note that the unaugmented FBR model is an ANOVA model because the design matrix contains only zeroes and ones (e.g., see equation

5.4). When the linear drift terms are added to the model, however, it becomes a mixed model that includes both ANOVA and regression terms (e.g., see equation 5.6). In contrast, the correlation model is a standard multiple regression model. One regressor is time (i.e., the linear drift term), and one or more regressors are the predicted BOLD responses.

### Parameter Estimation

Once we have specified our model, the next step is to estimate the parameters, which are the entries in the $\underline{\beta}$ vector. A famous result, called the Gauss–Markov theorem, guarantees that this is a simple problem, at least if the error terms are all uncorrelated and have equal variance.

**Gauss–Markov Theorem**   Within the GLM, if $\Sigma_\varepsilon = \sigma_\varepsilon^2 I$, then the method of least squares always produces minimum variance unbiased estimators (MVUEs) of $\underline{\beta}$.

If $\Sigma_\varepsilon = \sigma_\varepsilon^2 I$, then the error variance is the same on every TR, and so homogeneity of variance holds, and the covariance between errors (i.e., mispredictions by the model) in any two TRs is 0 (and so uncorrelated). These are standard assumptions in fMRI data analysis, but as we will see in a later section, their validity has been questioned.

Because MVUEs are the gold standard in the parameter estimation world, the Gauss–Markov theorem tells us that we need not bother with alternative estimation methods (e.g., the method of maximum likelihood). The method of least squares always produces the best possible estimators of $\underline{\beta}$. According to this method, the optimal estimator of $\underline{\beta}$ is the vector that minimizes the sum of squared errors, where an error is defined as the difference between an observed score and a score predicted by the GLM. The observed scores are cataloged in the vector $\underline{y}$, whereas the predicted scores according to the GLM are $X\underline{\hat{\beta}}$, where $\underline{\hat{\beta}}$ denotes an estimator of the vector $\underline{\beta}$ (i.e., $X\underline{\hat{\beta}}$ is an estimator of the expected value of the right side of equation 5.10). Therefore, the sum of squared errors, *SSE*, is equal to

$$SSE = (\underline{y} - X\underline{\hat{\beta}})'(\underline{y} - X\underline{\hat{\beta}}). \tag{5.11}$$

Differentiating with respect to $\underline{\hat{\beta}}$, setting the result equal to 0, and attempting to solve for $\underline{\hat{\beta}}$ produces

$$X'X\underline{\hat{\beta}} = X'\underline{y}. \tag{5.12}$$

These are known as the *normal equations*. If $X'X$ is nonsingular, as it will be in most fMRI applications, then the obvious solution to equation 5.12, and therefore the MVUEs of $\underline{\beta}$, is

$$\underline{\hat{\beta}} = (X'X)^{-1}X'\underline{y}. \tag{5.13}$$

Once the design matrix $X$ and the data vector $\underline{y}$ are defined, the MATLAB code that implements equation 5.13 is simply

```
beta = inv(X' * X) * X' * y
```

On the other hand, if $X'X$ is singular, as it is in standard ANOVA models, then $(X'X)^{-1}$ does not exist and as a result, there are no unique MVUEs of $\underline{\beta}$. Instead there are an infinite number of (equally good) MVUEs.

### Parameter Estimation in the FBR and Correlation Models

In both the FBR and correlation methods, an accurate estimate of $\beta$ is needed to identify voxels that show task-related activation. If there were an infinite number of equally good estimates, then such identification would be impossible because some estimates might suggest that a voxel shows task-related activation while other estimates do not. Thus, to proceed with either method, it is vital that $X'X$ is nonsingular (see previous section, "Parameter Estimation"). This is one main reason for adding jitter to the design, especially in the case of the FBR method (or using a partial-trials design). For example, we saw earlier that without jitter, two (or more) different $\beta_i$ can always appear together in the FBR equations in the form of a sum (e.g., $\beta_2 + \beta_4$). In this case, there may be a unique estimate of that sum, but there will be an infinite number of equally good estimates of each term in the sum. This indeterminacy will be inherent to the (jitter-free) model because $X'X$ will be singular. Adding jitter to the design should guarantee that $X'X$ is nonsingular. Therefore, in both the FBR and correlation methods, unique MVUEs of $\underline{\beta}$ can be found from equation 5.13 (i.e., assuming $\Sigma_\varepsilon = \sigma_\varepsilon^2 I$) when we substitute the vector of observed BOLD responses $\underline{B}$ for the observed-score vector $\underline{y}$

$$\hat{\underline{\beta}} = (X'X)^{-1}X'\underline{B}. \tag{5.14}$$

The standard procedure for adding jitter is to sample delays between successive events from some probability distribution (e.g., the truncated geometric distribution). This randomness can alter the invertability of the $X'X$ matrix. $X'X$ is a symmetric matrix, and any (real) symmetric matrix can be written in its so-called *diagonal form* as

$$X'X = QDQ',$$

where the columns of $Q$ are the eigenvectors of $X'X$, and $D$ is a diagonal matrix with entries on the main diagonal equal to the eigenvalues that correspond with the eigenvectors that define the columns of $Q$ (for a brief review of eigenvalues and eigenvectors, see appendix A). Now $(X'X)^{-1} = QD^{-1}Q'$, where

$$D^{-1} = \begin{bmatrix} \dfrac{1}{d_1} & 0 & \cdots & 0 \\ 0 & \dfrac{1}{d_2} & \cdots & 0 \\ \vdots & \vdots & \vdots & \vdots \\ 0 & 0 & \cdots & \dfrac{1}{d_N} \end{bmatrix}, \tag{5.15}$$

and $d_i$ is the $i^{th}$ eigenvalue of X'X. Therefore, if any of the eigenvalues equal zero, then X'X will be singular (i.e., have no inverse).

In practice, it is unlikely that random sampling of the interevent intervals will cause one or more of the eigenvalues of X'X to equal zero. However, it is possible that random sampling will produce an eigenvalue that is close to zero. Nonsingular matrices that have one or more eigenvalues near zero are said to be *ill conditioned*. It is difficult to compute the inverse of an ill-conditioned matrix accurately. This is because noise, or even rounding error, can slightly change the eigenvalues. When an eigenvalue near zero is perturbed, equation 5.15 makes it clear that $D^{-1}$ (and hence $X'X^{-1}$) can be significantly affected. For example, suppose $d_k = .002$. Then the $1/d_k$ term in $D^{-1}$ is 500. Suppose, though, that because of noise or rounding error, $d_k$ is perturbed by .001. In other words, instead of .002, suppose the estimated value of $d_k$ is .001. This changes the $1/d_k$ term from 500 to 1000. This will cause a major change in $X'X^{-1}$.

To avoid this problem, it is imperative that we create a design matrix for which X'X is not ill conditioned. One strategy is to generate many alternative design matrices by repeatedly sampling from the jitter distribution. For each one, the eigenvalues of X'X are computed, and of these, the eigenvalue nearest zero is recorded. Finally, the design matrix with the largest minimum eigenvalue is selected to use in the experiment. If this repeated sampling process proves ineffective, then the length of the longest delay in the jitter distribution (i.e., $N_{max}$ in equation 5.3) should be increased and the process repeated.

The Gauss–Markov theorem guarantees that if $\Sigma_\varepsilon = \sigma_\varepsilon^2$ I, then the equation 5.14 least squares estimator is the MVUE of β. Under these conditions, the only other parameter of the GLM is $\sigma_\varepsilon^2$. The Gauss–Markov theorem applies only to parameters in the β vector, and not to the error variance, so $\sigma_\varepsilon^2$ must be estimated using other methods. The standard method is to use the method of maximum likelihood. This produces a biased estimator of $\sigma_\varepsilon^2$. Even so, it is straightforward to correct this bias, which results in the estimator

$$\hat{\sigma}_\varepsilon^2 = \frac{1}{df_E}(\underline{B} - X\hat{\underline{\beta}})'(\underline{B} - X\hat{\underline{\beta}}), \tag{5.16}$$

where $df_E$ equals degrees of freedom error. In the current applications, $df_E$ equals[4] (e.g., Graybill, 1976)

$$df_E = (\text{\# of TRs}) - (\text{\# of parameters in } \underline{\beta}). \tag{5.17}$$

---

4. Technically the last term in equation 5.17 should be (# of free parameters in β). For example, in the one-way ANOVA model $y_{ij} = \mu + \tau_i + \varepsilon_{ij}$, the $\tau_i$ parameters are typically constrained to sum to 1. As a result, with $p$ treatments only $p - 1$ of the $\tau_i$ are free. Therefore, in this example β has $p + 1$ parameters (i.e., the $p$ $\tau_i$ plus $\mu$), but only $p$ of these are free, and $df_E$ in this model equals the number of data points minus $p$. In all models considered in this chapter, however, all entries in β are free parameters, so the simpler expression given here is correct.

Thus far, we have assumed that $\Sigma_\varepsilon = \sigma_\varepsilon^2\, \mathrm{I}$, or in other words that the error terms satisfy homogeneity of variance and independence. Within the fMRI literature, almost no attention has been directed at developing alternative approaches that assume heterogeneity of variance. In contrast, there have been many attempts to develop methods that allow for violations of independence. If the BOLD response at TR $n$ is greater than the value predicted by the model, then it seems plausible that the BOLD responses at TRs $n-1$ and $n+1$ will also be greater than predicted by the model. If so, then the mispredictions or errors of the model on successive TRs will be positively correlated, rather than independent. Unfortunately, these correlations considerably complicate parameter estimation and hypothesis testing within the GLM.

One approach to dealing with temporal correlations is to temporally smooth the data with a smoothing kernel that matches the hrf (Friston et al., 1995a; Worsley & Friston, 1995). Because this is a form of low-pass temporal filtering, it will reduce high-frequency (correlated) noise, and because of the matched filter theorem, it should also boost signal-to-noise ratio (see chapter 4).

An alternative approach, called *prewhitening*, is a standard option in FSL. The goal here is to estimate the correlation and then remove it from the data. For example, Bullmore et al. (1996) proposed first fitting the standard GLM (which assumes independence) to the data and then fitting an autoregressive model to the resulting error terms that models the temporal correlations. The correlations that are predicted by the best-fitting autoregressive model are then removed from the data. The resulting "independent" data are then reanalyzed with the standard (i.e., independent) GLM. This is an attractive approach because it preserves the statistical advantages that accrue from using a version of the GLM that assumes $\Sigma_\varepsilon = \sigma_\varepsilon^2\, \mathrm{I}$.

Finally, a third approach is to build a model that explicitly accounts for temporal correlations. For example, Lund, Madsen, Sidaros, Luo, and Nichols (2006) did this by including regressors in the GLM that modeled a number of effects thought to contribute to the temporal correlations often seen in fMRI data. Included in this list were low-frequency drift in the magnetic field strength, residual movement effects, respiration, and cardiac pulsation. Some versions of SPM use a similar but less detailed approach (e.g., Kiebel & Holmes, 2007). First, note that we expect the correlation between a pair of TRs to decrease as the TRs become more separated in time. A simple model that captures this phenomenon assumes

$$\Sigma_\varepsilon = \sigma_\varepsilon^2\, \mathrm{I} + \lambda \mathrm{Q}, \qquad\qquad\qquad (5.18)$$

where the entry in row $i$ and column $j$ of the matrix Q equals

$$Q_{ij} = \begin{cases} 0 & \text{if } i = j \\ e^{-|i-j|} & \text{if } i \ne j \end{cases}.$$

Note that according to this model,

$$
\Sigma_{\underline{\varepsilon}} = \begin{bmatrix}
\sigma_{\varepsilon}^2 & \lambda e^{-TR} & \lambda e^{-2TR} & \cdots \\
\lambda e^{-TR} & \sigma_{\varepsilon}^2 & \lambda e^{-TR} & \cdots \\
\lambda e^{-2TR} & \lambda e^{-TR} & \sigma_{\varepsilon}^2 & \cdots \\
\vdots & \vdots & \vdots & \ddots
\end{bmatrix}.
$$

Thus, all correlations are positive, the correlation is greatest between two successive TRs, and the correlation between two BOLD responses decreases exponentially with the number of TRs between them. This is a much more reasonable covariance structure than the model that assumes complete independence, and it only adds one extra free parameter to the model (i.e., $\lambda$). Nevertheless, as we will see in the next section, inference with this model is considerably more difficult than in the model that assumes independence.

### Hypothesis Testing via the Construction of Statistical Parametric Maps

In this chapter, we have seen how to design an experiment (i.e., add jitter so that $X'X$ is well conditioned), set up either an FBR model or a correlation model, and estimate the parameters of this model [i.e., via $\hat{\underline{\beta}} = (X'X)^{-1}X'\underline{B}$)]. We are now in a position to consider hypothesis testing, where our goal is to identify voxels that show task-related activation.

To begin, consider the correlation model that has as its $\underline{\beta}$ vector

$$
\underline{\beta} = \begin{bmatrix}
\theta_1 \\
\theta_2 \\
B_0 \\
\Delta
\end{bmatrix}.
$$

In this model there are two event types, and we have modeled baseline activation and a possible linear drift in the magnetic field properties of the scanner. Suppose we want to determine whether the voxel in question is participating in the processing of event type $E_1$. Then, we need to test the null hypothesis

$$
H_0 : \theta_1 = 0 \tag{5.19}
$$

against the alternative

$$
H_1 : \theta_1 > 0.
$$

In the case of an FBR model, the $\underline{\beta}$ vector might be

$$\underline{\beta} = \begin{bmatrix} \beta_1 \\ \beta_2 \\ \beta_3 \\ \beta_4 \\ \beta_5 \\ \beta_6 \\ B_0 \\ \Delta \end{bmatrix}.$$

Now it is not so clear how to state the null and alternative hypotheses. If the voxel shows task-related activity, then we expect the $\beta_i$ to be nonzero, and at least some to be positive. One possibility would be to pick the largest of the $\beta_i$. We could then test the hypothesis that this value is zero against the alternative that it is greater than zero. Unfortunately, there are distributional problems with this choice. As we will shortly see, the statistical estimators of each $\beta_i$ are normally distributed if the assumptions of the GLM hold. Despite this normality, the maximum of six random samples from a normal distribution is not normally distributed (nor is it a standard distribution). For example, suppose the voxel was from a brain region that did not participate in the task and that the expected value of each $\hat{\beta}_i$ is zero. In this case, unfortunately, the expected value of the largest of the six $\hat{\beta}_i$ will be greater than zero, so a standard t-test would be biased against the null hypothesis.

Another alternative is to choose the area under this estimated BOLD response curve. This is logically equivalent to computing the sum of the six $\hat{\beta}_i$. We could now test the hypothesis that this sum was zero against the alternative that it was greater than zero. The problem here is that an initial or late negative dip will decrease the sum and therefore bias the test against rejecting the null hypothesis. To avoid this problem, the first and last several $\hat{\beta}_i$ could be dropped from the sum. For example, we could construct the statistic $\hat{\beta}_2 + \hat{\beta}_3 + \hat{\beta}_4$. In this case, we would conclude that the voxel displayed task-related activation if we reject the null hypothesis

$$H_0 : \beta_2 + \beta_3 + \beta_4 = 0 \tag{5.20}$$

in favor of the alternative

$$H_1 : \beta_2 + \beta_3 + \beta_4 > 0.$$

If each $\hat{\beta}_i$ is normally distributed, then $\hat{\beta}_2 + \hat{\beta}_3 + \hat{\beta}_4$ will also be normally distributed, because the sum of normally distributed random variables is normally distributed. As a result, standard t-tests can be used to test the null hypothesis of equation 5.20.

Another, perhaps even better alternative is to compare these central $\hat{\beta}_i$ with the early and late $\hat{\beta}_i$. For example, if the BOLD response to an event is assumed to persist for 25 seconds and the TR is 2.5 seconds, then there will be 11 $\hat{\beta}_i$. In this case, to decide whether the voxel displays task-related activity, we could test the null hypothesis

$$H_0 : (\beta_2 + \beta_3 + \beta_4) - (\beta_1 + \beta_{10} + \beta_{11}) = 0 \qquad\qquad (5.21)$$

against the alternative

$$H_1 : (\beta_2 + \beta_3 + \beta_4) - (\beta_1 + \beta_{10} + \beta_{11}) > 0.$$

This more complex null hypothesis has several advantages over the simpler hypothesis specified by equation 5.20. Most importantly, a test of equation 5.21 uses more data than a test of equation 5.20 and makes stronger structural assumptions. For example, the equation 5.21 null hypothesis will tend to be rejected only if the BOLD response starts small, grows to a large value between 2.5 and 7.5 seconds after the stimulus event, and then decays back to a small value by 22.5 seconds after the event. Of course, we expect all these things to happen if the voxel is showing task-related activity. In contrast, the equation 5.20 null hypothesis will be rejected whenever the BOLD response between 2.5 and 7.5 seconds is large, regardless of whether the early and late BOLD responses have the properties we expect[5].

Note that the three null hypotheses specified by equations 5.19–5.21 can each be written in matrix form as

$$H_0 : \underline{c}'\underline{\beta} = 0,$$

where $\underline{c}'$ is a row vector of constants. In the case of the hypothesis specified in equation 5.19,

$$H_0 : \theta_1 = 0$$

---

5. Another possibility is to test for task-related activation with the null hypothesis

$$H_0 : \sum_{i=1}^{M} \beta_i^2 = 0$$

against the alternative

$$H_1 : \sum_{i=1}^{M} \beta_i^2 > 0,$$

where $M$ is the number of $\beta_i$ parameters in the FBR model. By proposition 5.2, if the null hypothesis is true then the resulting statistic will have an approximate $\chi^2$ distribution with $M$ degrees of freedom.

can be rewritten as

$$H_0 : [1 \quad 0 \quad 0 \quad 0] \begin{bmatrix} \theta_1 \\ \theta_2 \\ B_0 \\ \Delta \end{bmatrix} = 0,$$

and so

$$\underline{c}' = [1 \quad 0 \quad 0 \quad 0].$$

Similarly, the FBR hypothesis

$$H_0 : \beta_2 + \beta_3 + \beta_4 = 0$$

can be rewritten as

$$H_0 : [0 \quad 1 \quad 1 \quad 1 \quad 0 \quad 0 \quad 0 \quad 0] \begin{bmatrix} \beta_1 \\ \beta_2 \\ \beta_3 \\ \beta_4 \\ \beta_5 \\ \beta_6 \\ B_0 \\ \Delta \end{bmatrix} = 0,$$

and so

$$\underline{c}' = [0 \quad 1 \quad 1 \quad 1 \quad 0 \quad 0 \quad 0].$$

Finally, the $\underline{c}$ vector for the equation 5.21 null hypothesis equals

$$\underline{c}' = [-1 \quad 1 \quad 1 \quad 1 \quad 0 \quad 0 \quad 0 \quad 0 \quad 0 \quad -1 \quad -1 \quad 0 \quad 0].$$

Note that the hypothesis $H_0 : \beta_2 + \beta_3 + \beta_4 = 0$ is not a classical contrast because the sum of the coefficients on the $\beta_i$ do not equal 0. So, for example, this hypothesis would not be testable if the $\beta_i$ were treatment effects in a standard one-way ANOVA model. This raises the obvious question of whether such a hypothesis is testable in the current fMRI setting.

Within the GLM, a hypothesis $H_0: \underline{c}'\beta = 0$ is testable if and only if (e.g., see theorem 13.2.2, Graybill, 1976)

$$\text{rank}(X'X) = \text{rank}(X'X: \underline{c}), \tag{5.22}$$

where $(X'X: \underline{c})$ is the matrix $X'X$ augmented with an extra added column that contains the vector $\underline{c}$. Adding jitter to our experimental design guaranteed that $X'X$ is nonsingular. Therefore, $X'X$ is full row rank (i.e., all the rows of $X'X$ are linearly independent; see appendix A). Adding a new column to $X'X$ cannot reduce its rank, so equation 5.22 is satisfied *for any* vector $\underline{c}$. Therefore, so long as $X'X$ is nonsingular, every hypothesis that can be expressed as a linear combination of the entries in $\underline{\beta}$ is testable (i.e., not just contrasts).

Another common question with the correlation method is to ask whether a voxel is more responsive to event $E_1$ or to event $E_2$. In this case, we wish to test the null hypothesis

$$H_0 : \theta_1 = \theta_2$$

or equivalently,

$$H_0 : \theta_1 - \theta_2 = 0.$$

Note that in this case,

$$\underline{c}' = [1 \quad -1 \quad 0 \quad 0].$$

Likewise, it is straightforward to test whether a voxel is more responsive to event $E_1$ or $E_2$ using the FBR method. In this case, the null hypothesis can be written as

$$H_0 : \sum_{i=2}^{4} \beta_{1i} = \sum_{i=2}^{4} \beta_{2i},$$

or equivalently in matrix form as

$$H_0 : [0 \quad 1 \quad 1 \quad 1 \quad 0 \quad 0 \quad 0 \quad -1 \quad -1 \quad -1 \quad 0 \quad 0 \quad 0 \quad 0] \begin{bmatrix} \beta_{11} \\ \beta_{12} \\ \beta_{13} \\ \beta_{14} \\ \beta_{15} \\ \beta_{16} \\ \beta_{21} \\ \beta_{22} \\ \beta_{23} \\ \beta_{24} \\ \beta_{25} \\ \beta_{26} \\ B_0 \\ \Delta \end{bmatrix} = 0.$$

Therefore, to test any of these null hypotheses, we need to determine the sampling distribution of $\underline{c}'\underline{\beta}$, under the assumption that the null hypothesis is true. The following proposition solves this problem.

**Proposition 5.1**    Consider any version of the GLM that assumes homogeneity of variance and independence (i.e., so $\Sigma_\varepsilon = \sigma_\varepsilon^2\ I$). Suppose $\underline{c}'$ is a row vector of constants. Then under the null hypothesis $H_0 : \underline{c}'\underline{\beta} = 0$, the following statistic

$$t = \frac{\underline{c}'\underline{\hat{\beta}}}{\sqrt{\hat{\sigma}_\varepsilon^2\,\underline{c}'(X'X)^{-1}\underline{c}}},$$

has a t-distribution with degrees of freedom equal to

(# of TRs) − (# of parameters in $\underline{\beta}$).

The variance estimate is given by equation 5.16.

**Derivation**    Note that

$$\underline{c}'\underline{\hat{\beta}} = \underline{c}'(X'X)^{-1}X'\underline{B}.$$

The only random term on the right side is $\underline{B}$. But

$$\underline{B} = X\underline{\beta} + \underline{\varepsilon},$$

where $\underline{\varepsilon}$ has a multivariate normal distribution with mean vector $\underline{0}$ and variance-covariance matrix $\Sigma_\varepsilon = \sigma_\varepsilon^2\ I$. Thus, $\underline{B}$ is a linear transformation of a normal random vector and so is itself multivariate normally distributed with mean vector $X\underline{\beta}$ and variance-covariance matrix $\sigma_\varepsilon^2\ I$. Next note that $\underline{c}'\underline{\hat{\beta}}$ is a linear transformation of $\underline{B}$. Thus, $\underline{c}'\underline{\hat{\beta}}$ is univariate (because it is of order $1 \times 1$) and normally distributed. To finish, we need only find the mean and variance of $\underline{c}'\underline{\hat{\beta}}$. The mean or expected value of $\underline{c}'\underline{\hat{\beta}}$ is $\underline{c}'\underline{\beta}$ (because linear transformations of MVUEs are unbiased), which equals 0 under the null hypothesis. The variance of $\underline{c}'\underline{\hat{\beta}}$ is

$$\mathrm{Var}(\underline{c}'\underline{\hat{\beta}}) = \mathrm{Var}[\underline{c}'(X'X)^{-1}X'\underline{B}]$$

$$= [\underline{c}'(X'X)^{-1}X']\Sigma_\varepsilon[\underline{c}'(X'X)^{-1}X']'$$

$$= \sigma_\varepsilon^2\underline{c}'(X'X)^{-1}X'X(X'X)^{-1}\underline{c}$$

$$= \sigma_\varepsilon^2\underline{c}'(X'X)^{-1}\underline{c}.$$

The proposition follows directly from these results.                                                    ∎

Proposition 5.1 allows us to compute a *t*-statistic for every voxel in our experiment for the purpose of testing whether the FBR method or the correlation method has identified voxels that show task-related activation. Many fMRI experiments include hundreds of TRs. As a consequence, the resulting $t$ statistics will have hundreds of degrees of freedom. In this case, the $t$ distribution is approximately $z$ distributed (i.e., normal with mean 0 and variance 1). For example, the 95th percentile in a z distribution is 1.645, whereas the 95th percentile of a $t$ distribution with 200 degrees of freedom is 1.653. With differences this small it is not uncommon to assume the $t$-values have a z distribution for purposes of determining statistical significance. The set or map of all $t$-values (or $z$-values) that result from applying proposition 5.1 to every voxel in our region of interest is known as a *statistical parametric map*, which inspired the name of the software package SPM. In a typical fMRI experiment, there will be tens of thousands of such t-values, so any strategy for determining significance must avoid making an excessive number of type I errors (i.e., false-positive decisions). This is called the multiple comparisons problem. Because neighboring t-values are not independent, correcting for multiple comparisons is a serious problem that we consider in the next chapter.

Figure 5.5 illustrates an application of proposition 5.1 in a hypothetical block-design experiment in which two 5-minute task blocks are alternated with two 5-minute rest blocks and in which the TR is 2.5 seconds. The top panel shows the box-car model of the idealized neural activation expected from a task-responsive voxel in this experiment. The middle panel shows hypothetical BOLD responses that were generated by convolving the boxcar with an hrf (i.e., the same gamma function shown in figure 3.5), and then adding baseline activation, scanner drift, and noise. Specifically, the data were generated from the equation 5.8 version of the (correlation) GLM with $\theta = 2.9$, $B_0 = 40$, $\Delta = .01$, and $\sigma_\varepsilon^2 = 16$. Solving the normal equations with these data produced parameter estimates of $\hat{\theta} = 2.63$, $\hat{B}_0 = 40.14$, $\hat{\Delta} = 0.0096$, $\hat{\sigma}_\varepsilon^2 = 14.57$, which are all remarkably accurate.

The bottom panel of figure 5.5 shows the same observed BOLD response as in the middle panel (in gray) and the BOLD response predicted by this application of the GLM (in black). Finally, applying proposition 5.1 produces a t-statistic in this application of $t = 6.744$, which under the null hypothesis that this voxel is not task responsive has a t-distribution with 477 degrees of freedom [i.e., the number of TRs (480) minus the number of parameters in the GLM (3)]. This $t$-value should be highly significant, even with the most conservative methods for correcting for the multiple comparisons problem. MATLAB box 5.3 shows the MATLAB code that was used to produce figure 5.5. This code will create the $t$-statistics that can then be used to populate a statistical parametric map.

If the Friston et al. (1998) basis function model of the hrf (see chapter 3) is used in the correlation method, then in voxels that are not task-related, we expect $\theta_1 = \theta_2 = \theta_3 = 0$, or equivalently, that the sum of the squared $\theta_i$ equals zero. Thus, in this case we wish to test the null hypothesis

$$H_0 : \sum_{i=1}^{3} \theta_i^2 = 0,$$

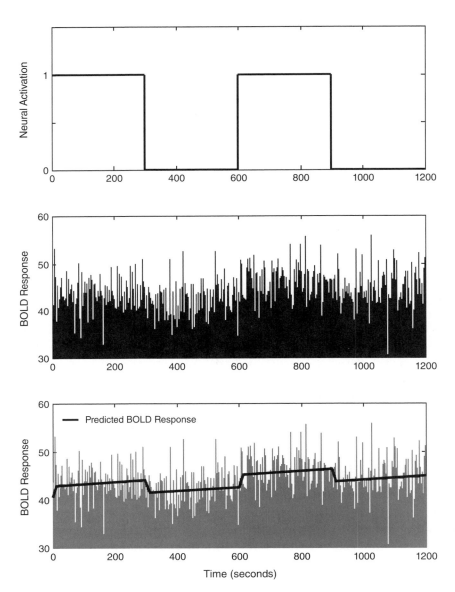

**Figure 5.5**
(Top) Boxcar model of the neural activation that might be expected from a task-responsive voxel in a block design with two 5-minute task blocks and two 5-minute rest blocks. (Middle) Hypothetical BOLD response in this experiment generated by convolving the boxcar with an hrf, and then adding baseline activation, scanner drift, and noise. (Bottom) The observed BOLD response (gray) and the BOLD response predicted by the GLM (black).

## MATLAB Box 5.3

Apply the correlation-based GLM to data (i.e., generate the t-statistic that fills a statistical parametric map; as in figure 5.5)

```
clear all; close all; clc;    % Clear all workspaces

% Define parameters, time, and the hrf
nTRs=480; theta=2.9; B0=40; delta=.01; beta=[theta; B0; delta];
t=0:.1:1200; T0=0; n=4; lamda=2;
hrf=((t-T0).^(n-1)).*exp(-(t-T0)/lamda)/((lamda^n)*factorial(n-1));

% Define and plot the boxcar
box=[ones(1,3000),zeros(1,3000),ones(1,3000),zeros(1,3001)];
subplot(3,1,1); plot(t,box); axis([0 1200 0 1.5]);

% Convolve the hrf and boxcar and discretize
B=conv(hrf,box)/10;
tp=0:.1:2400;
for i=1:480
   N(i)=B(i*25);
end;

% Fill the design matrix
X(:,1)=N'; X(:,2)=ones(nTRs,1); X(:,3)=linspace(1, nTRs, nTRs)';

% Create and plot the data
Bdat=X*beta+normrnd(0,4,[nTRs,1]);
Bdat_plot=zeros(1,12001);
for i=1:480
   Bdat_plot(i*25)=Bdat(i);
end;
subplot(3,1,2); plot(t,Bdat_plot); axis([0 1200 30 60]);

% Estimate the beta vector & error variance
beta_hat=inv(X'*X)*X'*Bdat
Var_e=(Bdat-X*beta_hat)'*(Bdat-X*beta_hat)/(nTRs-1-length(beta))

% Compute the t statistic
c=[1; 0; 0];
t_stat=c'*beta_hat/sqrt(Var_e*c'*inv(X'*X)*c)

% Plot predicted BOLD response
B_pred=X*beta_hat;
Bpred_plot=zeros(1,12001);
for i=1:480
   Bpred_plot((i-1)*25+1:i*25)=B_pred(i);
end;
subplot(3,1,3); plot(t,Bdat_plot); axis([0 1200 30 60]);
hold on; plot(t,Bpred_plot);
```

against the alternative

$$H_1 : \sum_{i=1}^{3} \theta_i^2 > 0.$$

Note that this null hypothesis cannot be written in the form $\underline{c}'\beta = 0$. Proposition 5.2 describes how to construct a $\chi^2$ map that tests this hypothesis.

**Proposition 5.2**    Consider a correlation model that assumes homogeneity of variance and independence (i.e., so $\Sigma_\varepsilon = \sigma_\varepsilon^2$ I). Define a matrix A such that

$$A\underline{\beta} = \underline{\theta} = \begin{bmatrix} \theta_1 \\ \theta_2 \\ \theta_3 \end{bmatrix}.$$

For example, if

$$\underline{\beta} = \begin{bmatrix} \theta_1 \\ \theta_2 \\ \theta_3 \\ B_0 \\ \Delta \end{bmatrix},$$

then

$$A = \begin{bmatrix} 1 & 0 & 0 & 0 & 0 \\ 0 & 1 & 0 & 0 & 0 \\ 0 & 0 & 1 & 0 & 0 \end{bmatrix}.$$

Under the null hypothesis that $\sum_{i=1}^{3} \theta_i^2 = 0$, the following statistic

$$\chi^2 = \frac{\underline{\hat{\theta}}'[A(X'X)^{-1}A']^{-1}\underline{\hat{\theta}}}{\hat{\sigma}_\varepsilon^2}$$

has an asymptotic $\chi^2$ distribution with 3 degrees of freedom[6].

---

6. It might seem counterintuitive that the use of a canonical hrf with no parameters (e.g., the gamma function) would result in $t$ statistics that each have hundreds of degrees of freedom (proposition 5.1), whereas the use of a basis function hrf with 3 free parameters results in $\chi^2$ statistics that each have three degrees of freedom. Recall however, that a $t$ statistic with hundreds of degrees of freedom is nearly $z$ distributed. Thus, an alternative way of viewing propositions 5.1 and 5.2 is that proposition 5.1 produces a $z$ statistic and proposition 5.2 produces the sum of three $z^2$ statistics (which is $\chi^2$ distributed).

**Derivation**  Note that $A\underline{\hat{\beta}} = \underline{\hat{\theta}}$ has a multivariate normal distribution under the null hypothesis with mean vector $\underline{0}$ (under the null hypothesis) and variance-covariance matrix

$$\Sigma_{\underline{\hat{\theta}}} = A\Sigma_{\underline{\hat{\beta}}}A' = \sigma_{\varepsilon}^2 A(X'X)^{-1}A'.$$

Next note that the statistic $\Sigma_{\underline{\hat{\theta}}}^{-\frac{1}{2}}\underline{\hat{\theta}}$ has a multivariate z distribution; that is, it is multivariate normally distributed (because linear transformations of normally distributed random vectors are multivariate normally distributed), it has mean $\underline{0}$ (because $\underline{\hat{\theta}}$ has mean $\underline{0}$ under the null hypothesis), and its variance-covariance matrix equals the identity (the variance-covariance matrix equals $\Sigma_{\underline{\hat{\theta}}}^{-\frac{1}{2}}\Sigma_{\underline{\hat{\theta}}}\Sigma_{\underline{\hat{\theta}}}^{-\frac{1}{2}} = \Sigma_{\underline{\hat{\theta}}}^{-\frac{1}{2}}\Sigma_{\underline{\hat{\theta}}}^{\frac{1}{2}}\Sigma_{\underline{\hat{\theta}}}^{\frac{1}{2}}\Sigma_{\underline{\hat{\theta}}}^{-\frac{1}{2}} = I$). Now if the $r \times 1$ vector $\underline{z}$ has a multivariate z-distribution, then $\underline{z}'\underline{z}$ has a $\chi^2$ distribution with $r$ degrees of freedom (e.g., theorem 4.1.1, Graybill, 1976). Therefore, the statistic

$$(\Sigma_{\underline{\hat{\theta}}}^{-\frac{1}{2}}\underline{\hat{\theta}})'(\Sigma_{\underline{\hat{\theta}}}^{-\frac{1}{2}}\underline{\hat{\theta}}) = \underline{\hat{\theta}}'\Sigma_{\underline{\hat{\theta}}}^{-1}\underline{\hat{\theta}}$$

$$= \underline{\hat{\theta}}'[\sigma_{\varepsilon}^2 A(X'X)^{-1}A']^{-1}\underline{\hat{\theta}}$$

$$= \frac{\underline{\hat{\theta}}'[A(X'X)^{-1}A']^{-1}\underline{\hat{\theta}}'}{\sigma_{\varepsilon}^2}$$

has a $\chi^2$ distribution with 3 degrees of freedom. However, because $\sigma_{\varepsilon}^2$ is unknown, it must be estimated from the data (i.e., via equation 5.16). Therefore, proposition 5.2 holds only for large sample sizes (i.e., many TRs).  ∎

Propositions 5.1 and 5.2 assume that the errors made by the GLM (i.e., the mispredictions) on any pair of TRs are uncorrelated (i.e., implied by the assumption that $\Sigma_{\underline{\varepsilon}} = \sigma_{\varepsilon}^2 I$ is diagonal). With real data this assumption will likely be violated. If so, then it is natural to ask how such violations will affect our ability to identify task-related voxels. Not surprisingly, the answer to this question depends on the method that is used to deal with the correlations. If the correlations are ignored, then the $t$- and $\chi^2$-statistics that are computed from propositions 5.1 and 5.2 will not have the t- and $\chi^2$-distributions described in those results. As a consequence, any method chosen to solve the multiple comparisons problem (see chapter 6) will produce an invalid threshold, and so the resulting true error rate will be unknown. If prewhitening is used to remove the temporal correlations (e.g., as in FSL), then the consequences are negligible, assuming the prewhitening was effective. In this case, the prewhitened data satisfy independence, so propositions 5.1 and 5.2 are now valid.

If the temporal correlations are explicitly modeled (e.g., as in the equation 5.18 covariance model), then valid inferences can be made, but the process is more complex than in propositions 5.1 and 5.2. For example, if $\Sigma_\varepsilon$ is not diagonal, then the $t$-statistic in proposition 5.1 is replaced by

$$t = \frac{\underline{c}'\hat{\beta}}{\sqrt{\underline{c}'(X'X)^{-1}X'\hat{\Sigma}_\varepsilon X(X'X)^{-1}\underline{c}}}.$$

The problem though is that because of the correlations, this statistic does not have a true t-distribution. Even so, its distribution can be approximated by a t distribution if the degrees of freedom are computed by the Satterthwaite approximation (Worsley & Friston, 1995). For more details, interested readers should see Worsley and Friston (1995) or Kiebel and Holmes (2007).

### Nonparametric Approaches to Hypothesis Testing

The validity of all statistical tests developed in the previous section depends strongly on the distributional assumptions of the GLM. In particular, the tests are valid only if the raw BOLD responses are normally distributed and we have correctly modeled the correlations that may or may not exist between BOLD responses on different TRs. An alternative approach to hypothesis testing that makes weaker distributional assumptions is to use nonparametric permutation methods that are based on a bootstrapping approach (e.g., Nichols & Holmes, 2001). A rigorous review will not be given here, but the basic ideas are conceptually straightforward.

In any approach to null hypothesis testing, the goal is to select a threshold for determining significance that controls the probability of a false-positive decision (i.e., a type I error). This requires a model of what the data would look like if the null hypothesis (e.g., the voxel is not task sensitive) was true. In the GLM, this model is constructed by making distributional assumptions about the data. In permutation approaches, the model is built from the existing data—essentially by randomly shuffling the TRs. To see why this makes sense, consider a voxel that shows a strong task-related response in a block design. In general, the BOLD response in this voxel will be greater during TRs in task blocks than during TRs in rest blocks, and because of this difference the observed BOLD response will correlate strongly with the BOLD response predicted in a task-sensitive voxel. If we shuffle the data before analysis, however (i.e., across TRs), then there is no longer any reason to expect a difference between the magnitudes of the BOLD responses during task versus rest blocks. The correlation with the predicted BOLD response should now be zero—exactly as in voxels containing only noise. But note that shuffling across TRs does not change the mean or variance of the data, so the shuffled data make an attractive model of what the BOLD response from this voxel might look like if it were not task sensitive. To implement a permutation test, the following steps are taken.

## Algorithm for Hypothesis Testing with a Permutation Test

*Step 1*   Follow the methods described earlier in this chapter to apply the GLM to the raw (unshuffled) data and create a $t$ (or $\chi^2$) statistic that tests the null hypothesis of interest. Call this value $t_{data}$.

*Step 2*   Randomly shuffle the data across TRs. Analyze these shuffled data using the same GLM as in step 1. Call the $t$-statistic that results from this analysis $t_1$.

*Step 3*   Repeat step 2 a total of $M$ times with a new random shuffle each repetition. Choose a large value for $M$ (e.g., 1000). At the end of this step, $M$ different $t_i$ values will exist.

*Step 4*   Compute the proportion of all the $t_i$ values that are greater than $t_{data}$. This proportion is the $p$-value for the permutation test of the null hypothesis.

This is a conceptually appealing algorithm. The main drawback may be computing time. Rather than running the GLM once for each voxel, as required by the standard GLM approach, permutation methods require running the GLM hundreds (or thousands) of times on each voxel. Also note that although this method creates null-hypothesis data with the same mean and variance as the real data, the shuffling operation changes the correlation between BOLD responses in adjacent TRs.

## Percent Signal Change

Absolute numerical values of the BOLD response have no obvious physical meaning. As a result, for purposes of communication they are often converted to a statistic known as *percent signal change*. The basic idea is that we typically do not care about the particular numerical value of the BOLD response that we record in an experiment. However, we do care how much the task we are studying affects this BOLD response. Percent signal change measures this effect on a percentage scale.

The easiest way to define and understand percent signal change is in a block design. Consider the simplest case where we alternate blocks of rest with blocks in which the subject continuously performs our task of interest. For example, we might alternate 90 seconds of rest with 90 seconds of finger tapping. Let $B_R(i)$ denote the BOLD response in the voxel or region of interest (ROI) on the i[th] TR in the experiment when the subject was resting, and let $B_T(i)$ denote the analogous BOLD response on the i[th] TR in the experiment when the subject was performing our task. Thus, all we have done here is separate out rest TRs from task TRs. The next step is to compute the mean of each of these vectors across all available TRs. In an experiment with $n$ total TRs, suppose half of these are part of rest blocks and half are part of task blocks (assuming $n$ is an even number). The two means we need to compute are therefore

$$\bar{B}_R = \frac{1}{\frac{n}{2}}\sum_{i=1}^{\frac{n}{2}} B_R(i) \quad \text{and} \quad \bar{B}_T = \frac{1}{\frac{n}{2}}\sum_{i=1}^{\frac{n}{2}} B_T(i).$$

Given these two means, the percent signal change induced by the task T is then defined as

$$Q_T = 100\left(\frac{\bar{B}_T - \bar{B}_R}{\bar{B}_R}\right)\%. \tag{5.23}$$

So $Q_T$ is literally the percentage of change in the baseline (i.e., resting) BOLD response that is caused by introducing the task T.

Note that $Q_T$ is negative if the task reduces the overall BOLD response and positive if the BOLD response is increased by the task. Also note that there is no theoretical upper limit on $Q_T$. For example, values above 100% are theoretically possible. In practice, however, percent signal change is usually small—most typically, below 1%. For example, a moderately sized percent signal change might be 0.5%.

Defining percent signal change in rapid event-related designs is considerably more difficult. The problem is that because of the sluggish nature of the BOLD response, it is not obvious how to compute $\bar{B}_R$ and $\bar{B}_T$. One common way to estimate $\bar{B}_R$ is to compute the mean of all BOLD responses collected in the entire experiment. If the task induces a positive percent signal change, then this will overestimate $\bar{B}_R$ because it will also include $\bar{B}_T$, which will be greater than $\bar{B}_R$. The GLM offers a better solution to this problem. From equation 5.5, we see that the mean BOLD response (i.e., the expected value) is $E(\underline{B}) = X\beta$.

Thus, computing the mean BOLD response across TRs is equivalent to computing the mean BOLD response that is predicted by the GLM across TRs. $\bar{B}_R$ is the mean BOLD response in the absence of the task. So to compute this, we can simply eliminate the terms in the GLM associated with the task and then compute the mean across TRs of what is left. This is most easily done by setting the parameter estimates in the $\beta$ vector associated with the task to 0, performing the multiplication $X\beta$, and then averaging across TRs.

As an example, consider the application of the FBR method illustrated in equation 5.6:

$$\underline{B} = X\begin{bmatrix} \beta_1 \\ \beta_2 \\ \beta_3 \\ \beta_4 \\ \beta_5 \\ B_0 \\ \Delta \end{bmatrix} + \underline{\varepsilon}.$$

The first step is to fit this model to the data. This is done by using the normal equations to estimate the entries in $\beta$ (i.e., equation 5.14). Next we compute the predicted BOLD responses in the absence of (i.e., without) the task by zeroing out all the $\beta_i$ estimates

$$\underline{B}_{\text{wo T}} = X \begin{bmatrix} 0 \\ 0 \\ 0 \\ 0 \\ 0 \\ \hat{B}_0 \\ \hat{\Delta} \end{bmatrix}, \tag{5.24}$$

where $\hat{B}_0$ and $\hat{\Delta}$ are the least squares estimates of $B_0$ and $\Delta$, respectively. Finally, we compute the mean of all entries in the $\underline{B}_{\text{wo T}}$ vector:

$$\bar{B}_R = \frac{1}{n} \sum_{i=1}^{n} \underline{B}_{\text{wo T}}(i). \tag{5.25}$$

If instead we had used the correlation model of equation 5.8

$$\underline{B} = X \begin{bmatrix} \theta \\ B_0 \\ \Delta \end{bmatrix} + \underline{\varepsilon},$$

then equation 5.24 would be replaced by

$$\underline{B}_{\text{wo T}} = X \begin{bmatrix} 0 \\ \hat{B}_0 \\ \hat{\Delta} \end{bmatrix} + \underline{\varepsilon}.$$

Unfortunately, computing $\bar{B}_T$ is not so straightforward. The obvious choice is to use the full model. In a block design, the observed BOLD response during task blocks includes activation due to the task plus activation due to all factors that would typically be present during rest blocks. So

$$\bar{B}_T = \frac{1}{n} \sum_{i=1}^{n} \underline{B}(i). \tag{5.26}$$

If this definition is used, note that the numerator of equation 5.23 (i.e., $\bar{B}_T - \bar{B}_R$) becomes the mean across TRs of the predicted task-related BOLD response, with all non-task-related parameters in $\beta$ set to 0. For example, in the correlation model $\bar{B}_T - \bar{B}_R$ is the mean of all entries in the vector

$$\underline{B} - \underline{B}_{\text{wo T}} = X \begin{bmatrix} \hat{\theta} \\ \hat{B}_0 \\ \hat{\Delta} \end{bmatrix} - X \begin{bmatrix} 0 \\ \hat{B}_0 \\ \hat{\Delta} \end{bmatrix} = X \begin{bmatrix} \hat{\theta} \\ 0 \\ 0 \end{bmatrix}. \tag{5.27}$$

Equation 5.26 is a standard way to define $\overline{B}_T$. Even so, methods that compute percent signal change with equations 5.23, 5.25, and 5.26 will underestimate percent signal change relative to the value that would be obtained from equation 5.23 in a block design that used the same task. This is easy to see from equation 5.27. The numerator of equation 5.23 computes the mean of the equation 5.27 vector across TRs (i.e., across the entries in the equation 5.27 vector). From equation 5.8 we see that this mean will equal

$$\overline{B}_T - \overline{B}_R = \frac{\hat{\theta}}{n} \sum_{i=1}^{n} x(i), \tag{5.28}$$

where, as before, $x(i)$ is the predicted BOLD response to the task on TR $i$ (computed by convolving the relevant boxcar function with an appropriate hrf). Thus, any factor that increases the mean of the $x(i)$ will increase this measure of percent signal change. Included in this list is the number of task-related TRs. This is because $x(i)$ will increase during the task and decrease during rest. So by this definition, an experimental design that includes many TRs when the subject is performing the task will report a larger percent signal change than a design that includes fewer task-related TRs, even if the change in the BOLD response induced by each application of the task is identical in the two experiments.

Figure 3.6 shows that as the duration of the boxcar increases, the predicted BOLD response $x(i)$ (the convolution of the boxcar and an hrf) also increases until it saturates at the height of the boxcar, where it remains until the boxcar is turned off. If we set the height of the boxcar at 1, this means that the predicted BOLD response will saturate at 1. In event-related designs, the boxcar duration will seldom be long enough to cause saturation in the predicted BOLD response, whereas this will happen routinely in block designs (because the duration of the boxcar will equal the duration of the block). Thus, values of $x(i)$ will typically be less than 1 in event-related designs and equal to 1 in block designs (i.e., during task blocks). As a result, using equation 5.27 to compute percent signal change in an event-related design will yield smaller values than one would expect in a block design with the same task.

One solution to this problem is to use the parameter estimates one obtains from fitting the GLM to data collected in an event-related design to estimate the $\overline{B}_T$ one would expect if a block design had been used instead. The key is to note that in a block design, the predicted task-related BOLD response should be at saturation (i.e., 1.0) for (almost) the entire duration of the block. In this case, equation 5.28 reduces to

$$\overline{B}_T - \overline{B}_R = \frac{\hat{\theta}}{n} \sum_{i=1}^{n} 1 = \hat{\theta}$$

and thus percent signal change equals

$$Q_T = \frac{\hat{\theta}}{\overline{B}_R} \times 100\%, \tag{5.29}$$

where $\overline{B}_R$ is computed using equation 5.25.

Unfortunately, there is no obvious analogue of equation 5.29 with the FBR GLM. This is because it is impossible to tell from the $\beta_i$ estimates what the saturation height will be of the predicted task-related BOLD response. Perhaps the best that one could do is to use

$$Q_T = \frac{(\hat{\beta}_2 + \hat{\beta}_3 + \hat{\beta}_4)/3}{\overline{B}_R} \times 100\%; \tag{5.30}$$

that is, we estimate the peak height of the predicted task-related BOLD response as the mean of the $\beta_2$, $\beta_3$, and $\beta_4$ estimates (e.g., see the discussion around equation 5.20). With rapid event-related designs, equation 5.30 should underestimate percent signal change, at least relative to equation 5.29. This is because the BOLD response to the task should not have time to saturate because of the rapidly changing nature of the design. As a result, the $\beta_i$ estimates should be smaller than what one would expect in a block design.

### Comparing the Correlation and FBR Methods

Both the correlation and FBR methods share some common assumptions, and they both make some unique assumptions. First, both methods assume macrolinearity; that is, that the BOLD responses from separate neural events add. As we saw in chapter 3, there is empirical evidence supporting this assumption, as long as the separate neural events are reasonably separated in time (e.g., Dale & Buckner, 1997). Second, both methods make all the statistical assumptions that define the GLM. Included in this list are that noise is additive, multivariate normally distributed, and stationary (i.e., the noise distribution does not change across TRs). These GLM assumptions are common to virtually all methods considered in this book, so at this time, they do not constitute a reason to shun the correlation or FBR methods in favor of other alternatives.

In addition to these common assumptions, the correlation and FBR methods each make their own unique assumptions. First, the FBR method assumes a fixed upper bound on the duration of the BOLD response. This upper bound determines the number of $\beta_i$ (or $\beta_{ij}$) to include in the model. Two types of errors are possible in this choice. One could set the bound higher than necessary by including more $\beta_i$ than are needed. This error should be apparent after data analysis, however, because the parameter estimates of the extra $\beta_i$ should all be near zero. In addition, the only cost incurred is negligible—degrees of freedom for the resulting $t$-map will be slightly reduced. The other type of error—underestimating the duration of the BOLD response—is more serious. In this case, there will be some residual BOLD response to an event $E_i$ that is not captured by the model's event $E_i$ parameters. As a result, this extra BOLD response will be absorbed by parameters that model events that occurred after $E_i$ or by the noise variance. In the former case, the parameter estimates of the $\beta_{ij}$ will be biased, and in the latter case the noise variance will be artificially inflated, which will unnecessarily reduce the magnitude of the resulting $t$-values. Because of this large asymmetry in the costs of the two types of errors, when using the FBR method one should always be conservative and include enough $\beta_{ij}$ to avoid underestimation of the duration of the BOLD response. If underestimation is avoided, then the FBR assumption that the duration of the BOLD response is known should be of little concern.

Second, the FBR method assumes that separate BOLD responses to identical stimulus events are always identical. This assumption is necessary because the GLM uses trial averaging to estimate its unknown parameters. In many experiments, it may be reasonable to assume that identical stimulus events always trigger identical BOLD responses, but there are certainly many experiments of interest in cognitive neuroscience for which this assumption is surely invalid. For example, we would expect the BOLD response to a particular stimulus to change over the course of a scanning session in any experiment in which subjects learn, or in which adaptation or sensitization occurs, or in which subjects might alter their strategy from trial to trial for responding to the stimulus. In chapter 11, we will consider a multivariate technique that does not assume the BOLD response to a particular event is invariant throughout the scanning session (i.e., independent component analysis).

In contrast with the FBR method, the correlation method makes a number of strong and unique assumptions. If any of these are wrong, the effects will be similar. In each case, an invalid assumption will cause the predicted BOLD response to differ from the observed BOLD response, which will cause $\theta$ to be underestimated and therefore make it more difficult to identify task-related activation. First, the correlation method assumes microlinearity (in addition to macrolinearity); that is, it assumes that the BOLD response to any event is equal to the convolution of the neural activation with the hrf. There is good evidence in support of this assumption for reasonably long-event durations (e.g., several seconds or longer), but this assumption is likely to be violated with rapid stimulus presentations (i.e., see chapter 3).

Second, the correlation method assumes that the duration of the neural activation induced by each stimulus event is known. This is actually a much stronger assumption than the analogous FBR assumption that the duration of the BOLD response is known. It is stronger because both types of errors—that is, both overestimation and underestimation of the true duration—are serious. In both cases, the duration of the predicted BOLD response will differ from the duration of the observed BOLD response, thereby decreasing the correlation between observed and predicted BOLD responses. On the other hand, although it is important to be accurate when predicting the onset and offset of neural activations when using the correlation method, unlike the FBR method, there is no requirement that these onsets and offsets are always the same (i.e., relative to the TR).

Third, the correlation method assumes that the form of all neural activations is known. The almost universal assumption is that these neural activations are all boxcar functions. In fact, we know that neural activations are not boxcars (e.g., Koch, 1999). At the very least, neural activation takes time to ramp up after a stimulus is presented, and it decays back to baseline after the stimulus disappears. In principle, it would be straightforward to replace the boxcar assumption in the correlation method with a more realistic model of neural activation (Ashby & Waldschmidt, 2008). This should increase the power of the correlation method.

Fourth, the correlation method assumes that the hrf is known. The seriousness of this assumption depends on which hrf option is chosen. The most common choice, and the one making the strongest assumptions, is to select a fixed hrf with no free parameters. There are two obvious problems with this approach. First, it is unlikely that any specific mathematical function (e.g., gamma) will exactly equal the true hrf in any brain region or subject. Second, there is good evidence that the hrf varies across subjects and brain regions. Choosing a flexible model of the hrf (e.g., a basis function model) alleviates the second problem, but not necessarily the first. An exception is the FIR model, which should alleviate both problems.

In summary, the FBR method makes weaker assumptions than the correlation method. These weaker assumptions, however, come at a cost. The FBR method has more free parameters that must be estimated, and it is more inflexible with respect to the predicted timing of neural events. For example, within-TR jittering is feasible only with the correlation method, as is adjusting the hypothesized duration of neural events from one presentation to the next based on the subject's response time.

# 6  The Multiple Comparisons Problem

In the previous chapter, we saw how to construct a statistical parametric map using either the FBR method or the correlation method. In this chapter, we discuss how to use this map to decide which voxels were responsive to the stimulus event or, alternatively, which voxels were more responsive to one type of stimulus event than to another. To keep the discussion concrete, we will assume throughout this chapter that the statistical parametric map we constructed is a $z$-map (or a $t$-map with a large number of degrees of freedom). When appropriate, we will comment on differences that arise if a statistic other than a $z$ is chosen. We will also assume one-tailed tests, or in other words, that our primary interest is in identifying voxels where the BOLD response is greater than we would expect from noise alone.

Regardless of the method used to construct the statistical map, such a map includes a statistic (e.g., a $z$-value) in every voxel of the ROI we are analyzing. Thus, in a whole-brain analysis, it would not be unusual to have a map with 100,000 or more $z$-statistics. Each one of these was constructed under the null hypothesis that the voxel was not responsive to the stimulus event or perhaps that the voxel was equally responsive to two different events. In other words, if the null hypothesis is true that the voxel did not show task-related activity, then the statistic we constructed for that voxel using the methods of chapter 5 should be a random sample from a z-distribution. If, on the other hand, the voxel was responsive to the stimulus, then the statistic will tend to have a value that is greater than we would expect to sample from a z-distribution. The question considered in this chapter is as follows: How do we decide what criterion to use to judge whether the observed $z$-value in a particular voxel is too large to be from a z-distribution?

Of course, if we only ask this question about a single voxel, then the answer is taught in every introductory statistics course. We first decide what type I error rate or false-positive rate we are willing to accept (i.e., choose a numerical value for $\alpha$). Next, from a z-table, we find the $z$-value that yields this value of $\alpha$. This $z$-value is our criterion. In other words, if the null hypothesis is true, then the probability is $\alpha$ that the observed $z$-value is greater than this criterion, and therefore judged falsely to be task sensitive.

If the probability of a false positive equals .05 for each test, then the first problem we face is that with 100,000 separate $z$-tests, we would expect 5000 false positives if none of these voxels were task sensitive. This is clearly unacceptable. For example, suppose the z-values from 6000 voxels are significant. This would mean that 5000 of these are false positives and only 1000 come from task-sensitive brain areas. But our problem would be that we would have no idea which 1000 of the 6000 significant values represented real activation. To avoid this problem, we must increase the criterion or threshold for deciding that each z-value is significant. This will reduce the number of false positives and therefore make it easier to identify task-related activation. Ideally, we would like to set the threshold on each z-value so that we control the probability that at least one false positive occurs in any of the voxels. This probability is typically called the *experiment-wise false-positive rate* and is denoted by $\alpha_E$. For example, if $\alpha_E = .05$ and if there is no task-related activation in any voxels, then (on average) we can expect zero type I errors in 19 of every 20 data sets. The classical statement of the multiple comparisons problem is therefore: How do we decide what criterion to use on each decision to guarantee that the experiment-wise false-positive rate is no greater than some value $\alpha_E$?

### The Sidak and Bonferroni Corrections

If all the separate tests are statistically independent, then an exact solution to the multiple comparisons problem is as follows.

**Proposition 6.1**   Suppose we are simultaneously performing $N$ separate and statistically independent tests. Let $\alpha_t$ equal the probability of a false-positive decision on any single test, and let $\alpha_E$ equal the probability of at least one false-positive decision in the whole set of $N$ tests. Then we can guarantee that $\alpha_E$ will equal any specific desired value by setting

$$\alpha_t = 1 - (1 - \alpha_E)^{1/N}. \tag{6.1}$$

Equation 6.1 is known as the Sidak correction for multiple comparisons.

**Derivation**   If all $N$ tests are independent and the null hypothesis is correct for all tests, then

$P(0 \text{ false positives}) = P(N \text{ correct decisions})$

$$= (1 - \alpha_t)^N.$$

Therefore,

$$\alpha_E = P(\text{at least 1 false positive}) = 1 - (1 - \alpha_t)^N. \tag{6.2}$$

To finish, we must solve for $\alpha_t$. First, note that

$$\alpha_E = 1 - (1 - \alpha_t)^N$$

implies that

$$(1 - \alpha_t)^N = 1 - \alpha_E,$$

which implies that

$$1 - \alpha_t = (1 - \alpha_E)^{1/N},$$

from which equation 6.1 immediately follows.                                                           ■

Thus, with 100,000 tests, if we want an overall $\alpha_E$ of .05, then we need to set the alpha level on each individual test to approximately $\alpha_t = .0000005$, which means our z-threshold for determining significance is 4.89. This is an extremely large value, and it raises the possibility that many true signals will be missed. One simple way to decrease this threshold is to increase the voxel size. For example, if we double the length of each edge of our voxels, the voxel volume will increase by a factor of 8, and as a result we will also decrease the number of voxels in our search volume by a factor of 8. So, for example, instead of 100,000 tests, we would have 12,500 tests. This drops the z-threshold to 4.46, which is better, but not by much. Another possibility is to decrease the number of comparisons by ignoring some voxels. This is common with ROI analyses. For example, rather than looking for significant voxels anywhere in the brain, a researcher might narrow the search to anywhere in the prefrontal cortex. This will greatly decrease $N$ in equation 6.2 and therefore significantly decrease the threshold for determining significance.

A computationally simpler alternative to equation 6.1, which closely approximates the $\alpha_t$ prescribed by the Sidak correction, is known as the Bonferroni correction,

$$\alpha_t = \alpha_E/N \doteq 1 - (1 - \alpha_E)^{1/N}, \tag{6.3}$$

where $\doteq$ means "is approximately equal to." The $\alpha_t$ suggested by the Bonferroni correction is very close to the true value of $\alpha_t$ computed from equation 6.1. Table 6.1 shows some values of $\alpha_t$ computed from both methods for different values of $N$, when the desired $\alpha_E$ is .05. Thus, the Bonferroni correction could be used to compute $\alpha_t$ quickly when $N$ independent tests are being simultaneously performed.

**Table 6.1**
A comparison of $\alpha_t$ values computed using the Sidak and Bonferroni corrections when $\alpha_E = .05$

| $N$ | Sidak $\alpha_t$ | Bonferroni $\alpha_t$ |
|------|--------|--------|
| 3 | .0170 | .0167 |
| 4 | .0127 | .0125 |
| 10 | .0051 | .0050 |
| 100 | .0005 | .0005 |
| 1000 | .00005 | .00005 |

The Sidak and Bonferroni corrections are useful only if the tests are all statistically independent. Unfortunately, this condition is not met with fMRI data. For example, if the $z$-value in one voxel is large, then it is likely that the $z$-values in neighboring voxels will also be large. Thus, the $z$-values from nearby voxels will be positively correlated, rather than independent as assumed by both the Sidak and Bonferroni corrections. There are a variety of reasons why such correlations should be expected. First, it is likely that nearby brain regions may be interconnected. Second, brain regions in neighboring voxels will tend to be oxygenated by similar vasculature. Third, the spatial smoothing that is routinely performed during preprocessing (see chapter 4) introduces positive spatial correlations between neighboring voxels.

Positive correlations between nearby voxels will cause the Sidak and Bonferroni corrections to be too conservative. In other words, if the Bonferroni correction is used on a statistical map, then the true probability of at least one false positive will be smaller than $\alpha_E$, and unfortunately, it will be smaller by an unknown amount. This is often a serious problem. The difference in the BOLD response in task-related voxels compared with voxels that do not respond to the stimulus is likely to be small (e.g., less than 2.0%). As a result, if the threshold for determining statistical significance is higher than necessary, it is likely that many true positives will be missed. It is for this reason that so much effort has been spent attempting to find the best possible threshold for determining significance. Unfortunately, none of the current methods for solving this problem are optimal. In most cases, they are too conservative. Different methods are popular because they make different assumptions and have different goals. In the remainder of this chapter, we consider the three most popular methods for solving the multiple comparisons problem: Gaussian random fields, false discovery rate, and permutation methods. The first two major sections consider methods where a separate decision is made for every voxel in the search region. After that, we consider methods that instead make separate decisions about clusters of voxels. Finally, at the end of the chapter, we briefly consider the permutation methods.

## Gaussian Random Fields

A random field is an ordered collection of random variables. In particular, an $n$-dimensional random field takes on a random value at every point in some $n$-dimensional region. For example, the surface height of the ocean could be modeled as a two-dimensional random field. Random fields are traditionally defined over continuous regions of space, but they can also be restricted to a lattice of points within a continuous region. For example, the BOLD responses collected on any trial of an fMRI experiment could be described as a random field over the lattice of points defined by the centers of each voxel in the search region. In a *Gaussian random field* (GRF), the random variables in the field have a joint multivariate normal distribution. GRFs are the most widely studied and best characterized of all random fields. For the applications considered here, the classic mathematical treatment of GRFs is by Adler (1981), whereas Worsley was most prominent in applying GRF theory to the multiple comparisons problems of fMRI (e.g., Worsley, 1995; Worsley et al., 1996; Worsley, Evans, Marrett, & Neelin, 1992; see also Friston, Frith, Liddle, & Frackowiak, 1991).

Multivariate normal distributions are briefly reviewed in appendix B. In brief, however, to assume that fMRI data have a multivariate normal distribution means that the BOLD response in each voxel is normally distributed across TRs and that the only statistical dependencies among BOLD responses in different voxels are pairwise linear relationships. Despite these restrictions, a GRF still possesses sufficient structure to model complex interrelationships. For example, a GRF can mimic any possible set of intervoxel correlations. Under the null hypothesis of no signal, the statistical parametric map we compute using the methods of chapter 5 should produce a random sample from a z-distribution in each voxel. Even so, neighboring z-values will be positively correlated. Ideally, we could model this z-map as a GRF, where the correlational structure of the GRF is constructed to mimic the actual correlations that exist between the BOLD responses from pairs of voxels in real fMRI data.

Let $z_i$ denote the z-value from this z-map in voxel $i$, and let $T$ denote our threshold for determining statistical significance. In other words, we will reject the null hypothesis that voxel $i$ is responding only to noise if $z_i > T$. If this condition is met, then our conclusion will be that voxel $i$ shows task-related activation. If none of the voxels respond to the task, then a type I error occurs if any of the $z_i$ are greater than $T$. Therefore, when the null hypothesis is true in every voxel, the experiment-wise type I error rate equals

$$\alpha_E = P\left(\max_{1 \le i \le N} z_i > T\right). \tag{6.4}$$

As a result, to control $\alpha_E$ using this approach, we need to determine the probability distribution of the maximum value within a GRF that accurately models z-values one would expect from the resting brain.

Unfortunately, there are two serious problems with this approach. First, no one has been able to characterize the nature of the spatial correlations that exist among activation values in the resting brain. Thus, it is unclear how to construct a suitable GRF. Second, the distribution of the maximum in an arbitrary GRF is unknown. As a result, even if an accurate model was found, it is likely that the tools of GRF theory could not be used to determine a suitable threshold $T$. Despite these problems, elegant solutions have been obtained for a certain restricted type of GRF that models at least some of the spatial correlations known to exist in real fMRI data. The remainder of this section focuses on this one special case.

Consider a GRF that is constructed in the following way. First, construct empty voxels that have the same size, orientation, and spatial configuration as the voxels in an fMRI experiment. Next, draw independent random samples from a standard normal z-distribution, and insert one of these samples into each empty voxel. A two-dimensional example of such an independent Gaussian field is shown in the top panel of figure 6.1. Finally, spatially smooth the values in these hypothetical voxels using exactly the same smoothing algorithm that was used during preprocessing of our fMRI data (see chapter 4). The bottom panel of figure 6.1 shows the result of smoothing the top panel.

As we saw in chapter 4, during preprocessing, spatial smoothing is commonly done with a Gaussian kernel for which the variance in directions $x$, $y$, and $z$ is equal to $\sigma_x^2$, $\sigma_y^2$, and $\sigma_z^2$, respectively. When we smooth the independent GRF with this same filter, note that the larger these variances, the smoother the resulting GRF. This is because large variances mean that more voxels make a significant contribution to the average. So $\sigma_i^2$ measures the width of the kernel in direction $i$. As we saw in chapter 4, another measure of width is the *full width at half maximum* (FWHM), which was illustrated in figure 4.11. The FWHM along direction $i$, denoted $FWHM_i$, is equal to the width of the interval between the points at which the height of the smoothing kernel along direction $i$ is exactly half its peak height. In figure 4.11, the peak height of the kernel is 1, so half this height is 0.5. The width of the kernel at height 0.5 therefore equals its FWHM. With a Gaussian kernel, $FWHM_i$ is equal to

$$FWHM_i = \sqrt{8 \log 2}\, \sigma_i. \tag{6.5}$$

The $FWHM_i$ values measure the width of the kernel and therefore the amount of smoothing that occurs in each direction. We can multiply these to create a measure of the amount of total smoothing that Worsley et al. (1992) called the *resel*, which is short for "resolution unit." Thus,

$$resel = FWHM_x \times FWHM_y \times FWHM_z. \tag{6.6}$$

Note that resels are in units of volume, and that if $V$ equals the total brain volume from which we have collected our data, then the total number of resels $R$ must equal

$$R = \frac{V}{resel} \tag{6.7}$$

Smoothing the independent GRF with a Gaussian filter introduces a spatial correlation. This is because smoothing is just a sophisticated form of averaging. Smoothing essentially replaces each voxel value with a weighted average of the values in all neighboring voxels. Thus, if one voxel in this neighborhood has an unusually large value, then the values in all neighboring voxels will be inflated by the smoothing process. In this way, smoothing causes values in nearby voxels to become positively correlated, and these correlations will decrease with the distance between those voxels (because the kernel weights decrease with distance). In addition, because the Gaussian smoothing we performed on the independent GRF is precisely the type of spatial smoothing that is routinely done during preprocessing,

Independent GRF

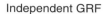

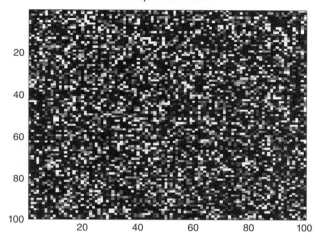

Smoothed with Gaussian Kernel

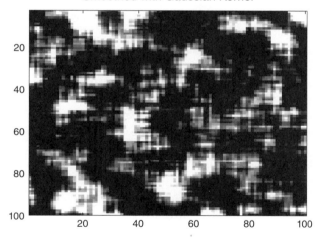

**Figure 6.1**
(Top) An independent GRF defined over a $100 \times 100$ (two-dimensional) lattice. (Bottom) The same GRF after smoothing with a Gaussian kernel. In both cases, larger numerical values are indicated by lighter shades of gray, abscissa values denote column number, and ordinate values denote row values.

we know that our fMRI data will possess exactly the same type of spatial correlation as the smoothed GRF. On the other hand, however, typical fMRI data will possess more spatial correlation than this type of GRF. In other words, the correlation in our smoothed GRF will be a subset of the correlation in the real fMRI data. To create the GRF, we smoothed independent data. During fMRI preprocessing, we smooth correlated data. Thus, this GRF approach to the multiple comparisons problem underestimates the true amount of correlation and as a result is likely to be too conservative. Even so, because it does model some spatial correlations, the GRF approach is much less conservative than the Bonferroni correction. The amount by which it is less conservative depends on the amount of smoothing. As the width or FWHM of the Gaussian kernel increases, the resulting spatial correlations extend for greater distances, and because of this increased correlation, the GRF threshold for determining significance will decrease. Thus, with no smoothing, the GRF threshold will equal the Sidak threshold (because without smoothing the GRF is independent). As the amount of smoothing increases (i.e., as *resel* increases), the GRF threshold decreases, whereas, of course, the Sidak threshold remains constant (as it does not take correlation into account). The bottom panel of figure 6.1 shows a two-dimensional GRF constructed from this process. Larger values are indicated by lighter shades of gray. Note that the GRF is patchy, with blobs occurring wherever, by chance, an unusually large sample was drawn from the z-distribution.

A solution to the multiple comparisons problem requires that we find a threshold $T$ that satisfies equation 6.4. Unfortunately, no exact solution to this problem is known. Even so, GRF theory makes it possible to find an approximate solution in the special case where the GRF is constructed by smoothing an independent $z$ GRF with a Gaussian kernel. The first step in this process is to define the *excursion set* of the GRF for the threshold $T$, which is the set of all $z$-values that exceed $T$. For example, if we treat the ocean's surface as a GRF and set the threshold $T$ at 2 m, then the excursion set would include all water that has an elevation 2 m or more above the mean surface height of the ocean.

The GRF method for correcting for multiple comparisons depends on a statistic of the excursion set called the *Euler characteristic*, which is denoted by $\chi_T$. The precise definition of the Euler characteristic is complex, but to a rough approximation

$$\chi_T \doteq \# \text{ of connected peaks (i.e., blobs)} - \# \text{ of valleys (or holes)}. \tag{6.8}$$

To gain an intuitive understanding of this definition, suppose an object is sitting on a table and that we pass a plane that is parallel to the table through the object. Suppose also that the plane is $T$ cm above the table, where $T$ is less than the height of the object. The excursion set includes all parts of the object that are above the plane. If the object is a sphere, then note that it will always have one peak in its excursion set and no valleys, so the Euler characteristic of a sphere is 1. In contrast, a doughnut always has one connected peak in its excursion set (i.e., a ring) and one hole, so its Euler characteristic is 0.

To see why the Euler characteristic is useful in solving the multiple comparisons problem, we need to think about what happens to it as the threshold $T$ is increased. In particular, note that as $T$ increases from an initially small value, any valleys that exist will tend to disappear before the peaks. For example, if the sea level on Earth were to increase substantially, the valleys would begin to disappear, and eventually a point would be reached where only mountain peaks would rise above the water. Thus, for a certain range of large values of $T$, the Euler characteristic $\chi_T$ is approximately equal to the number of peaks (i.e., because the number of valleys will be zero).

With fMRI data, the height at the center of each voxel is the voxel's $z$-value. Peaks exist at voxels where the $z$-value exceeds the significance threshold $T$. Under the null hypothesis of no signal, peaks therefore correspond with false positives. In other words, assuming the null hypothesis is true in all voxels (i.e., no task-related activation), then the probability of at least one false positive is equal to the probability that there is at least one peak in the excursion set. If in addition, the threshold is set high enough to eliminate all valleys, then the probability of at least one false positive equals the probability that the Euler characteristic is at least 1:

$$\alpha_E = P\left(\max_i z_i > T\right) \doteq P(\chi_T \geq 1). \tag{6.9}$$

As the value of $T$ increases even more, the peaks themselves begin to fall below the threshold, until eventually only the highest of all peaks is left. The highest summit on Earth (Mt. Everest) has an elevation of 29,029 ft, whereas the second highest peak (K2) has an elevation of 28,251 ft. Therefore, if sea level increased by more than 28,251 ft but less than 29,029 ft, there would be only a single connected peak rising above the earth's oceans. For these very high levels of $T$,

$$\chi_T = \begin{cases} 1 & \text{if } \max_i z_i > T \\ 0 & \text{if } \max_i z_i < T \end{cases} \tag{6.10}$$

Because $\chi_T$ takes on only two possible values for these large values of $T$, note that the mean or expected value of $\chi_T$ equals

$$E(\chi_T) = 0 \times P(\chi_T = 0) + 1 \times P(\chi_T \geq 1)$$

$$= P(\chi_T \geq 1).$$

By equation 6.9, therefore, we arrive at the fundamental result that makes it possible to use GRF theory to correct for multiple comparisons. Specifically, for sufficiently large values of $T$,

$$\alpha_E \doteq E(\chi_T). \tag{6.11}$$

This translation from $P(\chi_T \geq 1)$ in equation 6.9 to $E(\chi_T)$ in equation 6.11 is helpful because it turns out to be easier to estimate the expected value of $\chi_T$ than it is to compute the probability that $\chi_T \geq 1$. In fact, Worsley et al. (1996) showed that the expected value could be computed from

$$\alpha_E \doteq E(\chi_T) = \sum_{d=0}^{3} R_d(\text{ROI}) f_d(T), \qquad (6.12)$$

where $T$ is the threshold for determining significance, $R_d(\text{ROI})$ is the number of $d$-dimensional resels in the search region of interest (ROI), and $f_d(T)$ is the expected value of the Euler characteristic in one resel of dimension $d$ when the threshold is $T$. Worsley et al. (1996) provided equations for $f_d(T)$ for $z$, $t$, $\chi^2$, and $F$ maps. To make the current text self-contained, we reproduce those here.

$f_d(T)$ for $z$-maps:

$$f_0(T) = \int_T^\infty \frac{1}{(2\pi)^{\frac{1}{2}}} e^{-x^2/2} \, dx,$$

$$f_1(T) = \frac{(4\log_e 2)^{\frac{1}{2}}}{2\pi} e^{-T^2/2},$$

$$f_2(T) = \frac{(4\log_e 2)}{(2\pi)^{\frac{3}{2}}} e^{-T^2/2} T,$$

$$f_3(T) = \frac{(4\log_e 2)^{\frac{3}{2}}}{(2\pi)^2} e^{-T^2/2} (T^2 - 1).$$

$f_d(T)$ for $t$-maps (when degrees of freedom $v$ is greater than $d$):

$$f_0(T) = \frac{\Gamma\left(\frac{v+1}{2}\right)}{\sqrt{\pi v} \, \Gamma\left(\frac{v}{2}\right)} \int_T^\infty \left(1 + \frac{x^2}{v}\right)^{-\frac{1}{2}(v+1)} dx$$

$$f_1(T) = \frac{\sqrt{\log_e 2}}{\pi} \left(1 + \frac{T^2}{v}\right)^{-\frac{1}{2}(v-1)}$$

$$f_2(T) = \frac{4\log_e 2}{(2\pi)^{\frac{3}{2}}} \frac{\Gamma\left(\frac{v+1}{2}\right)}{\sqrt{\frac{v}{2}} \, \Gamma\left(\frac{v}{2}\right)} T \left(1 + \frac{T^2}{v}\right)^{-\frac{1}{2}(v-1)}$$

$$f_3(T) = \frac{2(\log_e 2)^{\frac{3}{2}}}{\pi^2}\left(1+\frac{T^2}{\nu}\right)^{-\frac{1}{2}(\nu-1)}\left(\frac{\nu-1}{\nu}T^2-1\right).$$

$f_d(T)$ for $\chi^2$-maps with $\upsilon$ degrees of freedom:

$$f_0(T) = \frac{1}{2^{\frac{\nu}{2}}\Gamma\left(\frac{\nu}{2}\right)}\int_T^\infty x^{\frac{1}{2}(\nu-2)}e^{-x/2}dx$$

$$f_1(T) = \frac{2\sqrt{\log_e 2}}{\sqrt{2\pi}}\frac{T^{\frac{1}{2}(\nu-1)}e^{-T/2}}{2^{(\nu-2)/2}\Gamma\left(\frac{\nu}{2}\right)}$$

$$f_2(T) = \frac{2\log_e 2}{\pi}\frac{T^{\frac{1}{2}(\nu-2)}e^{-T/2}}{2^{(\nu-2)/2}\Gamma\left(\frac{\nu}{2}\right)}(T-\nu+1)$$

$$f_3(T) = \frac{(4\log_e 2)^{\frac{3}{2}}}{(2\pi)^{\frac{3}{2}}}\frac{T^{\frac{1}{2}(\nu-3)}e^{-T/2}}{2^{(\nu-2)/2}\Gamma\left(\frac{\nu}{2}\right)}[T^2-(2\nu-1)T+(\nu-1)(\nu-2)].$$

$f_d(T)$ for $F$-maps with $\upsilon_1$ and $\upsilon_2$ degrees of freedom:

$$f_0(T) = \frac{\nu_2\Gamma\left(\frac{\nu_1+\nu_2-2}{2}\right)}{\nu_1\Gamma\left(\frac{\nu_1}{2}\right)\Gamma\left(\frac{\nu_2}{2}\right)}\int_T^\infty \left(\frac{\nu_2 x}{\nu_1}\right)^{\frac{1}{2}(\nu_2-2)}\left(1+\frac{\nu_2 x}{\nu_1}\right)^{-\frac{1}{2}(\nu_1+\nu_2)}dx$$

$$f_1(T) = \frac{2\sqrt{\log_e 2}}{\sqrt{\pi}}\frac{\Gamma\left(\frac{\nu_1+\nu_2-1}{2}\right)}{\Gamma\left(\frac{\nu_1}{2}\right)\Gamma\left(\frac{\nu_2}{2}\right)}\left(\frac{\nu_2 T}{\nu_1}\right)^{\frac{1}{2}(\nu_2-1)}\left(1+\frac{\nu_2 T}{\nu_1}\right)^{-\frac{1}{2}(\nu_1+\nu_2-2)}$$

$$f_2(T) = \frac{2\log_e 2}{\pi}\frac{\Gamma\left(\frac{\nu_1+\nu_2-2}{2}\right)}{\Gamma\left(\frac{\nu_1}{2}\right)\Gamma\left(\frac{\nu_2}{2}\right)}\left(\frac{\nu_2 T}{\nu_1}\right)^{\frac{1}{2}(\nu_2-2)}\left(1+\frac{\nu_2 T}{\nu_1}\right)^{-\frac{1}{2}(\nu_1+\nu_2-2)}\left[(\nu_1-1)\frac{\nu_2 T}{\nu_1}-(\nu_2-1)\right]$$

$$f_3(T) = \frac{2(\log_e 2)^{\frac{3}{2}}}{\pi^{\frac{3}{2}}}\frac{\Gamma\left(\frac{\nu_1+\nu_2-3}{2}\right)}{\Gamma\left(\frac{\nu_1}{2}\right)\Gamma\left(\frac{\nu_2}{2}\right)}\left(\frac{\nu_2 T}{\nu_1}\right)^{\frac{1}{2}(\nu_2-3)}\left(1+\frac{\nu_2 T}{\nu_1}\right)^{-\frac{1}{2}(\nu_1+\nu_2-2)}$$

$$\times\left[(\nu_1-1)(\nu_1-2)\left(\frac{\nu_2 T}{\nu_1}\right)^2-(2\nu_1\nu_2-\nu_1-\nu_2-1)\left(\frac{\nu_2 T}{\nu_1}\right)+(\nu_2-1)(\nu_2-2)\right].$$

One unfortunate complication is that the resel counts $R_d$ in equation 6.12 depend not only on the volume of the search region but also on its shape. Worsley et al. (1996) gave typical resel counts for a variety of brain regions along with the corresponding $t$-thresholds that result from applying equation 6.12. Some of those results are reprinted here in table 6.2.

Worsley et al. (1996) also provided an algorithm for computing resel counts that can be used if searching over some region that is not listed in table 6.2 or if considerable individual differences are expected (i.e., and normalization is not performed). This algorithm is described next.

**Worsley et al. (1996) Algorithm for Computing Resel Counts (i.e., $R_d$)**  The basic idea of this algorithm is to glue pairs of voxels together in various ways to create supervoxels (as illustrated in figure 6.2). Next we count how many of these supervoxels fit into our region of interest. The resel count for this region is then computed by adding and subtracting these supervoxel counts in specific ways. To begin, let ROI denote the search region, and suppose our voxels are of size $d_x \times d_y \times d_z$, where, for example, $d_i$ might be measured in millimeters. The first step is to redefine the voxels in a way that takes account of resel size. Specifically, we need to define new voxels that are each of size $r_x \times r_y \times r_z$, where $r_i = d_i/$ $FWHM_i$. The algorithm works on these new voxels.

The next step is to define the various supervoxel counts.

*0D Super Voxels*  This is just a single voxel (i.e., the centroid of a voxel is zero-dimensional), so the only relevant count is $A$ = total number of voxels in the ROI.

*1D Super Voxels*  Here we glue two voxels together. This can be done in three different ways (see figure 6.2). Note that the centroids of the two voxels define a line (which is one-dimensional).

*x-direction*  Glue two voxels together so that the resulting supervoxel is two voxels long in the $x$ direction. Let $B_x$ = total number of these voxels in the ROI.

*y-direction*  Glue two voxels together so that the resulting supervoxel is two voxels long in the $y$ direction. Let $B_y$ = total number of these voxels in the ROI.

*z-direction*  Glue two voxels together so that the resulting supervoxel is two voxels long in the $z$ direction. Let $B_z$ = total number of these voxels in the ROI.

*2D Super Voxels*  Now we glue four voxels in a way such that the voxel centroids define a plane. This can also be done in three different ways (see figure 6.2).

*xy-plane*  Glue four voxels together so that the resulting supervoxel is two voxels long in the $x$ direction and two voxels long in the $y$ direction (but only one voxel deep in the $z$ direction). Let $C_{xy}$ = total number of these voxels in the ROI.

*yz-direction*  Glue four voxels together so that the resulting supervoxel is two voxels long in the $y$ and $z$ directions (and only one voxel deep in the $x$ direction). Let $C_{yz}$ = total number of these voxels in the ROI.

*xz-direction*  Glue four voxels together so that the resulting supervoxel is two voxels long in the $x$ and $z$ directions. Let $C_{xz}$ = total number of these voxels in the ROI.

**Table 6.2**
Resel counts and GRF thresholds for various ROIs

| ROI | Volume (cc) | Resel Counts | | | | Threshold ($T$) for $\alpha_E =$ | | |
|---|---|---|---|---|---|---|---|---|
| | | $R_0$(ROI) | $R_1$(ROI) | $R_2$(ROI) | $R_3$(ROI) | .10 | .05 | .01 |
| Single voxel | 0 | 1 | 0 | 0 | 0 | 1.28 | 1.64 | 2.33 |
| Head of caudate | 7 | 0 | 6.18 | 4.63 | .65 | 2.75 | 3.02 | 3.55 |
| Putamen | 12 | 1 | 7.32 | 6.80 | 1.18 | 2.89 | 3.15 | 3.66 |
| Globus pallidus | 3 | 0 | 4.03 | 2.29 | .24 | 2.49 | 2.78 | 3.35 |
| Thalamus | 11 | 1 | 4.94 | 5.14 | 1.13 | 2.79 | 3.05 | 3.59 |
| Anterior cingulate | 9 | 1 | 8.20 | 5.79 | .86 | 2.86 | 3.11 | 3.63 |
| Posterior cingulate | 6 | 1 | 5.32 | 3.85 | .58 | 2.70 | 2.97 | 3.51 |
| Cingulate gyri | 15 | 0 | 12.89 | 9.63 | 1.44 | 3.03 | 3.27 | 3.77 |
| Superior frontal gyrus | 80 | 1 | 15.64 | 25.69 | 8.97 | 3.38 | 3.60 | 4.07 |
| Middle frontal gyrus | 57 | 1 | 14.89 | 21.14 | 6.23 | 3.31 | 3.53 | 4.00 |
| Inferior frontal gyrus | 37 | 1 | 11.22 | 14.25 | 4.06 | 3.17 | 3.41 | 3.89 |
| Precentral gyrus | 32 | 1 | 12.30 | 14.23 | 3.40 | 3.16 | 3.40 | 3.88 |
| Frontal gyri | 207 | 1 | 19.30 | 53.39 | 23.63 | 3.63 | 3.84 | 4.28 |
| Postcentral gyrus | 27 | 1 | 10.59 | 12.56 | 2.89 | 3.11 | 3.35 | 3.84 |
| Superior parietal lobule | 22 | 1 | 7.95 | 9.89 | 2.34 | 3.03 | 3.27 | 3.77 |
| Supramarginal gyrus | 19 | 1 | 7.27 | 7.72 | 2.00 | 2.95 | 3.21 | 3.72 |
| Angular gyrus | 20 | 1 | 6.56 | 8.20 | 2.14 | 2.96 | 3.22 | 3.73 |
| Paracentral lobule | 14 | 1 | 6.35 | 7.03 | 1.49 | 2.90 | 3.16 | 3.67 |
| Precuneus | 26 | 1 | 8.75 | 10.26 | 2.80 | 3.06 | 3.30 | 3.80 |
| Parietal lobe | 128 | 1 | 15.20 | 37.04 | 14.49 | 3.50 | 3.72 | 4.17 |
| Superior temporal gyrus | 40 | 0 | 13.75 | 16.70 | 4.24 | 3.22 | 3.45 | 3.93 |
| Middle temporal gyrus | 39 | 0 | 14.33 | 16.43 | 4.16 | 3.22 | 3.45 | 3.93 |
| Inferior temporal gyrus | 25 | 1 | 8.61 | 10.32 | 2.63 | 3.05 | 3.30 | 3.79 |
| Temporal gyri | 117 | 0 | 16.99 | 36.70 | 13.03 | 3.49 | 3.71 | 4.16 |
| Lateral occipitotemporal gyrus | 23 | −1 | 10.12 | 11.16 | 2.41 | 3.06 | 3.31 | 3.80 |
| Medial occipitotemporal gyrus | 5 | 1 | 3.96 | 2.93 | .44 | 2.58 | 2.86 | 3.42 |
| Occipital gyrus | 12 | 1 | 6.90 | 6.54 | 1.25 | 2.88 | 3.14 | 3.65 |
| Cuneus | 19 | 1 | 6.85 | 8.04 | 2.05 | 2.96 | 3.21 | 3.72 |
| Lingual gyrus | 6 | 1 | 4.86 | 3.69 | .59 | 2.68 | 2.95 | 3.49 |
| Occipital lobe | 65 | −1 | 10.68 | 23.11 | 7.17 | 3.32 | 3.55 | 4.02 |
| Whole brain | 1294 | 1 | 20.43 | 107.09 | 153.42 | 4.05 | 4.23 | 4.63 |

From Worsley et al., 1996). The volumes of smaller regions were computed from the atlas of Evans, Marrett, Torrescorzo, Ku, and Collins (1991).

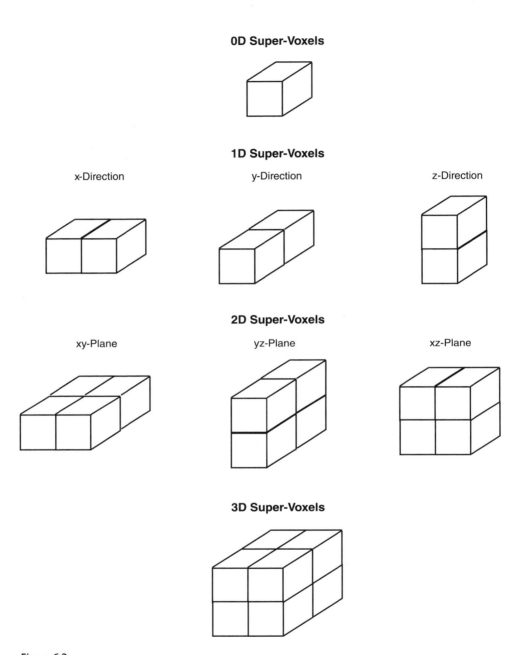

**Figure 6.2**
Various supervoxels that must be constructed to implement the Worsley et al. (1996) algorithm for computing resel counts (i.e., $R_d$).

*3D Super Voxels*   Now we glue eight voxels together in a way such that the voxel centroids define a cube. This can also be done in only one way. The resulting supervoxel is 2 voxels × 2 voxels × 2 voxels. Let $D$ = total number of these voxels in the ROI.

The resel counts can now be computed as

$$R_0(\text{ROI}) = A - (B_x + B_y + B_z) + (C_{xy} + C_{yz} + C_{xz}) - D$$

$$R_1(\text{ROI}) = (B_x - C_{xy} - C_{xz} + D)r_x + (B_y - C_{xy} - C_{yz} + D)r_y + (B_z - C_{xz} - C_{yz} + D)r_z$$

$$R_2(\text{ROI}) = (C_{xy} - D)r_x r_y + (C_{xz} - D)r_x r_z + (C_{yz} - D)r_y r_z \tag{6.13}$$

$$R_3(\text{ROI}) = D r_x r_y r_z. \qquad \blacksquare$$

Equation 6.12 depends on two especially important conditions. First, the null hypothesis of no signal must be true in every voxel. Second, the simple GRF is valid in which the only spatial correlation is induced by Gaussian smoothing. If equation 6.12 is used to set the threshold, rather than table 6.2, then an iterative process is used. First, a value of $T$ is selected, and then equation 6.12 is used to compute $\alpha_E$. If the resulting $\alpha_E$ is larger than desired, then $T$ is increased and the process is repeated. If instead $\alpha_E$ is smaller than desired, then $T$ is decreased. This process of setting and resetting $T$ is continued until the desired $\alpha_E$ is achieved.

### False Discovery Rate

The goal of the methods discussed so far has been to control $\alpha_E$, the probability that at least one false positive occurs in the entire set of tests. Benjamini and Hochberg (1995) suggested trying a qualitatively different approach. They argued that with many tests, a few false positives should not be feared. Thus, instead of trying to control $\alpha_E$, they argued that a more important goal should be to limit the proportion of significant results that are false positive. In other words, consider the set of all voxels for which the null hypothesis of no signal is rejected. Benjamini and Hochberg (1995) proposed a method that sets a limit of $q$ on what they called the *false discovery rate* (FDR); that is, the proportion of these voxels for which the null hypothesis was incorrectly rejected.

Consider an experiment with $N$ voxels. Suppose the null hypothesis of no signal is true in $N_0$ of these voxels, and $N_1$ voxels show task-related activation (i.e., a signal is present). Suppose some method is used to decide whether or not to reject the null hypothesis in each voxel and that the results shown in table 6.3 are obtained after all these tests are completed.

In this example, there are $V$ false positives. The standard approach is to try to control

$$\alpha_E = \text{P}(V \geq 1).$$

**Table 6.3**
Frequencies of all possible outcomes of $N$ tests of the null hypothesis of no signal

|  | Decision | | |
| --- | --- | --- | --- |
|  | Do not reject | Reject | Sum |
| $H_0$ true (no signal) | $U$ | $V$ | $N_0$ |
| $H_1$ true (signal) | $T$ | $S$ | $N_1$ |
| Sum | $W$ | $R$ | $N$ |

Instead, Benjamini and Hochberg (1995) suggested we control the FDR, which is defined as the expected value of $V/R$; that is,

$$FDR = \begin{cases} E\left(\dfrac{V}{R}\right) & \text{if } R > 0 \\ 0 & \text{if } R = 0. \end{cases} \tag{6.14}$$

In particular, the goal of FDR methods is to make decisions about the significance of each voxel in such a way that over all tests, we can be sure that $FDR \leq q$. Thus, the value $q$ plays the same role in FDR approaches that $\alpha_E$ plays in the Bonferroni and GRF approaches.

To guarantee that the FDR is less than or equal to $q$ for any desired value of $q$, Benjamini and Hochberg (1995) suggested the following algorithm.

**Benjamini and Hochberg (1995) Algorithm for Ensuring That $FDR < q$**

*Step 1*    Convert each of the $N$ $z_i$ (or $t_i$) to a $p$-value. Call the i[th] of such values $p_i$. In the case of activations, $p_i$ is the area under the $H_0$ distribution to the right of $z_i$, whereas in the case of deactivations, $p_i$ is the area under the $H_0$ distribution to the left of $z_i$.

*Step 2*    Rank order the $p_i$ from the smallest to the largest. Denote the k[th] smallest $p_i$ by $P[k]$. Therefore,

$$P[1] \leq P[2] \leq \cdots \leq P[N].$$

*Step 3*    The $z$-value with the k[th] smallest $p_i$ is significant if

$$P[k] < qk/N,$$

otherwise this $z$-value is not significant.                                                    ∎

This simple algorithm is illustrated graphically in figure 6.3. After the $p$-values are ordered in step 2, they are plotted in a graph where $i$ is the abscissa and $P[i]$ is the ordinate. Note that this plot must be nondecreasing. Next, a line is drawn on this graph with slope $q/N$ and intercept 0. All $p$-values below this line are significant. In figure 6.3, filled diamonds denote $p$-values associated with voxels that this algorithm judges to be significant (i.e., showing task-related activity), and open circles denote non-significant $p$-values.

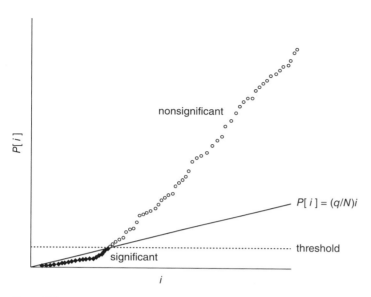

**Figure 6.3**
Illustration of the graphical algorithm used to control false discovery rate. Solid diamonds represent p-values of voxels judged to show task-related activity, whereas open circles represent p-values judged to be non-significant.

MATLAB box 6.1 shows code that produces a figure of this type and that will find the threshold associated with an FDR of $q$ for any set of data.

**Why This Algorithm Works** To see why this algorithm successfully controls the FDR, suppose that in our experiment described by table 6.3, all signals are strong—so strong in fact that their associated p-values are all near 0. Note that in this case, $T = 0$ and $N_1 = S$ because the null hypothesis will be rejected in all task-related voxels. According to table 6.3, $S$ signal voxels are judged significant as are $V$ no-signal voxels. Because the p-value on all signals is 0, the largest p-value of all voxels judged significant is equal to the p-value of the largest false positive, which in this example is $P[S + V]$. Thus, the step 3 threshold on the p-values for determining significance must be

$$p_T = P[S+V] = \frac{q}{N}(S+V). \tag{6.15}$$

In other words, all voxels for which the associated p-value is less than this value of $p_T$ are judged significant, and all voxels for which the p-value is greater than $p_T$ are judged non-significant. This situation is illustrated in figure 6.4. Next note that the p-value of all signal voxels is 0, and the p-value of all non-signal voxels should be greater than 0. Therefore, if the threshold is $p_T$, then the probability of randomly sampling a z-value from the $H_0$ distribution that is below this threshold is $p_T$. As a result,

**MATLAB Box 6.1**
Implementing false discovery rate (for a $1 \times N$ vector of z-values, Z, find the threshold $T$ that leads to false discovery rate $q$)

```
clear all; close all; clc;   % Clear all workspaces

% Define acceptable false discovery rate & number of tests
q=.05; N=120;

% Create (or read in) data (i.e., z- or t-values)
Z=[normrnd(0,1,[1,100]),normrnd(3,1,[1,20])];

% Convert data to P values, rank order, and plot
P=1-normcdf(Z,0,1);
P_rank=sort(P);
i=1:N; plot(i,P_rank,'o'); hold on;

% Plot criterion values
plot(i,q*i/N); axis([0 40 0 .02]); hold on;

% Find threshold
TT=0;
for j=1:N;
   if q*j/N > P_rank(j), TT=q*j/N; end;
end;

% Plot threshold
T=ones(1,N)*TT; plot(i,T);
```

$$p_T = \frac{V}{N_0}.$$  (6.16)

Equations 6.15 and 6.16 together imply that

$$\frac{V}{N_0} = \frac{q}{N}(S+V),$$

and therefore that

$$\frac{V}{S+V} = FDR = q\frac{N_0}{N} \leq q.$$

Thus,

$$FDR \leq q.$$                                                                                   ∎

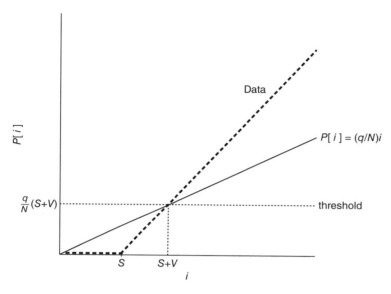

**Figure 6.4**
Conceptual illustration of why the Benjamini and Hochberg (1995) algorithm guarantees that the false discovery rate is no greater than $q$.

To illustrate the FDR algorithm and to compare it with a traditional method like Bonferroni, data were simulated from 20,000 voxels—19,000 of which contained only noise and 1000 of which were task sensitive. The $z$-values in the noise-filled voxels were independent random samples from a normal distribution with mean 0 and variance 1 (i.e., a z-distribution), and the $z$-values in the task-sensitive voxels were samples from a normal distribution with mean $\mu$ and variance 1. The value of $\mu$ was systematically varied from 1.5 to 8. For each value of $\mu$, 100 data sets were simulated, and both the FDR (with $q = 0.05$) and Bonferroni methods (with $\alpha_E = 0.05$) were used to compute the overall mean number of significant voxels, along with the number of false positives (type I errors) and misses (type II errors). Results are shown in table 6.4.

First note that because the samples in each data set were all drawn independently, the Bonferroni correction should be exact; that is, the expected number of false positives should be exactly .05. In other words, Bonferroni correction should produce only 1 false-positive voxel in roughly every 20 data sets. Table 6.4 verifies this prediction. The mean number of noise-filled voxels exceeding the Bonferroni threshold fluctuates around .05, regardless of the value of $\mu$. Note though that the price we pay for this low type I error rate is many type II errors. For example, even when the mean $z$-value in the task-sensitive voxels is 4, Bonferroni correction misses more than 700 of the 1000 task-sensitive voxels. The number of task-responsive voxels missed does not drop below 10% until the mean $z$-value rises to 6.

**Table 6.4**
Results of applying Bonferroni and false discovery rate methods of correcting for multiple comparisons to simulated data in which 19,000 voxels contained noise and 1000 voxels were task sensitive

| Mean $z$-Value in Task-Sensitive Voxels | Bonferroni | | | False Discovery Rate | | |
| --- | --- | --- | --- | --- | --- | --- |
| | Number Significant | False Positive | Misses | Number Significant | False Positive | Misses |
| 1.5 | 1.12 | .04 | 998.9 | 3.08 | .27 | 996.7 |
| 2 | 5.2 | .03 | 994.9 | 54.4 | 2.7 | 947.7 |
| 3 | 59.3 | .06 | 940.8 | 522.3 | 24.8 | 502.5 |
| 4 | 289.3 | .06 | 710.8 | 923.0 | 44.0 | 121.0 |
| 5 | 669.1 | .04 | 331.0 | 1034.8 | 48.0 | 13.3 |
| 6 | 923.6 | .03 | 76.5 | 1048.3 | 48.9 | .67 |
| 7 | 992.8 | .05 | 7.2 | 1050.4 | 50.4 | 0 |
| 8 | 999.9 | .09 | .26 | 1048.4 | 48.4 | 0 |

The FDR algorithm misses many fewer task-sensitive voxels. For example, note that it correctly identifies 88% of these voxels at a value of $\mu$ (i.e., 4) where Bonferroni correction only identified 29%. On the other hand, the cost of this greater power is a much higher false-positive rate. When the mean $z$-value in task-sensitive voxels is low, the number of false positives is well below the theoretical limit of 50 (i.e., 1000 task-sensitive voxels $\times q = .05$), but when this mean rises above 4, the algorithm is essentially making the maximum allowable number of false positives. The danger is that if these 50 false-positive voxels happened to cluster in some single brain region, then it is likely that a seriously incorrect inference would be made.

Regardless of how the data are generated, the FDR algorithm will almost always indicate a larger number of significant voxels than either the Bonferroni or GRF methods. But it must be remembered that these latter methods are controlling $\alpha_E$ rather than the FDR. Therefore, even if the assumptions of the various methods are all correct, the FDR method, by definition, will produce more false positives than the Bonferroni or GRF methods. For this reason, it is not appropriate to compare thresholds produced by the different methods.

It is also a mistake to assume that the FDR algorithm must be less conservative than the GRF method just because the FDR method will tend to identify more voxels as significant. The FDR algorithm is guaranteed to produce an FDR that is no greater than $q$. This is true regardless of the amount or type of correlations that exist in the SPM. In other words, the true FDR will be less than or equal to $q$ even with data that are as disadvantageous as possible. With more moderate data, the method will therefore be too conservative, in the sense that the true FDR will be strictly less than $q$. Unfortunately, as with the GRF method, there is no way to know how much less the true FDR will be when this method is used on fMRI data.

## Cluster-Based Methods

All of the methods considered thus far base their decisions on activation values of single voxels. There are several fundamental weaknesses inherent to such approaches. First, because there are many voxels, the threshold must be set high to correct for multiple comparisons. Second, single-voxel methods necessarily ignore activation values in neighboring voxels. One could imagine several scenarios in which this could be problematic, primarily because we might expect that if a brain region is participating in a task, then activation should be observed in a number of contiguous voxels. One reason for this expectation is that the spatial extent of the fMRI BOLD response is known to be greater than the electrophysiologic response of the underlying brain region (Disbrow, Slutsky, Roberts, & Krubitzer, 2000). For this reason, one might be suspicious of a single significant voxel in a region of a z-map that is surrounded on all sides by voxels with z-values near 0. Similarly, it seems likely that a large cluster of voxels, all with z-values just below the GRF threshold, is signaling task-related activity.

In this section, we consider two methods that base significance decisions on clusters of voxels. The first method, due to Friston, Worsley, Frackowiak, Mazziotta, and Evans (1994), identifies a cluster of activated voxels as significant if the number of voxels in that cluster, which we refer to as the cluster size or spatial extent, exceeds a threshold. The second method, due to Poline, Worsley, Evans, and Friston (1997), marks a cluster as significant if its spatial extent is large *or* if it contains a single voxel with high activation. The two methods are both based on GRF theory, and they both share many initial steps in common. Therefore, we will begin by considering the steps they have in common and then consider the computations that are unique to each method.

The first step in both methods is to form a standard statistical parametric map. Friston et al. (1994) and Poline et al. (1997) both assumed that this is a z-map. Even so, we will briefly consider extensions of the Friston et al. (1994) method to $t$-, $\chi^2$-, and $F$-maps. The second step in cluster-based methods is to set a preliminary threshold on the statistical map at some value $T$ in exactly the same manner as in the previous methods considered in this chapter. The one difference is that this threshold $T$ is selected to be large, but still smaller than in the single-voxel methods we have considered. For example, with a z-map, $T$ is typically chosen to equal 2.5 or 3. With $T$ in this range, there will be many voxels above threshold, even if the null hypothesis of no signal is true. The third step is to identify all clusters that are created by this thresholding process. A cluster is defined as a set of contiguous (i.e., touching) voxels that all have z-values above threshold. Finally, cluster-based methods decide whether or not each cluster is significant.

If the null hypothesis is true, and none of the voxels in the search region show task-related activity, then with $T = 3$ and, for example, 70,000 voxels, we expect around 95 voxels to be above threshold. Some but not all of these 95 voxels will be touching, which means, on average, that we should expect fewer than 95 clusters. The cluster-based methods then decide whether each of these clusters is or is not significant. Because we will make a decision about the significance of each cluster, this means we will have to contend with fewer than 95 multiple comparisons, rather than with the 70,000 tests required by the single-voxel methods discussed earlier in this chapter. This huge reduction in the number of multiple comparisons means that cluster-based methods do not need to be nearly as conservative as single-voxel methods.

On the other hand, one advantage of the single-voxel methods is that they always require a fixed number of comparisons (e.g., 70,000). With cluster-based methods, the number of comparisons is a random variable. For example, if we were to generate 100 separate $z$-maps (e.g., by repeatedly sampling from a z-distribution and then spatially smoothing using a Gaussian kernel) and threshold each map at $T = 3$, then the number of clusters, and consequently the number of comparisons, would vary across replications. So the first problem of cluster-based methods is to deal with the random number of comparisons they entail.

As in all methods, we first assume that the null hypothesis of no signal is true in every voxel. Now, if we know there are exactly $N$ clusters and these clusters occur independently of each other, then as in equation 6.2,

$$\alpha_E = P(\text{at least 1 false positive}) = 1 - (1 - \alpha_t)^N, \tag{6.17}$$

where $N$ equals the number of tests, which in this case also equals the number of clusters. The assumption that separate clusters are independent is made by both cluster-based methods considered in this chapter. Even so, it is important to realize that an assumption that activation in separate clusters is independent is considerably weaker than an assumption that activation in separate voxels is independent. We know there are strong spatial correlations in fMRI data, so activation in neighboring voxels will typically not be independent. By definition, however, separate clusters do not touch, so they must be separated by at least one voxel. Because we expect spatial correlations in fMRI to decrease with distance, it therefore follows that activation in neighboring voxels should be, on average, more strongly correlated that activation in neighboring clusters.

In equation 6.2, when we were deriving the Sidak correction, $N$ was a constant. In cluster-based methods, however, $N$ is a random variable. If we knew the probability that $N$ took on every possible value, then we could compute the overall $\alpha_E$ by weighting equation 6.17 for every value of $N$ by the probability of observing each of those values. In particular, this approach would produce

$$\alpha_E = \sum_{k=0}^{\infty} P(\text{false positive when } k \text{ clusters}) \times P(k \text{ clusters})$$

$$= \sum_{k=0}^{\infty} [1 - (1 - \alpha_t)^k] P(N = k). \tag{6.18}$$

Equation 6.18 requires that we know $P(N = k)$. Fortunately, Adler (1981; theorem 6.9.3) showed that $N$ has a Poisson distribution when the $z$-map is a GRF. The probability distribution of a Poisson distribution is given by

$$P(N = k) = \frac{\mu^k e^{-\mu}}{k!},\tag{6.19}$$

for $k = 0, 1, 2, \ldots \infty$. The single parameter $\mu$ is the mean of the distribution, which in the current case is the expected number of clusters. We have encountered this term before. Recall from GRF theory that when $T$ is large, the number of clusters above threshold equals the Euler characteristic. Therefore, from equation 6.12,

$$\mu = E(\chi_T) = \sum_{d=0}^{3} R_d(\mathrm{ROI}) f_d(T).$$

The $d = 0$, 1, and 2 terms correct for the possibility that a peak touches an edge of the search volume. The cluster-based methods do not correct for touching. As a result, the $d = 0$, 1, and 2 correction terms are not used, so

$$\mu \doteq R_3(\mathrm{ROI}) f_3(T).\tag{6.20}$$

Finally, we are in a position to combine equations 6.18 and 6.19 to arrive at a general expression for $\alpha_E$ in any cluster-based method. This result is expressed in the following proposition.

**Proposition 6.2**  Suppose the null hypothesis of no signal is true in every voxel. Consider a $z$-map constructed from an independent GRF that has been spatially smoothed with a Gaussian kernel (exactly as in the GRF section above). Let $\alpha_t$ denote the probability of a false positive at each cluster of a cluster-based method for correcting for multiple comparisons. Then the overall (or experiment-wise) probability of a false positive (i.e., $\alpha_E$ is equal to

$$\alpha_E = 1 - e^{-\mu \alpha_t},\tag{6.21}$$

and consequently

$$\alpha_t = \frac{-\log_e(1 - \alpha_E)}{\mu},\tag{6.22}$$

where $\mu$ is given by equation 6.20.

**Derivation**  Equation 6.21 is derived from the formula for the moment generating function of the Poisson distribution, $M_N(x)$, which is given by

$$M_N(x) = E(e^{xN}) = \sum_{k=0}^{\infty} e^{xN} P(N = k)$$

$$= \sum_{k=0}^{\infty} e^{xN} \frac{\mu^k e^{-\mu}}{k!} = e^{\mu(e^x - 1)}. \tag{6.23}$$

Combining equations 6.18 and 6.19 produces

$$\alpha_E = \sum_{k=0}^{\infty} [1 - (1 - \alpha_t)^k] \frac{\mu^k e^{-\mu}}{k!}$$

$$= \sum_{k=0}^{\infty} \frac{\mu^k e^{-\mu}}{k!} - \sum_{k=0}^{\infty} (1 - \alpha_t)^k \frac{\mu^k e^{-\mu}}{k!}$$

$$= 1 - \sum_{k=0}^{\infty} (1 - \alpha_t)^k \frac{\mu^k e^{-\mu}}{k!} \tag{6.24}$$

To take advantage of the equation 6.23 equality, we can rewrite $(1 - \alpha_t)^k$ as

$$(1 - \alpha_t)^k = e^{k \log_e (1 - \alpha_t)}.$$

Using this identity, equation 6.24 reduces to

$$\alpha_E = 1 - \sum_{k=0}^{\infty} e^{k \log_e (1 - \alpha_t)} \frac{\mu^k e^{-\mu}}{k!}$$

$$= 1 - \exp[\mu(e^{\log_e (1 - \alpha_t)} - 1)]$$

$$= 1 - e^{\mu(1 - \alpha_t - 1)}$$

$$= 1 - e^{-\mu \alpha_t}.$$

Equation 6.22 follows from solving equation 6.21 for $\alpha_t$. ∎

Proposition 6.2 holds for both cluster-based methods considered in this section. However, because the different methods use a different decision rule to decide the significance of each cluster, $\alpha_t$ will differ across methods. Thus, when we consider each method, our primary focus will be on determining how the method computes $\alpha_t$.

## Cluster-Based Methods Using a Spatial Extent Criterion

We begin with the method of Friston et al. (1994) that considers only the size of each cluster; that is, all large clusters are judged significant. Clusters smaller than the criterion on size are judged non-significant, regardless of how large their $z$-values. As before, we assume that the null hypothesis of no signal is true in every voxel and that we have completed the initial steps described above; that is, we have created a $z$-map, thresholded the map at $T$, and identified all of the clusters that result from this process. Let $S_T$ denote the size of one of these clusters selected at random (i.e., when the threshold is $T$). Note that $S_T$ will tend to increase as $T$ is decreased. Proposition 6.3 computes the $\alpha_t$ that results from applying this method.

**Proposition 6.3 (Friston et al., 1994)**   Suppose we threshold a $z$-map at a reasonably large value $T$, the null hypothesis of no signal is true in every voxel, the usual GRF assumptions are valid, and we decide that any cluster containing more than $S$ voxels is significant. Then the probability of a false positive at any cluster equals

$$\alpha_t = P(S_T > S) = e^{-\lambda S^{2/D}}, \tag{6.25}$$

where $D$ is the dimensionality of the search volume (usually $D = 3$), and

$$\lambda = \frac{\Gamma\left(\frac{D}{2}+1\right) R_3(\text{ROI}) f_3(T)}{VP(Z > T)}, \tag{6.26}$$

where $\Gamma(\ )$ is the gamma function.[1] The probability $P(Z > T)$ is just the single-voxel $p$-value associated with the threshold $T$, and, as before, $V$ is the volume of the ROI.

**Derivation**   Nosko (1969) showed that for large $T$, the random variable $S_T^{2/D}$ has an exponential distribution. Call the parameter of this distribution $\lambda$. Then for any non-negative value $x$,

$$1 - e^{-\lambda x} = P(S_T^{2/D} \leq x)$$

$$= P(S_T \leq x^{D/2}).$$

Next, let $S = x^{D/2}$. Note that this implies that $x = S^{2/D}$, and therefore that

$$P(S_T \leq S) = 1 - e^{-\lambda S^{2/D}},$$

which means that

$$P(S_T > S) = e^{-\lambda S^{2/D}}.$$

---

1. When $n$ is an integer, $\Gamma(n) = (n-1)!$. Other useful results are that $\Gamma\left(\frac{1}{2}\right) = \sqrt{\pi}$ and $\Gamma(x+1) = x\Gamma(x)$. Putting all these together, note that when $D = 3$, the term $\Gamma\left(\frac{D}{2}+1\right)$ in equation 6.26 reduces to

$\Gamma\left(\frac{3}{2}+1\right) = \frac{3}{2}\Gamma\left(\frac{1}{2}+1\right) = \left(\frac{3}{2}\right)\left(\frac{1}{2}\right)\Gamma\left(\frac{1}{2}\right) = \frac{3}{4}\sqrt{\pi}.$

Friston et al. (1994) showed that

$$\lambda = \frac{\Gamma\left(\frac{D}{2}+1\right)}{E(S_T)} = \frac{\Gamma\left(\frac{D}{2}+1\right)E(L_T)}{E(R_T)}, \tag{6.27}$$

where $L_T$ is the number of clusters in the search volume, and $R_T$ is the volume of all clusters above the threshold $T$.

Now the volume of all clusters above threshold is proportional to the $p$-value that is associated with $T$. In particular,

$$E(R_T) = VP(Z > T). \tag{6.28}$$

$E(L_T)$ is just $\mu$ from equation 6.20; that is,

$$\mu = E(L_T) \doteq R_3(V)f_3(T). \tag{6.29}$$

Combining equations 6.27–6.29 produces

$$\lambda = \frac{\Gamma\left(\frac{D}{2}+1\right)R_3(V)f_3(T)}{VP(Z > T)}. \qquad \blacksquare$$

In practical applications, we wish to use propositions 6.2 and 6.3 to select $S$ so that $\alpha_E$ has some desired value. Proposition 6.4 does just this.

**Proposition 6.4**  Under the conditions of propositions 6.2 and 6.3, the criterion on voxel size that controls the overall probability of a false positive at $\alpha_E$ is equal to

$$S = \left\{-\frac{1}{\lambda}\log_e\left[\frac{-\log_e(1-\alpha_E)}{\mu}\right]\right\}^{D/2}, \tag{6.30}$$

where the definitions of all terms are the same as in proposition 6.2.

**Derivation**  First note that from proposition 6.2

$$\alpha_t = P(S_T > S) = \frac{-\log_e(1-\alpha_E)}{\mu}.$$

Using the equation 6.25 substitution, this equality becomes

$$\exp(-\lambda S^{2/D}) = \frac{-\log_e(1-\alpha_E)}{\mu},$$

from which the result easily follows.  $\blacksquare$

To use the Friston et al. (1994) method therefore, we need to compute $\mu$ from equation 6.20, $\lambda$ from equation 6.26, and we need to decide on a desired value for $\alpha_E$. Next we substitute these values into equation 6.30 to determine $S$, our threshold on size. Finally, we compare the size of each cluster to $S$, and all clusters larger than $S$ are judged significant.

Cao (1999) extended these results to $\chi^2$-, $t$-, and $F$-maps. In these cases, proposition 6.2 still holds, but $\mu$ and $P(S_T > S)$ differ according to which type of SPM is constructed. In all cases,

$$\mu \doteq R_3(\text{ROI}) f_3(T).$$

However, $f_3(T)$ varies (as specified above) depending on whether a $\chi^2$-, $t$-, or $F$-statistic is used to construct the map, in just the same way it would in the standard GRF approach. On the other hand, $P(S_T > S)$ becomes considerably more complex with a $\chi^2$-, $t$-, or $F$-map. Interested readers should consult theorems 4.1 ($\chi^2$-map), 4.2 ($t$-map), and 4.3 ($F$-map) of Cao (1999) for details.

### Cluster-Based Methods Using a Criterion That Depends on Cluster Height and Spatial Extent

One weakness of methods that base significance decisions only on the spatial extent of a cluster is that they ignore cluster height. For example, consider a cluster that is one voxel smaller than the spatial extent criterion $S$. The previous method would judge this cluster to be non-significant, even if the $z$-values of all the voxels in this cluster were huge. Such a scenario seems unlikely to occur by chance in brain regions that do not exhibit task-related activation. Ideally, we would like a method that would decide a cluster is significant if its spatial extent was large *or* if its peak activation was large. We consider such a method in this section that was proposed by Poline, Worsley, Evans, and Friston (1997).

The idea behind this method is that we compute one $p$-value for the height of each cluster and one for the cluster's size. If either of these $p$-values is suitably small, then we will identify the cluster as significant. This sounds straightforward, but unfortunately, the height and size $p$-values are correlated because they depend on activation in the same voxels. In other words, even if the null hypothesis is true and all clusters were generated by noise, then any cluster with a small $p$-value for size (i.e., a large cluster) will also tend to have a small $p$-value for height (i.e., the largest $z$-value in the cluster will be large). This correlation considerably complicates the analysis.

The Poline et al. (1997) method is similar to the spatial extent method of Friston et al. (1994) that we considered in the previous section. Proposition 6.2 holds for both methods. Both methods begin by thresholding a $z$-map at a reasonably large value (e.g., $T = 2.5$ or 3). This thresholding process is used to identify the set of all possible clusters. The Poline et al. (1997) and Friston et al. (1994) methods both make a significance decision about each of these clusters. The methods differ because Friston et al. (1994) only consider the size of the cluster when determining significance, whereas Poline et al. (1997) consider both the size and the height.

As before, denote the size of a cluster chosen at random when the initial threshold is $T$ by $S_T$. Similarly, denote the largest $z$-value of all voxels in a random cluster, which we call the cluster height, by $H_T$. For each cluster, let $p_{size}$ denote the $p$-value of the size of the cluster, and let $p_{height}$ denote the $p$-value of the height of the cluster. Then the Poline et al. (1997) method is to decide that the cluster is significant if

$$\min(p_{size}, p_{height}) \leq \alpha_t$$

for some suitably chosen value of $\alpha_t$.

Note that this method defines height based on the single voxel with the largest $z$-value. Thus, the height of two clusters would be the same if the largest $z$-value in the two clusters is the same, regardless of the $z$-values of the other voxels in each cluster. Of course, we expect a task-related cluster to have more than one large $z$-value, so it might seem preferable to define height in some other way; for example, as the mean $z$-value of all voxels in the cluster. Whereas such alternatives might seem attractive, we will soon see that the mathematics of methods that combine extent and height is complex, and so, unfortunately, developing alternatives to the Poline et al. (1997) method is challenging.

To begin the Poline et al. (1997) method, let $S$ equal the threshold on cluster size for which $p_{size} = \alpha_t$, and let $H$ equal the threshold on cluster height for which $p_{height} = \alpha_t$. Then

$$\alpha_E = P(\text{cluster is significant})$$

$$= P(S_T > S, H_T > H) + P(S_T > S, H_T \leq H) + P(S_T \leq S, H_T > H)$$

$$= [P(S_T > S, H_T > H) + P(S_T > S, H_T \leq H)]$$

$$+ [P(S_T > S, H_T > H) + P(S_T \leq S, H_T > H)] - P(S_T > S, H_T > H)$$

$$= P(S_T > S) + P(H_T > H) - P(S_T > S, H_T > H).$$

Therefore, to apply this method, we must evaluate three terms: $P(S_T > S)$, $P(H_T > H)$, and $P(S_T > S, H_T > H)$.

*Evaluating $P(S_T > S)$*   This probability, which is given in equations 6.25 and 6.26, was derived in proposition 6.3.

*Evaluating $P(H_T > H)$*   Poline et al. (1997) showed that this probability equals

$$P(H_T > H) = \left(1 + \frac{H}{T}\right)^{D-1} \exp\left(-TH - \frac{H^2}{2}\right), \tag{6.31}$$

where, as before, $T$ is the initial threshold used to define the candidate clusters, and $D$ is the dimensionality of the search region.

*Evaluating $P(S_T > S, H_T > H)$* This computation is messy. For $D = 3$, Poline et al. (1997) showed that it equals

$$P(S_T > S, H_T > H) = \frac{T}{2^{2T^2/3} \Gamma\left(\frac{2T^2}{3}\right)} \int_H^\infty e^{-Th} \int_W^\infty u^{\frac{2T^2}{3}-1} e^{-\frac{u}{2}} \, du \, dh, \tag{6.32}$$

where

$$W = Ch^{3/2}$$

and

$$C = \frac{16R(\pi T)^{3/2} e^{T^2/2} P(Z < T)}{9S \log_e 2}.$$

As before, $R$ is the number of resels in the ROI, and $P(Z < T)$ equals the area under the z-distribution to the left of $T$. To see how these equations change when $D = 2$, see Poline et al. (1997). The double integral in equation 6.32 requires some rather sophisticated numerical integration.

Given that we now know how to compute these probabilities, we can finally implement the Poline et al. (1997) method.

### Poline et al. (1997) Method for Determining Cluster Significance Based on both Cluster Size and Height

*Step 1* Generate a z-map.

*Step 2* Threshold the map at $T = 2.5$ or 3.0.

*Step 3* Find all clusters (i.e., all contiguous voxels with z-values above $T$), and for each cluster, compute its size $s$ (i.e., number of voxels in the cluster) and its height $h$ (i.e., maximum z-value of all voxels in the cluster).

*Step 4* For each cluster, compute $P(S_T > s)$ (using equations 6.25 and 6.26) and $P(H_T > h)$ (using equation 6.31).

*Step 5* Set $p_{min}$ equal to

$$p_{min} = \min[P(S_T > s), P(H_T > h)].$$

*Step 6* If $P(H_T > h) = p_{min}$, then define a new value $h_0$ by setting $h_0 = h$. If $P(S_T > s) > p_{min}$, then find the value $s_0$ such that $P(S_T > s_0) = p_{min}$.

*Step 7* If $P(S_T > s) = p_{min}$, then define a new value $s_0$ by setting $s_0 = s$. If $P(H_T > h) > p_{min}$, then find the value $h_0$ such that $P(H_T > h_0) = p_{min}$. Poline et al. (1997) showed that the value of $h_0$ that (approximately) achieves this goal is

$$h_0 = \frac{-\log_e p_{\min}}{T}.$$

*Step 8*   Compute $P(S_T > s_0, H_T > h_0)$ from equation 6.32 (i.e., via numerical integration). Then compute a *p*-value for the cluster via

$$p_{cluster} = P(S_T > s_0) + P(H_T > h_0) - P(S_T > s_0, H_T > h_0)$$

$$= 2p_{\min} - P(S_T > s_0, H_T > h_0).$$

*Step 9*   The cluster is significant if

$$p_{cluster} < \alpha_t = \frac{-\log_e(1-\alpha_E)}{\mu} \quad \text{(from equation 6.22).}$$

Note that omitting $P(S_T > s_0, H_T > h_0)$ in step 8 makes the procedure conservative. Because this joint probability is never negative, omitting it when computing $p_{cluster}$ will cause an overestimation of this *p*-value. In other words, any cluster that is significant when $P(S_T > s_0, H_T > h_0)$ is omitted would also be significant if this probability was included in the calculations. For this reason and because $P(S_T > s_0, H_T > h_0)$ is not easy to compute, it is often omitted from step 8.

### Permutation-Based Solutions to the Multiple Comparisons Problem

The nonparametric permutation methods introduced in chapter 5 have also been applied to the multiple comparisons problem (Nichols & Holmes, 2001). Permutation methods can be used to correct either for multiple single-voxel decisions or for multiple cluster-based decisions. The algorithms in these two cases are as follows.

### Permutation-Based Algorithm for Finding the Threshold *T* That Leads to an Experiment-wise Error Rate of $\alpha_E$ When Decisions Are Made at the Single-Voxel Level

*Step 1*   Randomly shuffle the TRs. Reorder the BOLD responses in every voxel in the ROI so that the TRs agree with this shuffle. Apply the GLM to these shuffled data to produce a *z*-map. Find the maximum *z*-value in this SPM. Call this value $z_1^{\max}$.

*Step 2*   Repeat step 1 a total of *M* times with a new random shuffle on each repetition. Choose a large value for *M* (e.g., 1000). At the end of this step, *M* different $z_i^{\max}$ values will exist.

*Step 3*   Rank order the $z_i^{\max}$ from largest to smallest. Call the largest value $z_i^{\max}[1]$ and the smallest $z_i^{\max}[M]$. The threshold *T* associated with an experiment-wise error rate of $\alpha_E$ equals $T = z_i^{\max}[M\alpha_E + 1]$.                                                                        ∎

**Permutation-Based Algorithm for Finding the Threshold $S$ on Cluster Size That Leads to an Experiment-wise Error Rate of $\alpha_E$ When Cluster-Based Decisions Are Made**

*Step 1*  Randomly shuffle the TRs. Reorder the BOLD responses in every voxel in the ROI so that the TRs agree with this shuffle. Apply the GLM to these shuffled data to produce a $z$-map. Set an intermediate threshold at $T = 2.5$ or $3.0$ and find the largest cluster that results from this thresholding procedure. Call the size of this cluster $s_1$.

*Step 2*  Repeat step 1 a total of $M$ times with a new random shuffle on each repetition. Choose a large value for $M$ (e.g., 1000). At the end of this step, $M$ different $s_i$ values will exist.

*Step 3*  Rank order the $s_i$ from largest to smallest. Call the largest $s_i[1]$ and the smallest $s_i[M]$. The threshold $S$ on cluster size associated with an experiment-wise error rate of $\alpha_E$ equals $S = s_i[M\alpha_E + 1]$.  ∎

As with the permutation test considered in chapter 5, the main drawback of these algorithms is the considerable computation they require. One attractive feature of both algorithms though is that because the same shuffle is applied to every voxel, the shuffled data will display exactly the same spatial correlations as the raw data. To my knowledge, the permutation method is the only existing method for correcting for multiple comparisons that accurately models these correlations.

**Voodoo Correlations**

A topic of much recent debate is the problem of spuriously high correlations that can result from using a nonindependent criterion to select activated voxels (Vul, Harris, Winkielman, & Pashler, 2009). This is related to the multiple comparisons problem because they both are the result of having so many voxels of data to sift through during analysis. The voodoo correlation problem can occur because, given enough samples, pure noise can mimic almost anything. Because of this, great care must be taken to avoid a selection criterion that would be likely to discover positive results in pure noise.

For example, Vul et al. (2009) describe the case where outside of the scanner each subject is assessed in some way that results in a single score. For example, subjects might each complete a personality assessment. Next, in an attempt to determine whether this score is related to activation within some specific ROI, the outside-the-scanner scores are correlated with a $z$- or $t$-value from a single voxel within that ROI. In other words, for the first voxel within the ROI we have two values for each subject—an outside-the scanner score and a BOLD activation statistic (e.g., $t$ or $z$). The correlation between these two columns of numbers is computed. This process is then repeated for every voxel in the ROI, and all correlations exceeding some threshold are selected. The data from these voxels are then averaged together, and a final correlation with these averaged data is computed. If this correlation is high, then the tempting conclusion is that this ROI has some functional role in determining the behavioral score that was collected. The problem is that high correlations can occur from this process even with fMRI data that are pure noise (Vul et al., 2009).

These spurious correlations occur because the criterion used to select voxels is the same as the criterion used to test the research hypothesis (i.e., a correlation between the behavioral measure and the BOLD response)—a condition called the nonindependence error by Vul et al. (2009). The validity of the nonindependence error is not in question. However, its prevalence and importance is highly controversial (e.g., Lieberman, Berkman, & Wager, 2009; Nichols & Poline, 2009; Poldrack & Mumford, 2009). To avoid this error, the criterion used to select voxels should be independent of the research question. For example, the ROI could be defined anatomically using a standard atlas (see chapter 4), then within that ROI the 20 (or some other number) most active voxels could be identified. The $z$-values from these voxels would then be averaged and the across-subject correlation would be computed between these averaged z-values and the behavioral measure.

### Conclusions

In this chapter, we reviewed many methods for solving the multiple comparisons problem. The very fact that a variety of methods are popular implies that no optimal method exists. If the test statistics (e.g., $z$-values) from all possible pairs of voxels were statistically independent, then the Sidak correction would be optimal—at least if the goal was to control the overall rate of false positives. But in fact we know that test statistics from neighboring voxels are positively correlated, and this correlation makes the Sidak correction too conservative. The problem is that the true correlational structure is unknown. As a result, an exact method for correcting for these correlations is unknown. This is the main reason that so many alternative approaches have been proposed.

All of the current methods that attempt to build a parametric model of the spatial correlations present in statistical parametric maps are based on GRF theory. These approaches have the advantage of assuming a correlational structure that is known to exist in fMRI data—at least as long as spatial smoothing is done during preprocessing. However, the GRF approaches all assume that spatial smoothing is the only source of correlation. This assumption is clearly false, which is why GRF approaches are also not optimal. Even so, these methods have the advantage of making specific and known assumptions about spatial correlation. The cluster-based methods are based on GRFs, but they have two advantages over the single-voxel GRF method. First, because they make significance decisions about clusters rather than individual voxels, they require many fewer comparisons (and therefore a larger $\alpha_t$). Second, they exploit the reasonable assumption that task-related activation should usually occupy more than a single voxel.

# 7 Group Analysis

The design of every fMRI experiment includes a decision about how many subjects to run. This choice typically requires a trade-off between the cost in both money and time of collecting the data and the ability to generalize the results to some larger population. In some experiments, the subjects have some unique ability or feature that makes their particular results of special interest, but in most cases subjects are chosen in the belief that they are somehow typical of the larger population from which they were drawn. In this case, our primary interest in a subject is that his or her results should be somehow typical and therefore that by running the experiment we have learned something new about this population.

All analyses thus far discussed in this book assume that our data came from a single subject. For example, chapter 5 describes how to construct a statistical parametric map from a single data set. This chapter addresses the problem of how to integrate results from multiple subjects, how to make inferences to the population from which those subjects were sampled, and how to determine the number of subjects that should be included in the experiment.

The standard methods for group analysis require at least two stages or levels of analysis. In the first stage, some version of the GLM is fitted to the data of each individual subject in exactly the way as described in chapter 5. The end result of the first stage is a statistical parametric map for each subject. No attempt is made at this stage to correct for multiple comparisons because no significance decisions are made about data from any single subject. The second stage of a group analysis combines these various statistical maps into a single group map. Significance decisions are now made on this group map.

## Individual Differences

To make an inference from a sample of subjects to a population, we must use a statistical method that accurately models the variation within this population. The standard statistical models for group analysis of fMRI data all assume that there are no structural differences across subjects and that functionally the data from different subjects who ran in the same conditions are statistically identical except for noise. Structural differences across subjects or systematic individual differences in functional activation are therefore violations of the standard statistical model.

If the brain structures of two subjects are different, then a voxel at a certain physical location within the scanner may lie in different functional brain regions in the two subjects. The popular statistical methods of group analysis are designed to determine, for example, whether there is more activation in a particular voxel across the group than would be expected from noise alone. If this voxel is in different brain regions for different subjects, then such an analysis, even if successful, is functionally meaningless. For this reason, it is crucial that normalization (i.e., see chapter 4) is successfully performed on all subjects before any group analysis is attempted. Ideally, after normalization is complete, structural differences across subjects will no longer exist. In other words, every voxel will have the same relative position within the same functional brain region in every subject.

Normalization can eliminate structural differences across subjects, but not functional differences. Individual differences in how subjects perform a task are potentially a more serious problem in fMRI experiments than in psychological or cognitive science experiments that collect purely behavioral measures such as response time or response accuracy. This is because a variety of different cognitive strategies could yield statistically similar response times and accuracies, but almost by definition, if the strategies are different, then the underlying neural activations should also be different. This means that the greatest advantage of fMRI research, namely the unprecedented observability it offers, can sometimes complicate the data analysis.

Miller et al. (2009) specifically looked at the reproducibility of functional brain activity by scanning 14 subjects in two fMRI sessions separated by several months. During each session, subjects performed an episodic memory retrieval task, a semantic memory retrieval task, and a working memory task. Some results from the episodic retrieval task are shown in figure 7.1. The group map, which was constructed by methods described later in this chapter, is shown in the upper left corner. The rest of the figure shows the two scans from each of the 14 subjects. The number in the middle of each individual subject panel is the correlation (i.e., across voxels) between the two statistical maps from that subject. Although these values vary significantly across individuals—ranging from .186 to .742— overall they are reasonably high, suggesting that the same subject tended to produce similar BOLD responses in sessions that were separated in time by a month. The numbers in the lower right and left corners of each subject panel are the correlations between the individual subject maps and the group map. With only one exception, these are all lower than the within-subject correlations, and usually much lower. For example, 8 of the 14 within-subject correlations are greater than .40, whereas the highest correlation between the group map and the map of any single subject is only .287. Thus, in this experiment individual differences were significantly larger than within-subject variability. In fact, Miller et al. (2009) reported that activity patterns of the same individual performing different tasks were more similar than activity patterns of different individuals performing the same task.

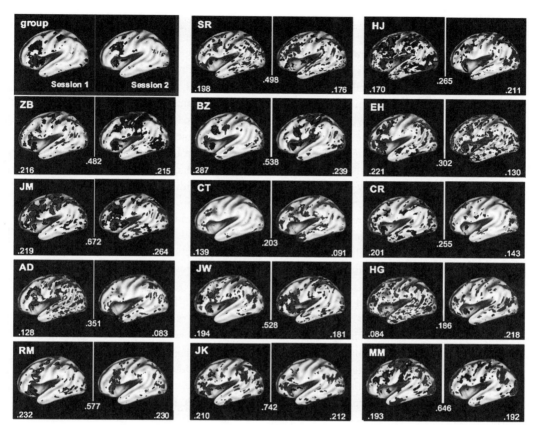

**Figure 7.1**
Statistical parametric maps (left hemisphere) of 14 subjects in an episodic retrieval task. Two letter codes are subject identifiers. The number in the middle of each individual subject panel is the correlation (i.e., across voxels) between the two statistical maps from that subject. The numbers in the lower right and left corners are the correlations between the individual subject maps and the group map. (Reprinted from Miller, Donovan, Van Horn, German, Sokol-Hessner, & Wolford, "Unique and persistent individual patterns of brain activity across different memory retrieval tasks," *NeuroImage*, 2009, *48*, 625–635, with permission from Elsevier.)

Not all tasks studied in fMRI experiments would be expected to show such large individual differences (e.g., finger tapping). Even so, the Miller et al. (2009) results suggest that individual differences in functional activation across subjects may be large. Given this, it is important to distinguish between two different types of individual difference: qualitative and quantitative. A qualitative difference in functional activation occurs when two subjects use different strategies to solve the same task. Presumably, different strategies will recruit different neural networks. If so, then the activation patterns of these subjects will differ qualitatively. If a subject population includes many subjects who use different strategies, then the distribution of activation patterns observed in an experiment will often be discontinuous. Some subjects will show an activation pattern consistent with one strategy, and other subjects will show a different pattern consistent with some other strategy. Few if any subjects will show patterns in between.

Quantitative differences result when different subjects use the same strategy. Different subjects who recruit the same neural network will not produce identical activation patterns because of many small individual differences. Theoretically, these differences will add together to produce a continuous distribution of activation patterns across the subject population.

The standard statistical models account for quantitative differences across subjects but not qualitative differences. Thus, a successful group analysis requires either that all qualitative differences have been eliminated or that subjects have been grouped according to the strategy they used. In the latter case, a separate group analysis could then be run on each group. The use of qualitatively different strategies can be reduced via careful attention to the tasks, instructions, and/or experimental methods that are used. In addition, the behavioral data should always be probed for individual differences. For example, one might fit a variety of quantitative models to the accuracy or response time data that each assumes a different task strategy. Subjects could then be grouped according to the best-fitting model, and each resulting group would then receive its own analysis.

In summary, the rest of this chapter assumes that normalization has been performed successfully on all subjects so that all structural differences have been eliminated and that there are either no qualitative differences or else subjects have been grouped according to the strategy they used to perform the task that is being studied.

### Fixed versus Random Factors in the General Linear Model

Often the goal of a group analysis is to make an inference from the sample of subjects included in the experiment to the larger population from which these subjects were selected. In the GLM, such an inference is possible only if we treat subject-related effects as *random factors*, rather than as *fixed factors*.

One way to understand the difference between random and fixed factors is to imagine replicating an experiment that has just been completed. If exactly the same levels of an experimental factor are used again in the replication, then the factor is fixed. In this case, the levels are usually carefully chosen to have some specific properties. If instead, the levels are determined by random sampling and each replication uses a different random sample, then the factor is random. For example, an experiment that looked at the effects of three different dopamine antagonists on working memory performance would likely use the same three drugs in any future replication, but different subjects. If so, then drugs is a fixed factor and subjects is a random factor.

If every replication uses exactly the same levels of a factor, then the results of the experiment can only tell us about those specific levels. It has little or nothing to say about other possible levels of the factor that were not included in the study. However, if the levels are chosen by blind, random sampling, then usually they are meant to be somehow representative of the larger population from which they were drawn. If so, then we expect our results also to hold for other members of that population. In other words, we expect our results to generalize from the sample to the larger population.

In most experiments, subjects is a random factor because the participants are selected from a subject pool in a pseudo-random fashion, and our goal is to learn something about this population. In some experiments, however, subjects is a fixed factor. This is the case, for example, in experiments that are run on special neuropsychological patients who are so unique that a replication would have to include the same patients.

Mathematically, the GLM treats fixed and random factors very differently. For example, consider the simplest possible correlation-based model from chapter 5,

$$B_i(TR_j) = x(TR_j)\theta_i + \varepsilon_{ij}, \tag{7.1}$$

where $B_i(TR_j)$ represents the BOLD response from subject $i$ in the voxel of interest on TR $j$, $x(TR_j)$ is the predicted BOLD response (obtained by convolving an hrf with a suitable boxcar function), $\theta_i$ is a measure of how strongly this voxel responds to the stimulus event in subject $i$, and $\varepsilon_{ij}$ is noise. Typically, $\varepsilon_{ij}$ is assumed to be normally distributed with mean 0 and variance $\sigma_W^2$. The subscript W emphasizes that $\sigma_W^2$ measures within-subject variance; that is, how variable this subject's responses are across TRs.

In chapter 5, we treated $\theta_i$ as a constant, which means that the GLM assumed it was a fixed effect. If subjects is a random factor, however, then under replication, subject $i$ would be a different person and the numerical value of $\theta_i$ would therefore change. This *random effects model* treats $\theta_i$ as a random variable. Although there are several ways to do this, one convenient way is to assume

$$\theta_i = \theta_G + \varepsilon_G, \tag{7.2}$$

where $\theta_G$ is the average group response in this voxel, and $\varepsilon_G$ is a noise term that models individual difference. The standard model assumes $\varepsilon_G$ is normally distributed with mean 0 and variance $\sigma_G^2$, where $\sigma_G^2$ measures the variability in the average response of this voxel across subjects.

Note that this random effects model makes stronger assumptions about how subjects differ than the fixed effects model. In the fixed effects model, the $\theta_i$ parameters in equation 7.1 can take on any values. Thus, any type of qualitative or strategic differences across subjects can be accommodated in a fixed effects analysis.

In the random effects model, however, the $\theta_i$ parameters are constrained to be normally distributed. Normality should be a reasonable assumption if we were successful at preventing or eliminating qualitative differences across subjects (e.g., by grouping according to strategy used). The normal distribution assumes that subjects should produce a continuous range of $\theta_i$'s with values near $\theta_G$ most likely. Suppose, however, that our subjects include two subpopulations each of which is using a different strategy to perform the task. In that case, some voxels will show activation in one subpopulation but not the other. Because of this, the true $\theta_i$ will have a bimodal distribution across subjects; that is, subjects in which this voxel is recruited for the task will show a large $\theta_i$, and subjects in which this voxel is not recruited will show a small $\theta_i$. The normal distribution will provide a poor model in this case. As a result, if individual differences in strategy are expected, and there is no known way to group subjects by strategy, then a fixed effects analysis may be more appropriate than a random effects analysis. The cost of the extra flexibility provided by the fixed effects model is that the results provide no basis for generalization to a larger subject population.

### A Fixed Effects Group Analysis

To understand the differences between fixed and random effects analyses, consider the data shown in table 7.1. In this hypothetical experiment, 10 samples of data were collected from each of eight subjects. These data were generated from the model shown in figure 7.2. First, a population of subjects was created by defining a normal distribution with a mean of 2 and a group variance of $\sigma_G^2 = 16$. This distribution, which is assumed to model individual differences, is denoted in figure 7.2 by the broad, black curve. Eight hypothetical subjects were identified by drawing eight random samples from the group distribution and then creating eight normal distributions with means equal to these eight sample values and with all within-subject variances equal to $\sigma_W^2 = 0.25$. These eight distributions are denoted in figure 7.2 by the narrow, light-gray curves. The top row of table 7.1 shows the means of these eight individual subject distributions. Each individual subject distribution represents the population of all possible samples that could be collected from that subject. Finally, the 10 samples from each subject were generated by drawing 10 random samples from that subject's individual distribution. These 80 sample values are shown both numerically in table 7.1 and graphically in figure 7.2. One fMRI-related interpretation of these data is that each sample value represents a $t$- or $z$-value from some ROI in a different functional run. The group mean of 2 indicates that this ROI is moderately task responsive, but the large group variance ($\sigma_G^2 = 16$) suggests there is significant individual difference.

**Table 7.1**
Hypothetical data from an experiment with eight subjects

| | Subject | | | | | | | |
|---|---|---|---|---|---|---|---|---|
| | 1 | 2 | 3 | 4 | 5 | 6 | 7 | 8 |
| Population mean | 9.69 | 5.36 | 0.06 | 5.99 | 2.59 | 6.02 | −1.09 | −4.31 |
| Sample 1 | 9.44 | 6.15 | −0.86 | 6.22 | 2.73 | 6.61 | −0.66 | −4.28 |
| Sample 2 | 9.13 | 6.25 | 0.09 | 5.90 | 2.84 | 6.90 | −0.66 | −3.62 |
| Sample 3 | 9.48 | 5.11 | −0.23 | 6.27 | 2.73 | 6.00 | −1.14 | −4.57 |
| Sample 4 | 9.66 | 5.83 | −0.53 | 6.23 | 2.15 | 6.36 | −0.38 | −4.98 |
| Sample 5 | 10.95 | 5.79 | −0.26 | 6.40 | 3.78 | 5.92 | 0.06 | −4.23 |
| Sample 6 | 9.79 | 5.61 | −0.64 | 6.10 | 1.84 | 6.56 | −2.36 | −5.33 |
| Sample 7 | 9.36 | 5.63 | −0.24 | 5.60 | 2.71 | 6.41 | −0.67 | −5.11 |
| Sample 8 | 9.88 | 4.48 | 0.02 | 6.00 | 2.26 | 5.67 | −1.15 | −5.01 |
| Sample 9 | 9.61 | 4.81 | 0.37 | 6.01 | 2.58 | 5.78 | −0.95 | −4.64 |
| Sample 10 | 10.12 | 5.11 | 0.63 | 5.22 | 1.52 | 7.00 | −0.77 | −3.86 |
| Sample mean | 9.74 | 5.48 | −0.17 | 6.00 | 2.51 | 6.32 | −0.87 | −4.56 |
| Sample variance | 0.26 | 0.34 | 0.21 | 0.12 | 0.38 | 0.36 | 0.41 | 0.31 |

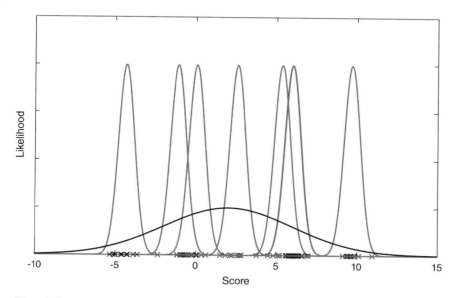

**Figure 7.2**
Model used to generate the hypothetical data shown in table 7.1. First, eight mean subject scores were sampled randomly from the broad, black group distribution. Next, 10 scores were randomly sampled from each narrow, gray individual subject distribution. Likelihoods were rescaled to aid visual display.

A fixed effects analysis essentially treats the different subjects in this experiment in exactly the same way it would treat different stimulus events presented to the same subject. In this analysis, a unique parameter is assigned to every column mean, so the only source of unexplained variance is within-subjects noise. The fixed effects model assumes that all differences between numbers in the same column in table 7.1 are due to this noise. As a result, the sample variance of each column is an unbiased estimator of within-subject variance. A more powerful (i.e., less variable) estimator is created by pooling together the eight sample variances. Because the sample sizes are the same for each subject, the pooled estimator of within-subject variance is just the mean of the eight sample variances shown in the bottom row. The fixed-effects test statistic of the null hypothesis that the mean across subjects is zero is a *t*-statistic in which the numerator is the mean of the eight sample means (second to last row in table 7.1) and the denominator is the pooled standard deviation (i.e., the square root of the pooled variance) divided by the square root of 80 (i.e., the number of samples per subject × the number of subjects). Under the null hypothesis that the mean equals zero, this statistic has 72 degrees of freedom (the number of subjects, 8, times the degrees of freedom per subject, 9). In table 7.1, this *t*-statistic has a numerical value of 400.1, which is highly significant (i.e., $p < .0001$).

In matrix form, the fixed effects GLM assumes

$$\underline{B}_i = X_i \underline{\beta}_i + \underline{\varepsilon}_i, \tag{7.3}$$

where $\underline{B}_i$ is an $n \times 1$ vector containing the BOLD responses from subject $i$ on each of the $n$ TRs (i.e., in this voxel), $X_i$ is the design matrix for subject $i$, $\underline{\beta}_i$ is the beta vector, and $\underline{\varepsilon}_i$ is the within-subject error vector. Most applications assume that $\underline{\varepsilon}_i$ has a multivariate normal distribution with mean vector $\underline{0}$ and variance-covariance matrix $\Sigma_i = \sigma_W^2 I$ (see appendix B for a review of multivariate normal distributions). In other words, it is standard to assume homogeneity of variance and that the BOLD responses in successive TRs are independent. Modeling temporal correlations (i.e., so that $\Sigma_i$ is not diagonal) is as challenging here as it was in the single-subject GLM analyses that we considered in chapter 5. Nevertheless, a number of the methods described there for dealing with temporal correlation have been extended to group analyses (e.g., Beckmann, Jenkinson, & Smith, 2003; Mumford & Nichols, 2008).

Note that even if every subject undergoes exactly the same experimental conditions, different subjects will usually have different design matrices because of random jittering. Even so, we assume that each subject receives the same number of TRs and that the GLM for each subject is constructed from the same parameters (although the parameter estimates will differ across subjects). Neither of these assumptions is critical. They mainly just simplify the bookkeeping. Note that equation 7.3 is identical to equation 5.5, except a subscript $i$ has been added to each term to denote the subject number. Thus, the GLM considered in chapter 5 assumed all factors were fixed.

In a group analysis, we are usually interested in whether, on average, some combination of parameters in the $\underline{\beta}_i$ vector equals zero, where the average is taken across subjects. To facilitate answering questions of this type, it helps to define a group beta vector

$$\underline{\beta}_G = \frac{1}{M} \sum_{i=1}^{M} \underline{\beta}_i. \tag{7.4}$$

Thus, the estimate of $\underline{\beta}_G$ is just the mean of the estimates of each $\underline{\beta}_i$ that are obtained from the GLMs that were fitted to the data from each individual subject.

As in chapter 5, suppose we want to test a null hypothesis of the form

$$H_0 : \underline{c}'\underline{\beta}_G = 0, \tag{7.5}$$

where $\underline{c}$ is a vector of constants. Note that any linear combination of the entries in the $\underline{\beta}_G$ vector can be written in this form. For example, consider a task with two stimulus events and a correlation-based model that also accounts for a nonzero baseline and linear drift in magnetic field strength. In this case, the $\underline{\beta}_G$ vector would be

$$\underline{\beta}_G = \begin{bmatrix} \theta_{1G} \\ \theta_{2G} \\ B_{0G} \\ \Delta_G \end{bmatrix}.$$

A natural hypothesis to test is

$$H_0 : \theta_{1G} - \theta_{2G} = 0.$$

This hypothesis asks whether, on average, this voxel or ROI responds more strongly to event type 1 than to event type 2 across all of our subjects. Note that this hypothesis can be rewritten in the equation 7.5 form with $\underline{c}' = [1 \ -1 \ 0 \ 0]$.

As proposition 7.1 will show, the equation 7.5 null hypothesis is tested with a $t$-test. The numerator of the $t$-statistic is our best estimate of $\underline{c}'\underline{\beta}_G$, which is just the mean of the estimates of each $\underline{c}'\underline{\beta}_i$ that were obtained from the GLMs that were fitted to the data from each individual subject. The denominator includes lots of constants as well as our best estimate of the only source of unexplained variance in the fixed effects model; namely, within-subject variance $\sigma_W^2$. As mentioned above, the key is to realize that the fixed effects model treats subjects the same as any other independent variable. Thus, the best estimate of $\sigma_W^2$ is computed in exactly the same way as $MS_{error}$ in standard ANOVA. Remember that in this analysis, we first run the GLM separately on the data from each individual subject. Each of these analyses produces an estimate of $\sigma_W^2$. Denote the estimate of $\sigma_W^2$ from subject $i$ by $\hat{\sigma}_i^2$. Pooling these separate estimates together creates the best estimator. The pooled estimate is a weighted sum of the separate estimates where the weights reflect the amount of data collected from each subject (so subjects with more data are given greater weight). If every subject completes the same number of TRs, then the pooled estimate of $\sigma_W^2$ is just the mean of the separate $\sigma_W^2$ estimates obtained from each subject (as in table 7.1). Proposition 7.1 describes this t-test more formally.

**Proposition 7.1**   Consider the fixed effects model

$$\underline{B}_i = X_i \underline{\beta}_i + \underline{\varepsilon}_i \tag{7.6}$$

where $\underline{\varepsilon}_i$ has a multivariate normal distribution with mean vector $\underline{0}$ and variance-covariance matrix $\Sigma_i = \sigma_W^2 I$. Under the null hypothesis $H_0 : \underline{c}'\beta_G = 0$, the statistic

$$t_{FX} = \frac{\underline{c}'\hat{\beta}_G}{\dfrac{\hat{\sigma}_W}{M}\sqrt{\underline{c}'\displaystyle\sum_{i=1}^{M}(X_i'X_i)^{-1}\underline{c}}} \tag{7.7}$$

has a t-distribution with $M(n - r)$ degrees of freedom, where $r$ is the number of parameters in each $\beta_i$ vector of the GLM, $M$ is the number of subjects, and $n$ is the number of TRs for each subject. The within-subject standard deviation is estimated from the pooled sample variance

$$\hat{\sigma}_W^2 = \frac{1}{M}\sum_{i=1}^{M}\hat{\sigma}_i^2, \tag{7.8}$$

where $\hat{\sigma}_i^2$ is the variance estimate from the first-level GLM analysis of the data of subject $i$. The numerator of the equation 7.7 $t$-statistic equals

$$\underline{c}'\hat{\beta}_G = \frac{1}{M}\sum_{i=1}^{M}\underline{c}'\hat{\beta}_i = \frac{1}{M}\sum_{i=1}^{M}\underline{c}'(X_i'X_i)^{-1}X_i'\underline{B}_i. \tag{7.9}$$

**Derivation**   To begin, construct the supervectors $\underline{B}$ and $\underline{\beta}$ and the super design matrix $X$ as follows:

$$\underset{Mn\times1}{B} = \begin{bmatrix} \underline{B}_1 \\ \underline{B}_2 \\ \vdots \\ \underline{B}_M \end{bmatrix}, \quad \underset{Mr\times1}{\beta} = \begin{bmatrix} \underline{\beta}_1 \\ \underline{\beta}_2 \\ \vdots \\ \underline{\beta}_M \end{bmatrix}, \quad \text{and} \quad \underset{Mn\times Mr}{X} = \begin{bmatrix} X_1 & 0 & \cdots & 0 \\ 0 & X_2 & \cdots & 0 \\ \vdots & \vdots & \ddots & \vdots \\ 0 & 0 & \cdots & X_M \end{bmatrix},$$

where $0$ is a matrix of all zeros. Similarly, define

$$\underset{Mn\times1}{\underline{\varepsilon}_W} = \begin{bmatrix} \underline{\varepsilon}_1 \\ \underline{\varepsilon}_2 \\ \vdots \\ \underline{\varepsilon}_M \end{bmatrix} \quad \text{and} \quad \underset{Mr\times1}{\underline{c}_G} = \frac{1}{M}\begin{bmatrix} \underline{c} \\ \underline{c} \\ \vdots \\ \underline{c} \end{bmatrix}.$$

Given these definitions, note that the model can be rewritten as

$$\underline{B} = X\underline{\beta} + \underline{\varepsilon}_W. \tag{7.10}$$

The least squares estimator of $\underline{\beta}$ is

$$\hat{\underline{\beta}} = (X'X)^{-1}X'\underline{B}. \tag{7.11}$$

Expanding the right side of equation 7.11 produces

$$\hat{\underline{\beta}} = \begin{bmatrix} (X_1'X_1)^{-1} & 0 & \cdots & 0 \\ 0 & (X_2'X_2)^{-1} & \cdots & 0 \\ \vdots & \vdots & \ddots & \vdots \\ 0 & 0 & \cdots & (X_M'X_M)^{-1} \end{bmatrix} \begin{bmatrix} X_1' & 0 & \cdots & 0 \\ 0 & X_2' & \cdots & 0 \\ \vdots & \vdots & \ddots & \vdots \\ 0 & 0 & \cdots & X_M' \end{bmatrix} \begin{bmatrix} \underline{B}_1 \\ \underline{B}_2 \\ \vdots \\ \underline{B}_M \end{bmatrix}$$

$$= \begin{bmatrix} (X_1'X_1)^{-1}X_1'\underline{B}_1 & 0 & \cdots & 0 \\ 0 & (X_2'X_2)^{-1}X_2'\underline{B}_2 & \cdots & 0 \\ \vdots & \vdots & \ddots & \vdots \\ 0 & 0 & \cdots & (X_M'X_M)^{-1}X_M'\underline{B}_M \end{bmatrix}. \tag{7.12}$$

Next note that

$$\underline{c}_G'\hat{\underline{\beta}} = \frac{1}{M}[\underline{c}' \quad \underline{c}' \quad \cdots \quad \underline{c}'] \begin{bmatrix} \hat{\underline{\beta}}_1 \\ \hat{\underline{\beta}}_2 \\ \vdots \\ \hat{\underline{\beta}}_M \end{bmatrix}$$

$$= \frac{1}{M}\sum_{i=1}^{M}\underline{c}'\hat{\underline{\beta}}_i$$

$$= \underline{c}'\left[\frac{1}{M}\sum_{i=1}^{M}\hat{\underline{\beta}}_i\right]$$

$$= \underline{c}'\hat{\underline{\beta}}_G. \tag{7.13}$$

Combining equations 7.12 and 7.13 produces equation 7.9.

The variance of $\underline{c}'\hat{\beta}_G$ is equal to

$$
\mathrm{Var}(\underline{c}'\hat{\beta}_G) = \mathrm{Var}\left[\frac{1}{M}\sum_{i=1}^{M}\underline{c}'(X_i'X_i)^{-1}X_i'\underline{B}_i\right]
$$

$$
= \frac{1}{M^2}\sum_{i=1}^{M}\mathrm{Var}[\underline{c}'(X_i'X_i)^{-1}X_i'\underline{B}_i]
$$

$$
= \frac{1}{M^2}\sum_{i=1}^{M}\underline{c}'(X_i'X_i)^{-1}X_i'\Sigma_i X_i(X_i'X_i)^{-1}\underline{c}
$$

$$
= \frac{1}{M^2}\sum_{i=1}^{M}\underline{c}'(X_i'X_i)^{-1}X_i'[\sigma_W^2 I]X_i(X_i'X_i)^{-1}\underline{c}
$$

$$
= \frac{\sigma_W^2}{M^2}\sum_{i=1}^{M}\underline{c}'(X_i'X_i)^{-1}(X_i'X_i)(X_i'X_i)^{-1}\underline{c}
$$

$$
= \frac{\sigma_W^2}{M^2}\sum_{i=1}^{M}\underline{c}'(X_i'X_i)^{-1}\underline{c}. \tag{7.14}
$$

The denominator of the $t$-statistic is the square root of this value with $\sigma_W^2$ replaced by its pooled estimator (equation 7.8). As in standard applications of the GLM, the number of degrees of freedom equals the number of data points (i.e., $Mn$) minus the number of parameters in the $\underline{\beta}$ vector (i.e., $Mr$).                                                                              ■

Proposition 7.1 assumes the same number of TRs for each subject. If this assumption is false, then the equation 7.7 $t$-statistic has $\sum_{i=1}^{M}(n_i - r)$ degrees of freedom, where $n_i$ is the number of TRs for subject $i$. Similarly, equation 7.8 is replaced by a weighted sum of the $\hat{\sigma}_i^2$, where the weight on the $i^{th}$ sample variance is

$$
\frac{(n_i - r)}{\sum_{i=1}^{M}(n_i - r)}.
$$

### A Random Effects Group Analysis

A random effects analysis of the data in table 7.1 computes a $t$-statistic that uses the same numerator as the $t$-statistic in the fixed effects analysis. The only difference is the denominator. The random effects model includes two sources of unexplained variance: within-subjects and between-subjects. The within-subjects variance is the same as in the fixed effects model. The between-subjects variance is the variance of the population from which the subjects were sampled. In the case of table 7.1, the between-subjects variance is the variance of the broad, group distribution shown in figure 7.2 (which has a population value of $\sigma_G^2 = 16$), and the within-subjects variance is the variance of the narrow, individual subject distributions (which each have a population value of $\sigma_W^2 = 0.25$). A simple way to account for both sources of variance is to compute the sample variance of the eight sample (i.e., column) means in table 7.1. To see this intuitively, note that both sources of variance will cause the sample means of different subjects to be different from each other. Thus, the random effects analysis of the table 7.1 data simply performs a one-sample $t$-test on the column means. In this case, the resulting $t$-statistic has 7 degrees of freedom. In table 7.1, the numerical value of this $t$-statistic is 1.84, which yields a $p$-value of .054. Recall that a fixed effects analysis of these same data produced a $t$-statistic equal to 400.1 with 72 degrees of freedom, and therefore a $p$-value less than .0001. In the current case, this huge difference occurs because the between-subject or group variance (i.e., 16) is much larger than the within-subject variance (i.e., 0.25). In other words, if subjects is a random factor then the conclusions that can be drawn from these data must be tentative because there is so much individual difference (i.e., between-subject variance is large) that a replication could include subjects who produce very different results. In contrast, if subjects is a fixed factor then a replication must include exactly these same subjects. Each of these subjects produces such highly reliable data (i.e., within-subject variability is low) that our confidence in the present results can be high. MATLAB box 7.1 shows the code that was used to produce figure 7.2 and table 7.1 and also to compute the fixed and random effects $t$-statistics.

More formally, the random effects GLM assumes

$$\underline{B}_i = X_i\underline{\beta}_i + \underline{\varepsilon}_i \tag{7.15}$$

$$\underline{\beta}_i = \underline{\beta}_G + \underline{\varepsilon}_{G_i}, \tag{7.16}$$

where $\underline{B}_i$ is an $n \times 1$ vector containing the BOLD responses from subject $i$ on each of the $n$ TRs (i.e., in this voxel), $X_i$ is the design matrix for subject $i$, $\underline{\beta}_i$ is the subject $i$ beta vector, and $\underline{\varepsilon}_i$ is the within-subject noise vector. Note that even if every subject undergoes exactly the same experimental conditions, different subjects will usually have different design matrices because of random jittering. Finally, the vector $\underline{\beta}_G$ contains the group means of every parameter, and $\underline{\varepsilon}_{G_i}$ denotes the group noise for subject $i$. Note that equation 7.15 and 7.16 can be combined to produce

$$\underline{B}_i = X_i\underline{\beta}_G + X_i\underline{\varepsilon}_{G_i} + \underline{\varepsilon}_i. \tag{7.17}$$

Technically, this will usually be a *mixed effects model*, even if we treat subjects as a random factor. This is because there will typically be parameters in the beta vectors that would be associated with fixed effects. For example, the linear drift in magnetic field strength that was included in the chapter 5 models would typically be considered a fixed

**MATLAB Box 7.1**
Fixed effects and random effects analysis of group data (as in figure 7.2 and table 7.1)

```
clear all; close all; clc;    % Clear all workspaces
nsubs=8;                      % Select number of subjects
ntrials=10;                   % Select number of trials per subject

% Create (or read in) the data
% Set the individual subject means by sampling from the group distribution
group=2+4*randn(1,nsubs);

% Sample the ntrials scores from each subject
for i=1:nsubs;
    x(:,i)=group(i)*ones(ntrials,1)+.5*randn(ntrials,1);
end;

% Compute the individual subject mean and standard deviation
M=mean(x)
s=std(x)

% Compute the fixed effects t-statistic
variance=s.^2;   pooledvar=mean(variance);
sfixed=sqrt(pooledvar);    tfixed=mean(M)/sqrt(pooledvar/nsubs)

% Compute the random effects t-statistic
srandom=std(M);    trandom=mean(M)/(srandom/sqrt(nsubs))

% Plot everything
tx=[-10:.01:15]; k=1/sqrt(2*pi);
for i=1:nsubs;
    pdf=.5*(k/.5)*exp(-(tx-group(i)).^2/(2*.25));
    plot(tx,pdf); hold on;
    scatter(x(:,i),zeros(1,10),84,'x','k');
end;
pdfg=(k/4)*exp(-(tx-2).^2/(2*16));
plot (tx,pdfg); axis([-10 15  0 .5]);
```

effect. Equations 7.15–7.17 can accommodate fixed effects simply by setting the variance term associated with that effect in equation 7.16 to 0.

As with the fixed effects model, suppose we want to test the null hypothesis described by equation 7.5:

$$H_0 : \underline{c}'\underline{\beta}_G = 0.$$

Proposition 7.2 establishes the test of this null hypothesis.

**Proposition 7.2**  Consider the random effects model

$$\underline{B}_i = X_i \underline{\beta}_i + \underline{\varepsilon}_i \tag{7.18}$$

$$\underline{\beta}_i = \underline{\beta}_G + \underline{\varepsilon}_{G_i}, \tag{7.19}$$

where $\underline{\varepsilon}_i$ and $\underline{\varepsilon}_{G_i}$ both have multivariate normal distributions with mean vector $\underline{0}$ and variance-covariance matrices $\Sigma_i = \sigma_W^2 \, I$ and $\Sigma_{G_i} = \sigma_G^2 \, I$, respectively. Under the null hypothesis $H_0 : \underline{c}'\underline{\beta}_G = 0$, the statistic

$$t = \frac{\underline{c}'\hat{\underline{\beta}}_G}{\sqrt{\dfrac{S^2_{\underline{c}'\hat{\underline{\beta}}_i}}{M}}} \tag{7.20}$$

has a t-distribution with $M-1$ degrees of freedom. The term $S^2_{\underline{c}'\hat{\underline{\beta}}_i}$ denotes the sample variance of the $M$ separate values of $\underline{c}'\hat{\underline{\beta}}_i$ (i.e., one for each subject). As in proposition 7.1, the numerator of this t-statistic equals

$$\underline{c}'\hat{\underline{\beta}}_G = \frac{1}{M}\sum_{i=1}^{M} \underline{c}'\hat{\underline{\beta}}_i = \frac{1}{M}\sum_{i=1}^{M} \underline{c}'(X_i'X_i)^{-1}X_i'\underline{B}_i. \tag{7.21}$$

The expected value of the terms inside the radical in the denominator equals

$$E\left(\frac{S^2_{\underline{c}'\hat{\underline{\beta}}_i}}{M}\right) = \frac{\sigma_G^2}{M}\underline{c}'\underline{c} + \frac{\sigma_W^2}{M^2}\underline{c}'\sum_{i=1}^{M}(X_i'X_i)^{-1}\underline{c}. \tag{7.22}$$

**Derivation**  To begin, construct the same supervectors $\underline{B}$, $\beta$, $\underline{\varepsilon}_W$, and $\underline{c}_G$, and the same super design matrix $X$ as in proposition 7.1. In addition, define the two new supervectors

$$\underset{Mr\times 1}{\underline{\varepsilon}_G} = \begin{bmatrix} \underline{\varepsilon}_{G_1} \\ \underline{\varepsilon}_{G_2} \\ \vdots \\ \underline{\varepsilon}_{G_M} \end{bmatrix} \quad \text{and} \quad \underset{Mr\times 1}{\underline{\beta}_{Group}} = \begin{bmatrix} \underline{\beta}_G \\ \underline{\beta}_G \\ \vdots \\ \underline{\beta}_G \end{bmatrix}.$$

Given these definitions, note that the model can be rewritten as

$$\underline{B} = X\underline{\beta} + \underline{\varepsilon}_W. \tag{7.23}$$

$$\underline{\beta} = \underline{\beta}_{Group} + \underline{\varepsilon}_G \tag{7.24}$$

The variance-covariance matrix of $\underline{B}$ is

$$\Sigma_{\underline{B}} = \sigma_G^2(XX') + \sigma_W^2 I, \tag{7.25}$$

and the least squares estimate of $\underline{\beta}$ is

$$\hat{\underline{\beta}} = (X'X)^{-1}X'\underline{B}. \tag{7.26}$$

Because $E(\underline{\varepsilon}_G) = \underline{0}$, note that the best estimator of $\underline{\beta}_{Group}$ is $\hat{\underline{\beta}}$. Therefore, following the derivation in equation 7.12 of proposition 7.1,

$$\hat{\underline{\beta}}_{Group} = \begin{bmatrix} (X_1'X_1)^{-1}X_1'\underline{B}_1 & 0 & \cdots & 0 \\ 0 & (X_2'X_2)^{-1}X_2'\underline{B}_2 & \cdots & 0 \\ \vdots & \vdots & \ddots & \vdots \\ 0 & 0 & \cdots & (X_M'X_M)^{-1}X_M'\underline{B}_M \end{bmatrix}. \tag{7.27}$$

As in the fixed effects model, $\underline{c}_G'\hat{\underline{\beta}}_{Group} = \underline{c}'\hat{\underline{\beta}}_G$. Combining this result with equation 7.27 produces equation 7.21.

Next, note that $E(\underline{c}'\hat{\underline{\beta}}_i) = \underline{c}'\underline{\beta}_G$. Therefore, the statistic $S_{\underline{c}'\hat{\underline{\beta}}_i}^2/M$ is an unbiased estimator of the population variance of $\underline{c}'\hat{\underline{\beta}}_G$. In other words,

$$E\left(\frac{S_{\underline{c}'\hat{\underline{\beta}}_i}^2}{M}\right) = \mathrm{Var}(\underline{c}'\hat{\underline{\beta}}_G).$$

The derivation of this variance is the same as in proposition 7.1 up to line 3 of equation 7.14. From there,

$$\mathrm{Var}(\underline{c}'\hat{\underline{\beta}}_G) = \frac{1}{M^2}\sum_{i=1}^{M}\underline{c}'(X_i'X_i)^{-1}X_i'\Sigma_{\underline{B}_i}X_i(X_i'X_i)^{-1}\underline{c}$$

$$= \frac{1}{M^2}\sum_{i=1}^{M}\underline{c}'(X_i'X_i)^{-1}X_i'[\sigma_G^2 XX' + \sigma_W^2 I]X_i(X_i'X_i)^{-1}\underline{c}$$

$$= \frac{1}{M^2}\sum_{i=1}^{M}[\sigma_G^2\underline{c}'\underline{c} + \sigma_W^2\underline{c}'(X_i'X_i)^{-1}\underline{c}],$$

from which the result easily follows.                                                   ∎

More general versions of proposition 7.2 are possible that allow for temporal correlations between successive BOLD responses and for correlations between group level effects (Beckmann et al., 2003; Mumford & Nichols, 2008).

### Comparing Fixed and Random Effects Analyses

Whether one uses the fixed effects model or random effects model, the following steps will form the group map that would be used to test the null hypothesis $H_0 : \underline{c}'\beta_G = 0$. First, run the GLM separately on each subject in every voxel. Second, compute $\underline{c}'\hat{\beta}_i$ for each subject in every voxel. At the end of step 2, note that in every voxel there will be $M$ values of $\underline{c}'\hat{\beta}_i$—one for every subject. The first two steps together comprise the first level of analysis. The second level of analysis begins with step 3. In this step, a group map is formed from the $M$ individual subject maps by using either proposition 7.1 or 7.2 to compute one group $t$-value in every voxel. The final step of the group analysis is to choose some method of solving the multiple comparisons problem and then make significance decisions about each voxel in the group map. These five steps were used to create the group map shown in the upper left part of figure 7.1.

Propositions 7.1 and 7.2 show that to test the equation 7.5 null hypothesis $H_0 : \underline{c}'\beta_G = 0$, a $t$-test is used in both a fixed effects and random effects analysis. Furthermore, in both cases the numerator of the $t$-statistic is the same (i.e., $\underline{c}'\hat{\beta}_G$). The two $t$-tests differ only in the denominators of their $t$-statistics. The expected value of the squared denominator of the fixed effects $t$-statistic is

$$E(\text{FX denominator}^2) = \frac{\sigma_W^2}{M^2}\underline{c}'\sum_{i=1}^{M}(X_i'X_i)^{-1}\underline{c},$$

whereas the expected value of the squared denominator of the random effects $t$-statistic is

$$E(\text{RX denominator}^2) = \frac{\sigma_G^2}{M}\underline{c}'\underline{c} + \frac{\sigma_W^2}{M^2}\underline{c}'\sum_{i=1}^{M}(X_i'X_i)^{-1}\underline{c}.$$

Note that

$$E(\text{RX denominator}^2) = \frac{\sigma_G^2}{M}\underline{c}'\underline{c} + E(\text{FX denominator}^2),$$

and therefore that, on average, the denominator of the fixed effects $t$-test will be smaller than the denominator of the random effects $t$-test and that this difference increases with the magnitude of the individual differences (i.e., with $\sigma_G^2$). The results of Miller et al. (2009) suggest that within-subject variance is often considerably less than the group (i.e., between-subject) variance, although typically this difference will be less than in table 7.1. Often when designing an fMRI experiment, one must choose whether to invest in longer sessions for fewer subjects or shorter sessions for more subjects. Increasing either the length of each session (i.e., the number of TRs) or the number of subjects will decrease both the fixed and random effects denominators. Increasing the number of subjects increases $M$, which decreases every term in both denominators. Increasing the number of TRs increases $n$, which decreases the within-subject variance terms but has no effect on the contribution of the group or between-subject variance in the random effects model. Therefore, if $\sigma_G^2$ is substantially larger than $\sigma_W^2$, as in the Miller et al. (2009) experiments, then the most effective use of scanning resources might be to run more subjects for fewer TRs.

Another difference between the fixed-effects and random-effects $t$-tests is in their degrees of freedom. Note that in most cases, the degrees of freedom in the random-effects $t$-test (i.e., $M - 1$) will be far less than in the fixed-effects $t$-test [i.e., $M(n - r)$]. In the table 7.1 example, the random-effects $t$-test had 7 degrees of freedom, whereas the fixed-effects $t$-test had 72 degrees of freedom. As a result, the significance threshold will be considerably higher in the random-effects $t$-test. This is the price that must be paid for the ability to generalize the results from the sample of subjects run in the experiment to the population to which they belong.

## Multiple Factor Experiments

Group analysis on more complex experiments with multiple factors is performed in a similar manner. The first step is always to run a standard GLM analysis on the data from each individual subject. The result is a statistical parametric map for each subject that specifies a statistic (e.g., a $t$-statistic or percent signal change) in every voxel. The second step is to run a group-level ANOVA on the SPM values in each separate voxel. This will create separate group maps for each statistic in the relevant ANOVA summary table.

As an example, consider the experiment of Calvo-Merino, Glaser, Grèzes, Passingham, and Haggard (2005). In this study, three groups of subjects viewed two types of video during scanning. The videos showed professional dancers performing either classical ballet or capoeira (an Afro-Brazilian dance form) dance movements. One group of subjects consisted of professional ballet dancers, one group was composed of professional capoeira dancers, and the third group of subjects included non-expert controls. Thus, the experiment used a $2 \times 3$ factorial design with repeated measures on the video-type factor.

The data from every subject were first analyzed using the correlation-based GLM, as described in chapter 5. The results included two $t$-maps for every subject—one for each video type. The $t$-statistics from each voxel in these SPMs were then entered into a $2 \times 3$ repeated-measures ANOVA. The result of this second-stage group analysis is three $F$-statistics for every voxel—one that measures the main effect of dance or video type, one that measures the main effect of subject type, and one that measures the video-type $\times$

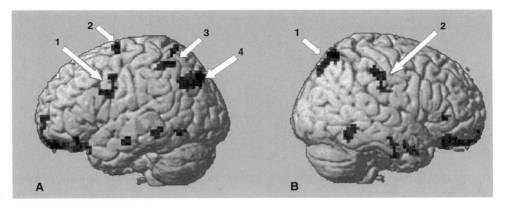

**Figure 7.3**
A group interaction map. (A) Left hemisphere, (B) right hemisphere. Arrows and numbers indicate regions of significant activation that are predicted by theory. (Reprinted from Calvo-Merino, Glaser, Grèzes, Passingham, & Haggard, "Action observation and acquired motor skills: An fMRI study with expert dancers," *Cerebral Cortex*, 2005, *15*, 1243–1249, with permission from Oxford University Press.)

subject-type interaction. Each of these could be used to construct their own statistical map. Figure 7.3 shows the interaction map. Voxels showing significance here indicate regions where the two dance types were viewed differently by the three groups of subjects.

A standard application of this 2 × 3 ANOVA would treat group type as a fixed factor. This is because a replication of the experiment would presumably again include a control group and two groups of dancers who are professionals in the two dance types depicted in the videos. In addition, the results of the experiment would be used to make inferences about differences in the neural basis of action observation between novices and experts, but it seems unlikely that there would be strong motivation to generalize results to intermediate skill levels. In contrast, video type or dance type could be interpreted as either a fixed or random factor. If a replication again used videos of ballet and capoeira, and if no attempt was made to generalize the results to other dance types, then video type should be treated as a fixed factor. However, one could imagine that a replication might randomly sample two dance types from the population of all possible dance types, and that the results would be used to make an inference about watching any type of dance. In this case, video type should be treated as a random factor.

Suppose we choose to treat video type and group type both as fixed factors. Then in what sense have we performed a random effects analysis? As in our simpler examples, the critical issue is how we estimate variability within each of the six cells in the 2 × 3 design. A standard ANOVA on the individual subject statistical maps would effectively compute the variance of all *t*-values within each cell. The numerical value of this statistic increases with both within- and between-subject variance. Thus, this method treats subjects as a random

**Table 7.2**
Possible outcomes when testing a null hypothesis

|  |  | Decision | |
|---|---|---|---|
|  |  | Do Not Reject $H_0$ | Reject $H_0$ |
| State of Nature | $H_0$ is True | Correct decision<br>Probability = $1 - \alpha$ | Type I error<br>Probability = $\alpha$ |
|  | $H_1$ is True | Type II error<br>Probability = $\beta$ | Correct decision<br>Probability = power = $1 - \beta$ |

factor, even though the other factors in the experiment are fixed. An analysis that treats subjects as a fixed factor would estimate within-cell variance by averaging the error-variance estimates from the initial GLM analysis that was run on each individual subject. This statistic increases with within-subject variance but is not affected by between-subject variance.

**Power Analysis**

Consider again null and alternative hypotheses of the form

$$H_0 : \underline{c}'\underline{\beta} = 0$$

$$H_1 : \underline{c}'\underline{\beta} > 0.$$

The four possible outcomes associated with this test are illustrated in table 7.2. Note that there are two possible correct decisions and two possible errors. The power of the test is the probability of a correct rejection. By convention, this probability is denoted by $1 - \beta$, where $\beta$ is the probability of a type II error (not to be confused with the beta vector in the GLM). In fMRI experiments, power is the probability of detecting a true task-related activation.

In traditional null hypothesis testing, we have direct control over the type I error rate (i.e., $\alpha$). If the outcome of a test is to reject the null hypothesis, then the only error that is possible is a type I error. In this case, the power of the test is relatively unimportant.

On the other hand, if the decision is to not reject the null hypothesis, then the only possible error is a type II error. The probability of a type II error (i.e., $\beta$) is not directly controlled during hypothesis testing, and without knowing the numerical value of this probability, it is impossible to interpret a decision to not reject $H_0$. For example, suppose $\alpha = .10$ and power is so low that $1 - \beta$ only equals .20. In other words, when $H_0$ is true, the probability of not rejecting is .90, and when $H_0$ is false, the probability of not rejecting is .80. Before we even collect the data therefore, we know that non-significance is very likely, regardless of whether the null hypothesis is true or false. If we now run this experiment and fail to reject $H_0$, then we have learned very little about the validity of $H_0$. For this reason, before any decision of non-significance can be interpreted, it is vital to know something about the power of the test.

In virtually every statistical parametric map, many voxels will fail to reach significance, regardless of how the multiple comparisons problem is solved. Thus, to interpret the results of these many non-significant tests, it is important to have some idea about the power of the experiment. The other time when power computations are important is during experimental design. Running fMRI experiments is expensive, and it is critical to know beforehand whether the proposed experiment is powerful enough to detect the effect that the experiment was designed to study. Naturally enough, this question is also of great interest to grant-reviewing agencies. Almost every grant proposal should include a power analysis of each proposed fMRI experiment.

Power can only be computed if a numerical value is specified for the alternative hypothesis. Power is the probability of rejecting $H_0$ when it is false. The null hypothesis assumes that a voxel does not respond to the stimulus event we are studying, so when $H_0$ is false, the voxel does respond to the stimulus. Obviously, we are more likely to reject $H_0$ correctly when the voxel responds strongly to the stimulus than when it responds weakly. In the former case power is large, and in the latter case power is small.

Consider the null and alternative hypotheses

$$H_0 : \underline{c}' \underline{\beta}_G = 0$$

$$H_1 : \underline{c}' \underline{\beta}_G = K \tag{7.28}$$

for some numerical value $K$. Proposition 7.2 states that if $H_0$ is true, then the random-effects $t$-statistic given in equation 7.20 has a t-distribution with $M-1$ degrees of freedom. If instead $H_1$ is true, then the same statistic has a noncentral t-distribution (e.g., Mumford & Nichols, 2008) with $M-1$ degrees of freedom and noncentrality parameter equal to

$$\delta = \frac{K}{\sqrt{\dfrac{\sigma_G^2}{M} \underline{c}'\underline{c} + \dfrac{\sigma_W^2}{M^2} \underline{c}' \sum_{i=1}^{M} (X_i'X_i)^{-1} \underline{c}}}. \tag{7.29}$$

Given numerical values for $\alpha$, $\delta$, and degrees of freedom, power can be computed from MATLAB box 7.2, from noncentral t-tables (e.g., Winer et al., 1991), or from a variety of software packages.

To compute $\delta$, some numerical value of $K$ must be chosen. This is the value of the contrast that is expected in a task-sensitive voxel. When designing our experiment, we should plan for enough subjects and TRs to detect a specific value of $K$ with reasonably high probability (e.g., $1 - \beta = .80$). But what value of $K$ is reasonable? Desmond and Glover (2002) attempted to answer this question empirically. They estimated percent signal change in a Sternberg (1966) memory-scanning task in 3024 voxels from 9 ROIs across 12 subjects. From these data, they estimated a mean percent signal change of 0.48% and on this basis concluded that percent signal change might often fall somewhere in the range from 0.25% to 0.75%. Thus, following Cohen (1992), we might tentatively define a small effect size (i.e., $K$ in equation 7.29) as a 0.25% signal change, a moderate effect size as a 0.50% signal change, and a large effect size as a 0.75% signal change. Given these definitions, when planning an experiment, we might therefore want to include enough subjects to ensure that a moderate effect of 0.50% signal change is likely to be detected. A common statistical choice for "likely" is with probability $1 - \beta = .80$.

Computing the noncentrality parameter in equation 7.29 requires not only specifying a numerical value of $K$ but also numerical values of $\sigma_G^2$ and $\sigma_W^2$. Desmond and Glover (2002) also estimated both of these parameters. Since effect size (i.e., $K$) is measured in units of percent signal change, $\sigma_G$ and $\sigma_W$ must be measured in these same units. Desmond and Glover (2002) estimated that in their memory scanning experiment $\sigma_G$ was approximately 0.5% signal change and $\sigma_W$ was approximately equal to 0.75% signal change.

MATLAB box 7.2 computes power for a block design with two alternating block types for any values of $\alpha$, $K$, $\sigma_W$, $\sigma_B$, $M$, and $n$ (i.e., number of TRs). Figure 7.4 shows some results produced from this code using the parameter estimates of Desmond and Glover (2002). The two panels show power plotted as a function of the number of subjects (i.e., $M$) for a variety of different percent signal changes (i.e., $K$) and two different values of $\alpha$. Both panels assume a one-tailed test and 200 TRs in each block type (i.e., so $n = 400$). The top panel shows that when $\alpha = .05$, 8 subjects are sufficient to guarantee a power of .80 when the effect size is moderate (i.e., when $K = 0.50\%$). In other words, in an experiment with 8 subjects, the probability of detecting task-related activation that is of moderate intensity is .8 when $\alpha = .05$ (i.e., in any single voxel). Of course, because of the multiple comparisons problem, an $\alpha$ of .05 is only appropriate for single-voxel decisions. The bottom panel of figure 7.4 shows the effects of decreasing $\alpha$ as a result, for example, of correcting for multiple comparisons. For example, with 12,500 separate independent tests, the Bonferroni correction that produces an experiment-wise error rate of $\alpha_E = .05$ sets the singe–test type I error rate to $\alpha_t = .000004$. Figure 7.4 shows that with this much smaller level of $\alpha$, 38 subjects are needed to detect a moderate effect with a power of .8. This sample size is considerably larger than in most published studies, which suggests that it may be common to have relatively low power when performing group-level whole-brain analyses. This limitation is offset somewhat by the large number of voxels that would typically be expected to show task-related activation in most studies. For example, suppose there are 1000 task-sensitive voxels across the brain and that power in any voxel

**MATLAB Box 7.2**

Compute the power of the t-test in which the null hypothesis is that there is no difference in activation between task and rest blocks and the alternative hypothesis is that the difference between task and rest is K% signal change.

```
clear all; close all; clc;   % Clear all workspaces

% Set the effect size K (i.e., the value of the alternative hypothesis)
K=0.50;

% Set the standard deviation of within-subject noise
sigW=0.75;

% Set the standard deviation of between-subject noise
sigG=0.75;

% Set the total number of TRs
% (half are from task blocks; half from rest blocks)
n=400;

% Set the alpha level (single voxel, one-tailed test)
alpha=.05;

% Select the number of subjects
M=16;

% Compute the noncentrality parameter
delta=K/sqrt((sigG*sigG/M) + ((sigW*sigW)/(M*n)));

% Compute the critical value of the t-test
tc=icdf('t',1-alpha,M-1);

% Compute the power using the normal approximation to the area under the
% noncentral t
X=(tc-delta)/sqrt(1+ ((tc*tc)/(2*(M-1))));
power=1-normcdf(X,0,1)

% if the following commands are available, then power can be computed
% exactly
powerNCT=1-cdf('nct',tc,M-1,delta);
```

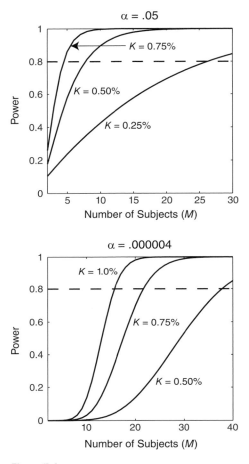

**Figure 7.4**
Power curves for different values of $\alpha$ (one-tailed) and for different percent signal changes (i.e., $K$). In all cases, the number of TRs per condition is 200, $\sigma_W = 0.75\%$ signal change, and $\sigma_G = 0.5\%$ signal change.

is only .5. Note that even in this case, we would still expect to find significance in 500 voxels, on average.

It should be emphasized that the curves shown in figure 7.4 depend strongly on the assumptions that the number of TRs per condition is 200, $\sigma_W = 0.75\%$ signal change, and $\sigma_G = 0.5\%$ signal change. A change in any of these values will change the power of the test. For example, an increase in $\sigma_G$ from 0.50% to 0.75% signal change doubles the sample size needed to detect a moderate task-related effect (i.e., $K = 0.50\%$) with probability .8 when $\alpha = .05$ (i.e., from $M = 8$ to $M = 16$). For this reason, it is vital that power computations are done with parameter values chosen to describe the proposed experiment as accurately as possible. With a fixed effects analysis, power should be significantly higher than in figure 7.4. First, there will be more degrees of freedom, so the critical value will be less extreme for the same level of $\alpha$. Second, as described earlier, the denominator of the group $t$-statistic will be smaller for the fixed effects analysis than with random effects. The cost, of course, is an inability to generalize the results to a larger subject population. The consensus in the field is that this cost is too high. As a result, many journals and reviewing agencies expect to see a random effects analysis, despite the lower power.

# 8  Coherence Analysis

Chapter 5 reviewed GLM-based methods for constructing a statistical parametric map. In these approaches, the GLM is applied separately to every voxel in the ROI. Chapter 6 described methods for deciding which of the resulting $z$- or $t$-statistics are significant, and chapter 7 reviewed methods for combining these results across a group of subjects. In this and the next chapter, we consider methods that help researchers interpret the results of all these analyses. For example, suppose an application of the methods described in chapters 5–7 reveals strong task-related activation in the dorsolateral prefrontal cortex and in the dorsal striatum. Because these two significance decisions were based on independent applications of the GLM, we have no basis to conclude that these areas are functionally connected in the task we are studying. It could be that they are both part of independent neural networks that just happened to both be activated at similar times. The methods described in this and the next chapter address this problem. This phase of the fMRI data analysis process, where an attempt is made to identify functionally connected neural networks that are mediating performance in the task under study, is known as *connectivity analysis*.

The idea underlying connectivity analysis is that a standard GLM analysis identifies clusters (or voxels) that show task-related activation, but it does not specify whether any pair of these clusters is part of the same or different neural networks. If two clusters are part of the same network, then they should be functionally connected, in the sense that activation in one might cause activation in the other, or at least the separate activations in the two clusters should be correlated. If instead the clusters are in separate neural networks, then we would not expect either of these two conditions to hold. Connectivity analysis, then, is done after a GLM analysis, with the goal of determining which ROIs in the task-related activation map are functionally connected. In chapters 10 and 11, we will consider multivariate approaches that attempt to answer the significance and functional connectivity questions at the same time while also completely avoiding the multiple comparisons problem. The trick is that multivariate approaches identify task-related networks, rather than task-related clusters.

An obvious method for testing whether two brain regions are functionally connected in a particular cognitive task is to measure the correlation between the BOLD responses in the two regions across TRs in an experiment where the task is performed. Regions that work together to mediate performance in the task should have correlated neural activations; that is, they should both be active while the task is being performed, and they should both be inactive during rest periods. An obvious choice for measuring such a correlation would be to compute the standard Pearson correlation coefficient between the separate BOLD responses across time (i.e., across TRs).

This approach has several weaknesses, however. First, the neural activations in the two regions could be highly correlated, but because their vasculature is different, the two regions might be characterized by significantly different hrfs. In this case, if superposition holds, the observed BOLD responses would equal the convolution of two similar neural activations with two dissimilar hrfs. The result, unfortunately, would be two dissimilar BOLD responses, and therefore a low correlation. A second problem is that independent noise in the two regions would also lower their Pearson correlation coefficient.

Both of these problems are illustrated in figure 8.1. Two identical neural activations are convolved with two slightly different hrfs. The top panel shows the results of the two convolution operations in the absence of noise, and the bottom panel shows the results when independent noise is added to each result. In the absence of noise, the squared Pearson correlation between the two BOLD responses is .532, and when noise is added this squared correlation drops to .212. Of course, in a real application, the neural activations in the two regions would not be identical, even if they were functionally connected. Figure 8.1 illustrates the difficulty in identifying functional connectivity from the standard Pearson correlation coefficient.

In this chapter, we consider an alternative method for assessing functional connectivity called *coherence analysis*. Basically, coherence analysis computes a correlation between two BOLD responses, but in the frequency domain, rather than the time domain. The measure of correlation that results from this method is called coherence. As we will see, a major advantage of coherence analysis is that the coherence between two BOLD responses equals the coherence between the neural activations that elicited those BOLD responses, even if the two regions are characterized by different hrfs. In addition, coherence is mostly unaffected by the presence of (high frequency) independent noise in the separate regions. Thus, coherence analysis avoids both of the problems that plague standard correlation techniques.

## Autocorrelation and Cross-Correlation

Consider two regions of interest, or two single voxels. Let $B_j(T)$ and $B_k(T)$ denote the BOLD responses in these two regions when the TR equals $T$ (which in this chapter we assume is a random variable). The fundamental statistics that coherence analysis operates on are the *autocorrelation functions* for regions $j$ and $k$ and the *cross-correlation function* between the two regions.

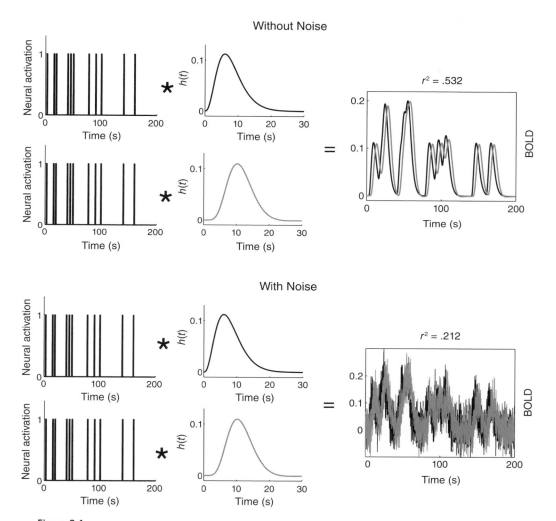

**Figure 8.1**
Two separate BOLD responses (right column) generated by convolving identical neural activations (left column) with slightly different hrfs (middle column). The top panel shows the results in the absence of any noise. The bottom panel is identical except independent noise was added to both BOLD responses at each time point (normally distributed with mean = 0 and standard deviation = .04).

The autocorrelation function for region $j$, denoted by $R_j(t)$, is defined as

$$R_j(t) = E[B_j(T + t)B_j(T)], \tag{8.1}$$

where, as before, $E$ denotes expected value. Note that

$$R_j(0) = E\{[B_j(T)]^2\}.$$

This is relevant because the variance of a random variable $X$ is defined as

$$\sigma_X^2 = E(X - \mu_X)^2.$$

So if $\mu_X = 0$, then

$$\sigma_X^2 = E(X)^2.$$

Therefore, if the data have been standardized so that the mean across TRs is 0 (i.e., so $E[B_j(t)] = 0$; data standardized in this way are said to be mean centered), then

$$R_j(0) = \sigma_{B_j}^2.$$

Similarly, the covariance between two random variables $X$ and $Y$ is defined as

$$\mathrm{Cov}(X, Y) = E[(X - \mu_X)(Y - \mu_Y)],$$

so if $\mu_X = \mu_Y = 0$, then

$$\mathrm{Cov}(X, Y) = E(XY).$$

Thus, with mean-centered data,

$$R_j(t) = \mathrm{Cov}[B_j(T + t), B_j(T)].$$

Finally, the correlation between random variables $X$ and $Y$ is defined as the standardized covariance

$$\rho_{XY} = \frac{\mathrm{Cov}(X, Y)}{\sigma_X \sigma_Y}.$$

As a result, if the data have also been standardized to have unit variance, then $R_j(t)$ is the correlation coefficient between $B_j(T + t)$ and $B_j(T)$ for all different values of $t$. This property, of course, is the reason that $R_j(t)$ is called the autocorrelation function.

Figure 8.2 shows a hypothetical BOLD response and its autocorrelation function. The BOLD response was generated by convolving a neural activation constructed as a series of boxcar functions with the gamma function hrf shown in the top of figure 8.1 and then add-

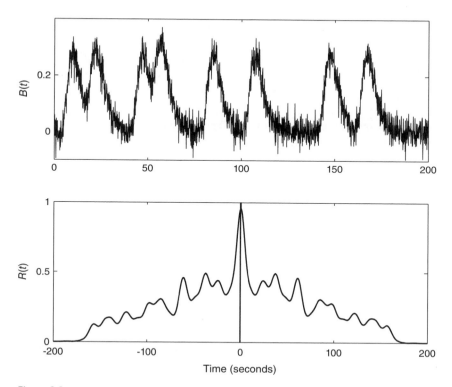

**Figure 8.2**
A hypothetical BOLD response (top) and its autocorrelation function (bottom). The BOLD response was generated by convolving a neural activation with the gamma function hrf shown in the top panel of figure 8.1 and then adding Gaussian noise (mean = 0, standard deviation = .03).

ing Gaussian noise (i.e., with mean zero and standard deviation = .03). The boxcar modeled eight separate stimulus presentations each of which was presented for one TR (i.e., 2.5 seconds). The BOLD response was then normalized to have 0 mean and unit variance, so the autocorrelation function shows the correlation coefficient between the BOLD responses at all different temporal lags.

Several features of the autocorrelation function should be noted. First, when $t = 0$, note that $R_j(0) = 1.0$. This is because any function is perfectly correlated with itself. Second, note that $R_j(t)$ tends to decrease as $t$ moves away from 0. In fact, $R_j(t)$ must take on its greatest value when $t = 0$, even if the data are not standardized (e.g., Papoulis, 1965). With standardized data, $R_j(t)$ equals the correlation between $B_j(T)$ and a version of itself that has been shifted in time by an amount $t$. Because a shifted version of $B_j(T)$ is not identical to itself, this correlation will be less than one, and in general, the greater the shift in time, the greater the drop in the correlation. Third, note that this drop in correlation as the shift or lag increases is not monotonic. Instead, there are some dramatic scallops in $R_j(t)$ as $t$ moves away from 0. This is because the BOLD response to each successive neural activation (i.e., boxcar) is identical. Thus, if the time $T$ occurs at one of the peaks of the BOLD response shown in the top panel of figure 8.2, then when the function is shifted by an amount $t$ that happens to coincide with another peak in the BOLD response, the correlation will be high. In other words, the figure 8.2 BOLD response is roughly periodic, and the autocorrelation of any function that is approximately periodic will be scalloped. Finally, note that $R_j(t)$ is symmetric about zero. This is a general property of all autocorrelation functions and is true because

$$R_j(t) = E[B_j(T)B_j(T + t)] = E[B_j(T + t)B_j(T)] = R_j(-t). \tag{8.2}$$

The cross-correlation function, $R_{jk}(t)$, is defined in a similar way to the autocorrelation function, except it describes the correlation between a pair of BOLD responses at all possible lags. In particular,

$$R_{jk}(t) = E[B_j(T + t)B_k(T)]. \tag{8.3}$$

As with the autocorrelation, if the data are mean centered and standardized to have unit variance, then $R_{jk}(t)$ equals the Pearson correlation between $B_j(T)$ and $B_k(T)$ at all possible lags.

Figure 8.3 shows two hrfs, two BOLD responses, and their cross-correlation function. The BOLD responses were generated from two neural activations (each a series of boxcars) that were identical except that the first lagged 10 seconds behind the second. These two neural activations were then convolved with the two hrfs shown in the top panel. Finally, independent Gaussian noise (with mean zero and standard deviation = .03) was added to the results of these two convolutions to produce the hypothetical BOLD responses shown in the middle panel. Note that although the neural activations are temporal shifts of each other, each peak of $B_j(T)$ is higher and narrower than the corresponding peak in $B_k(T)$. This is because the (difference-in-gamma-functions) hrf used to generate $B_j(T)$ (shown in gray in the top panel) is higher and narrower than the (gamma function) hrf used to generate $B_k(T)$ (in black). Finally, the BOLD responses were both mean centered and standardized to have unit variance before the cross-correlation was computed.

Note that the cross-correlation in figure 8.3 looks very much like the autocorrelation in figure 8.2 except that it is shifted to the left by 10 seconds. Because the neural activations that produced these BOLD responses were identical except for a 10-second lag, note that shifting $B_j(T)$ earlier in time by 10 seconds will maximize its correlation with $B_k(T)$. For example, $B_j(60)$ is almost the same as $B_k(50)$. This is the reason $R_{jk}(t)$ has its peak at $t = -10$ (because $R_{jk}(-10) = E[B_j(T - 10)B_k(T)]$).

The figure 8.3 cross-correlation $R_{jk}(t)$ is lower than the figure 8.2 autocorrelation $R_j(t)$ because the two BOLD responses were generated from different hrfs, and independent

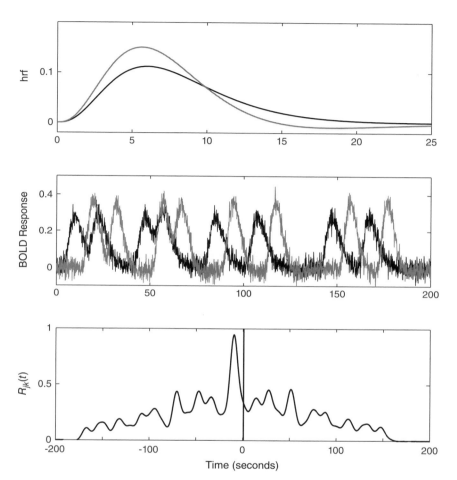

**Figure 8.3**
Two hrfs (top), two hypothetical BOLD responses (middle), and their cross-correlation function (bottom). The BOLD responses were generated from two neural activations that were identical except that one lagged 10 seconds behind the other. These two neural activations were then convolved with the two hrfs shown in the top panel. Finally, independent Gaussian noise (mean = 0, standard deviation = .01) was added to the results of these two convolutions to produce the predicted BOLD responses shown in the middle panel.

noise was added to each. The different hrfs cause the shape of each peak in $B_j(T)$ and $B_k(T)$ to differ, which lowers the correlation, even following a shift of $-10$ seconds. When the same hrf is used to generate $B_j(T)$ and $B_k(T)$ and no noise is added, then the figure 8.3 cross-correlation $R_{jk}(t)$ is identical to the figure 8.2 autocorrelation $R_j(t)$, except for a 10-second shift to the left. This is true, however, only because identical neural activations were used to generate $B_j(T)$ and $B_k(T)$. If the neural activations differ in any way, then the cross-correlation must necessarily always be less than the autocorrelation (i.e., following any shift needed to align their peaks). MATLAB box 8.1 shows code that will generate figures 8.2 and 8.3.

**MATLAB Box 8.1**
Compute and plot an autocorrelation function (as in figure 8.2) and a cross-correlation function (as in figure 8.3)

```
clear all; close all; clc;    % Clear all workspaces

% Create the hrf
n=4; lamda=2; n2=7; lamda2=2; a=.3;
t=0:.1:200;
hrf=(t.^(n-1)).*exp(-t/lamda)/((lamda^n)*factorial(n-1));
h2=(t.^(n2-1)).*exp(-t/lamda2)/((lamda2^n2)*factorial(n2-1));
hrf2=(hrf-a*h2)/(sum(hrf-a*h2)*.1);

% Create the boxcar
n=zeros(1,2001);
n(26:50)=ones(1,25); n(151:175)=ones(1,25); n(401:425)=ones(1,25);
n(501:525)=ones(1,25); n(776:800)=ones(1,25);
n(1001:1025)=ones(1,25);
n(1401:1425)=ones(1,25); n(1601:1625)=ones(1,25);
n2=[zeros(1,100),n(1:1901)];

% Convolve hrf & boxcar, then add noise
B=conv(hrf,n)/10; B2=conv(hrf2,n2)/10;
B=B(1:2001)+.03*randn(1,2001); B2=B2(1:2001)+.03*randn(1,2001);
subplot(4,1,1); plot(t,B); axis([0 200 -.1 .4]);

% Compute autocorrelation function & plot
[R_B,lags]=xcorr(B,'coeff');
subplot(4,1,2); plot(lags/10,R_B); axis([-200 200 0 1]);

% Plot both BOLD responses
subplot(4,1,3); plot(t,B,t,B2); axis([0 200 -.1 .4]);

% Compute cross-correlation function & plot
[R12,lags]=xcorr(B,B2,'coeff');
subplot(4,1,4); plot(lags/10,R12); axis([-200 200 0 1]);
```

## Power Spectrum and Cross-Power Spectrum

The introduction to this chapter mentioned that coherence analysis computes the correlation between $B_j(T)$ and $B_k(T)$ in the frequency domain. The autocorrelation and cross-correlation functions are defined exclusively in the time domain. The transition to the frequency domain is accomplished via Fourier analysis of these temporal functions. In one of the most famous results in all of mathematics, Fourier showed that almost any mathematical function can be written as a weighted sum of cosine waves. Thus, a function of time can be expressed in its usual temporal form or in its Fourier, or frequency, form. The Fourier representation of a function requires specifying two values for every cosine-wave frequency—the weight or amplitude of that frequency, and its phase shift, or the amount that the cosine wave is shifted to the right or left of zero. Thus, the Fourier transform of a function includes a record of the amplitude and phase of each frequency.

The *power spectrum* of $B_j(t)$, denoted by $P_j(f)$, is defined as the Fourier transform of the autocorrelation function $R_j(t)$,

$$P_j(f) = \Im[R_j(t)] = \int_{-\infty}^{\infty} e^{-i2\pi ft} R_j(t)\, dt,$$

where $f$ is cosine-wave frequency in cycles per second (i.e., hertz; Hz), and $i = \sqrt{-1}$. In general, a Fourier transform is a complex-valued function. Any complex number $z$ can be expressed as $z = x + iy$, where $x$ is the real part and $y$ is the imaginary part. A famous and powerful result in complex variables, called Euler's formula, states that

$$e^{ix} = \cos(x) + i\sin(x).$$

Note that by using this identity, the power spectrum $P_j(f)$, can be rewritten as

$$P_j(f) = \Im[R_j(t)] = \int_{-\infty}^{\infty} e^{-i2\pi ft} R_j(t)\, dt$$

$$= \int_{-\infty}^{\infty} \cos(2\pi ft) R_j(t)\, dt - i \int_{-\infty}^{\infty} \sin(2\pi ft) R_j(t)\, dt. \qquad (8.4)$$

From equation 8.4 we can see that the first integral on the last line denotes the real part of $P_j(f)$ and the second integral denotes the imaginary part.

For each frequency $f$ in a Fourier transform, the amplitude and phase of the corresponding cosine wave can be found by writing the imaginary number that is the result of the Fourier integral in polar coordinates. Thus, the amplitude, also called the modulus of $z = x + iy$, equals

$$|z| = \sqrt{x^2 + y^2} \, , \tag{8.5}$$

and the phase, also called the argument of $z$, is equal to (when $x > 0$)

$$\phi = \arg[z] = \tan^{-1}\left(\frac{y}{x}\right). \tag{8.6}$$

In summary, virtually any mathematical function can be written as a weighted linear combination of cosines. In this sum, each cosine frequency is scaled up or down by some amount (i.e., the amplitude of that frequency) and is shifted forward or backward in time by some amount (i.e., the phase of that frequency). Mathematically, the Fourier transform of a function is a complex-valued function of frequency. Evaluating the Fourier transform at any particular frequency produces a complex number $z$. The modulus of that number, $|z|$, specifies the amplitude of the cosine wave of that frequency, and the argument, $\arg(z)$, specifies the phase of that frequency.

An intuitive description of equation 8.4 is as follows. Consider any particular frequency $f$. For example, suppose $f = 1$ Hz. The first integral computes a kind of correlation between a cosine wave with a frequency of 1 Hz and $R_j(t)$, whereas the second integral computes the correlation between a sine wave of the same frequency and $R_j(t)$. From equation 8.5, we see that the amplitude of this frequency in the Fourier representation of $R_j(t)$ is determined by the sum of the squares of these two correlations. In other words, if $R_j(t)$ is roughly periodic with peaks that are about 1 Hz apart, then one or both of the correlations of $R_j(t)$ with cosine and sine waves of 1 Hz will be large.

Next, from equation 8.6, note that if the imaginary part is 0, then the phase is 0 [i.e., because $\tan(0) = 0$]. So the imaginary part of a Fourier transform determines whether any phase shifts are needed. Now a cosine function is symmetric about zero, whereas a sine function is shifted to the right by a quarter of a cycle. It turns out that the Fourier transform of any function that is symmetric about zero (called an even function in mathematics) has no imaginary component (i.e., it is strictly real). Because the autocorrelation $R_j(t)$ is symmetric about zero, its Fourier transform (given in equation 8.4) is therefore real. In other words, the autocorrelation shown in figure 8.2 (as well as every other autocorrelation function) can be written as a weighted sum of (nonshifted) cosines.

The Fourier transform of the autocorrelation function is called the *power spectrum*.[1] The power spectrum measures the power in the BOLD response at each temporal frequency. Figure 8.4 shows the BOLD response from figure 8.2 along with its power spectrum. MATLAB box 8.2 shows the code that generates this figure.

---

1. To compute the power spectrum of a raw signal, the amplitude of the Fourier transform is squared. However, note that the autocorrelation function is already in units of squared signal. Thus, in this case the squaring operation is not needed.

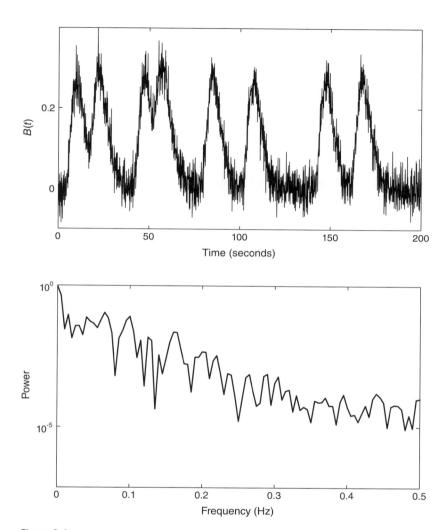

**Figure 8.4**
The BOLD response from figure 8.2 (top) and its power spectrum (bottom).

**MATLAB Box 8.2**
Compute the power spectrum of a BOLD response (as in figure 8.4)

```
clear all; close all; clc;    % Clear all workspaces

ntime=2000;                   % number of time points
T=200;                        % time interval in seconds
t=T*[0:ntime-1]/ntime;        % define time

% Create the hrf
n=4; lamda=2; n2=7; lamda2=2; a=.3;
hrf=(t.^(n-1)).*exp(-t/lamda)/((lamda^n)*factorial(n-1));

% Create the boxcar
n=zeros(1,ntime); n(26:50)=ones(1,25); n(151:175)=ones(1,25);
n(401:425)=ones(1,25); n(501:525)=ones(1,25); n(776:800)=ones(1,25);
n(1001:1025)=ones(1,25); n(1401:1425)=ones(1,25);
n(1601:1625)=ones(1,25);

% Convolve hrf & boxcar, add noise, then plot
B=conv(hrf,n)/10; B=B(1:ntime)+.03*randn(1,ntime);
subplot(2,1,1); plot(t,B); axis([0 200 -.1 .4]);

[R_B,lags]=xcorr(B,'coeff');   % Compute autocorrelation function
P_B=abs(fft(R_B))/(ntime/2);   % Absolute value of the fft
P_B=P_B(1:ntime/2);            % Compute power for positive frequencies
freq=[0:ntime/2-1]/T;          % Define frequency in Hz

% Plot on semilog scale
subplot(2,1,2); semilogy(freq,P_B); axis([0 .5 0 1]);
```

The *cross-spectral density* of two BOLD responses $B_j(T)$ and $B_k(T)$, denoted by $S_{jk}(f)$, is defined as the Fourier transform of their cross-correlation function $R_{jk}(t)$:

$$S_{jk}(f) = \Im[R_{jk}(t)] = \int_{-\infty}^{\infty} e^{-i2\pi ft} R_{jk}(t) \, dt. \tag{8.7}$$

Despite the similarity of the mathematical equations that define $P_j(f)$ and $S_{jk}(f)$, they are qualitatively different because $P_j(f)$ is purely real, whereas $S_{jk}(f)$ will generally have a nonzero imaginary component. This is because $R_j(t)$ is always symmetric about the point $t = 0$, whereas $R_{jk}(t)$, in general, is not symmetric. For example, the cross-correlation function shown in figure 8.3 is not symmetric around 0, and therefore some phase shifts are required to write it as a weighted sum of cosines. Thus, unlike $P_j(f)$, which is real, the *cross-spectral density* $S_{jk}(f)$ is a complex-valued function. We will use the phase information inherent in $S_{jk}(f)$ later in this chapter. For now though, we focus on the amplitude of $S_{jk}(f)$, which is defined[2] as the cross-power spectrum of $B_j(T)$ and $B_k(T)$; that is, as

$$P_{jk}(f) = |S_{jk}(f)|. \tag{8.8}$$

The cross-power spectrum of the BOLD responses shown in figure 8.3 looks very similar to the power spectrum shown in figure 8.4. This is because the major difference between the two figure 8.3 BOLD responses is a 10-second shift in time. Such a shift affects the phase spectrum of the cross-spectral density, but not the cross-power spectrum. In other words, the 10-second shift affects the phase of the cosine terms that make up the Fourier transform of the figure 8.3 cross-correlation, but not their amplitude.

## Coherence

We are finally in a position to define the coherence of two BOLD responses. As we will see, coherence focuses exclusively on the amplitude of frequencies in the cross-spectral density and the power spectrum and ignores all phase information. Later in this chapter, we will consider an alternative measure of connectivity that uses the phase shifts of the cross-spectral density.

To begin, recall that the squared correlation coefficient between two random variables $X$ and $Y$, typically denoted by $\rho_{XY}^2$, is defined as

$$\rho_{XY}^2 = \frac{[\text{Cov}(X, Y)]^2}{\sigma_X^2 \sigma_Y^2}.$$

The squared correlation coefficient, which must fall in the range $0 \leq \rho_{XY}^2 \leq 1$, measures the strength of the linear relationship between $X$ and $Y$.

The coherence between $B_j(T)$ and $B_k(T)$, which we denote by $C_{jk}(f)$, has exactly the same form as the squared correlation coefficient, except it operates in the frequency domain, rather than the time domain. Specifically, for a given frequency $f$,

$$C_{jk}(f) = \frac{[P_{jk}(f)]^2}{P_j(f)P_k(f)}. \tag{8.9}$$

As with the squared correlation coefficient, coherence is also restricted to the range $0 \leq C_{jk}(f) \leq 1$. Also like the correlation coefficient, coherence is a measure of the linear

---

2. Note that we could have defined the equation 8.4 integral as the spectral density of $B_j(T)$, denoted by $S_j(f)$, and then defined the power spectrum of $B_j(T)$ as $|S_j(f)|$. However, because $S_j(f)$ is real, $|S_j(f)| = S_j(f)$. So the spectral density of $B_j(T)$ is the same as the power spectrum of $B_j(T)$. It should also be noted that not all authors use the terms *cross-spectral density* and *cross-power spectrum* as they are defined here. For example, Papoulis (1965) refers to equation 8.7 as the *cross-power spectrum*.

relationship between $B_j(T)$ and $B_k(T)$, except coherence focuses on the frequency domain, whereas correlation is in the time domain. Coherence is sensitive to linear relationships because it is based on the Fourier transform of the cross-correlation function, and the cross-correlation measures the linear relationship between $B_k(T)$ and all possible shifted versions of $B_j(T)$.

The denominator of equation 8.9 can be considered a normalizing term, so $C_{jk}(f)$ essentially is a measure of the power (or amplitude) of frequency $f$ in the cross-correlation function between $B_j(T)$ and $B_k(T)$. If $C_{jk}(f)$ is large, then the cross-correlation function is quasi-periodic at frequency $f$, which means that every shift of $B_j(T)$ by $1/f$ seconds results in a large correlation with $B_k(T)$. In other words, $B_j(T)$ and $B_k(T)$ rise and fall in a synchronized fashion.

The bottom panel of figure 8.5 shows the coherence of the two hypothetical BOLD responses shown in the middle panel. The BOLD responses were generated from two neural activations that were identical except that one lagged 300 milliseconds behind the other. Next, the slower neural activation was convolved with the hrf shown in gray in the top panel of figure 8.5, and the faster neural activation was convolved with the hrf shown in black. Independent Gaussian noise (with mean zero and standard deviation = .03) was then added to the results of these two convolutions to produce the predicted BOLD responses.

The coherence function shown in the bottom panel of figure 8.5 was generated with the cohere command that is a standard part of the MATLAB signal processing toolbox. MATLAB box 8.3 shows the code that implements this command and that creates figure 8.5.

In figure 8.5, the correlation between the two BOLD responses shown in the middle panel is only 0.548, but note from the bottom panel that the coherence is around 0.9 or higher for frequencies below .12 Hz. Above .12 Hz, coherence quickly decreases. As we will see later in this chapter, for the purposes of establishing connectivity, coherence is most meaningful at lower frequencies. For example, at higher frequencies, coherence is strongly affected by noise.

The high coherence values at low frequencies seen in figure 8.5 suggest that coherence may be preferable to standard correlation analysis. To fully appreciate the advantages that coherence has over more traditional time-based correlation techniques, however, requires that we understand how the hrf affects coherence. The remainder of this section addresses this problem.

Consider the BOLD responses $B_j(t)$ and $B_k(t)$ recorded from two separate voxels or regions of interest, denoted by the subscripts $j$ and $k$. Denote the neural activation in these two regions by $N_j(t)$ and $N_k(t)$. Suppose superposition (i.e., microlinearity) holds in both regions so that the BOLD responses are the convolution of the neural activations and an hrf. In this analysis, however, we will allow for the possibility that the two regions have different hrfs, denoted by $h_j(t)$ and $h_k(t)$. In other words, we are assuming that

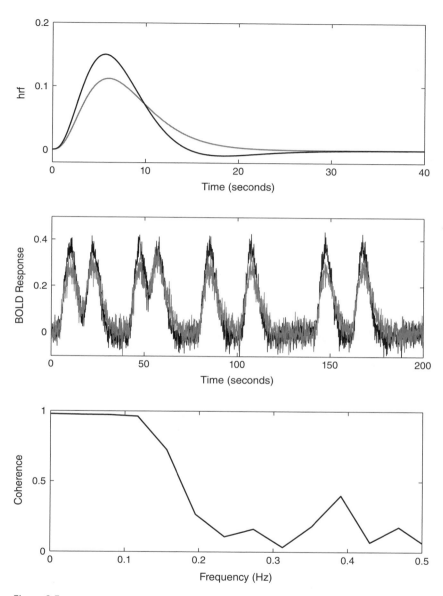

**Figure 8.5**
Coherence (bottom) of the two BOLD responses shown in the middle panel. The BOLD responses were generated from two neural activations that were identical except that one lagged 300 milliseconds behind the other. Next, the slower neural activation was convolved with the hrf shown in gray in the top panel, and the faster neural activation was convolved with the hrf shown in black. Independent Gaussian noise (mean = 0, standard deviation = .03) was then added to the results of these two convolutions to produce the predicted BOLD responses shown in the middle panel.

**MATLAB Box 8.3**
Compute coherence between two BOLD responses (as in figure 8.5)

```
clear all; close all; clc;      % Clear all workspaces

ntime=2000;                     % number of time points
T=200;                          % time interval in seconds
t=T*[0:ntime-1]/ntime;          % define time

% Create the hrfs & plot
n=4; lamda=2; n2=7; lamda2=2; a=.3;
hrf=(t.^(n-1)).*exp(-t/lamda)/((lamda^n)*factorial(n-1));
h2=(t.^(n2-1)).*exp(-t/lamda2)/((lamda2^n2)*factorial(n2-1));
hrf2=(hrf-a*h2)/(sum(hrf-a*h2)*.1);
subplot(3,1,1); plot(t,hrf,t,hrf2); axis([0 25 -.02 .2]);

% Create the boxcars
n=zeros(1,ntime);
n(26:50)=ones(1,25); n(151:175)=ones(1,25); n(401:425)=ones(1,25);
n(501:525)=ones(1,25); n(776:800)=ones(1,25); n(1001:1025)=ones(1,25);
n(1401:1425)=ones(1,25); n(1601:1625)=ones(1,25);
n2=[zeros(1,3),n(1:1997)];

% Convolve hrf & boxcar, add noise, then plot
B=conv(hrf,n)/10; B2=conv(hrf2,n2)/10;
B=B(1:ntime)+.03*randn(1,ntime); B2=B2(1:ntime)+.03*randn(1,ntime);
subplot(3,1,2); plot(t,B,t,B2); axis([0 200 -.1 .5]);

[C12,freq]=cohere(B,B2,[],[]);   % Compute coherence

% freq runs from 0 to 1. Our sampling rate is ntime/T samples per sec.
% Nyquist rate is half this value. So in hz, frequencies run from 0
% to one-half of ntime/T.
freq=freq*ntime/(T*2);

subplot(3,1,3); plot(freq, C12); axis([0 0.5 0 1]);   % Plot
```

$$B_j(t) = N_j(t) * h_j(t)$$  (8.10)

and

$$B_k(t) = N_k(t) * h_k(t).$$  (8.11)

In chapter 3, we saw that the Fourier transform of both sides of equation 8.10, for example, is equal to

$$\Im[B_j(t)] = \Im[N_j(t) * h_j(t)]$$

$$= \Im[N_j(t)] \times \Im[h_j(t)]$$

$$= \Im[N_j(t)] \times H_j(f),$$  (8.12)

In linear systems theory, the Fourier transform of the impulse response function is often called the transfer function (e.g., Chen, 1970). So here, we denote the transfer function that corresponds with the hrf $h_j(t)$ by $H_j(f)$. Proposition 8.1, which is the major result of this chapter, uses equation 8.12 to establish the relationship between the coherence of $B_j(t)$ and $B_k(t)$ and the coherence of $N_j(t)$ and $N_k(t)$.

**Proposition 8.1**   Suppose BOLD responses $B_j(t)$ and $B_k(t)$ are recorded from two brain regions $j$ and $k$, and let $N_j(t)$ and $N_k(t)$ denote the neural activations in those regions. If superposition (i.e., microlinearity) holds, then the coherence between $B_j(t)$ and $B_k(t)$ (when nonzero) equals the coherence between $N_j(t)$ and $N_k(t)$, even if the hrfs are different in the two regions.

**Derivation**   The proof of proposition 8.1 depends on two identities that relate the power spectrum and cross-power spectrum of $B_j(t)$ and $B_k(t)$ to the power spectrum and cross-power spectrum of $N_j(t)$ and $N_k(t)$ and to the two transfer functions $H_j(f)$ and $H_k(f)$. Derivations of both identities can be found in Papoulis (1965). The first identity relates the power spectrum of $B_j(t)$ to the power spectrum of $N_j(t)$ and the transfer function $H_j(f)$,

$$P_j(f) = P_{N_j}(f)|H_j(f)|^2,$$  (8.13)

where $P_{N_j}(f)$ is the power spectrum of the neural activation $N_j(t)$. Of course, an equation analogous to equation 8.13 holds for region $k$. The second identity relates the cross-power spectrum of $B_j(t)$ and $B_k(t)$ to the cross-power spectrum of $N_j(t)$ and $N_k(t)$ and to the two transfer functions $H_j(f)$ and $H_k(f)$,

$$P_{jk}(f) = P_{N_j N_k}(f)|H_j(f)| |H_k(f)|,$$  (8.14)

where $P_{N_j N_k}(f)$ is the cross-power spectrum of $N_j(t)$ and $N_k(t)$.

From equations 8.13 and 8.14, it follows that

$$C_{jk}(f) = \frac{[P_{jk}(f)]^2}{P_j(f)P_k(f)}$$

$$= \frac{[P_{N_jN_k}(f)|H_j(f)||H_k(f)|]^2}{[P_{N_j}(f)|H_j(f)|^2][P_{N_k}(f)|H_k(f)|^2]}$$

$$= \frac{[P_{N_jN_k}(f)]^2}{P_{N_j}(f)P_{N_k}(f)}$$

$$= C_{N_jN_k}(f),$$

which proves the result. ∎

Proposition 8.1 describes the main advantage of coherence analysis over more traditional correlation methods. In fact, evidence suggests that the hrf differs across brain regions (e.g., Schacter et al., 1997). Such differences significantly reduce the Pearson correlation coefficient between BOLD responses collected from two regions, even if the neural activations are identical. However, proposition 8.1 tells us that the coherence between these BOLD responses is unaffected by the difference in hrfs.

This powerful property of coherence is illustrated in figure 8.6. The bottom panel shows the coherence of two BOLD responses (not shown) that were generated by convolving the same neural activation (shown in the top panel) with two different hrfs (shown in the middle panel). The squared correlation coefficient between the two resulting BOLD responses is .914. Note though that for frequencies below 0.3 Hz, the coherence is nearly 1. The reason it is not exactly 1 is that in figure 8.6, coherence was computed (using MATLAB's "cohere" command) from a discrete sample of BOLD values—in this case, 1 every 100 milliseconds for 200 seconds. For this reason, the relevant Fourier transforms were not exact.

Figure 8.7 shows the effects of adding noise to each BOLD response. The BOLD responses shown in the top panel of figure 8.7 are identical to those used to produce figure 8.6, except independent, zero-mean Gaussian noise (with standard deviation .04) was added to each BOLD value (i.e., every 100 milliseconds). Now the squared correlation coefficient between the two BOLD responses is only .670. Note though that coherence is still nearly 1 for all frequencies below around .1 Hz. Thus, the main effect of noise is to reduce coherence at higher frequencies.

Proposition 8.1 holds only when the coherence between $B_j(t)$ and $B_k(t)$ is nonzero. More specifically, the derivation assumed that

$$|H_j(f)| > 0 \quad \text{and} \quad |H_k(f)| > 0$$

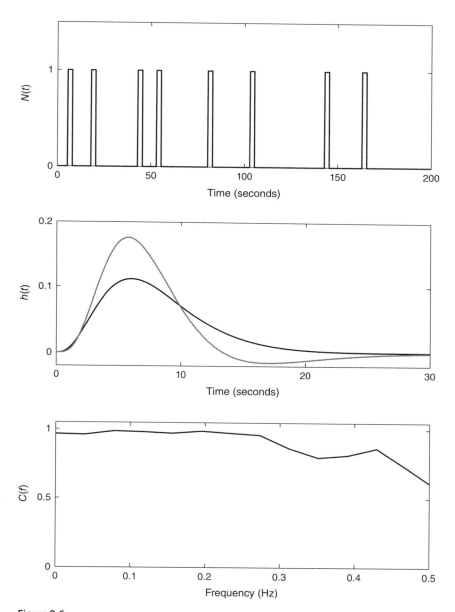

**Figure 8.6**
Coherence (bottom) of BOLD responses generated by convolving the same neural activation (top) with two different hrfs (middlel).

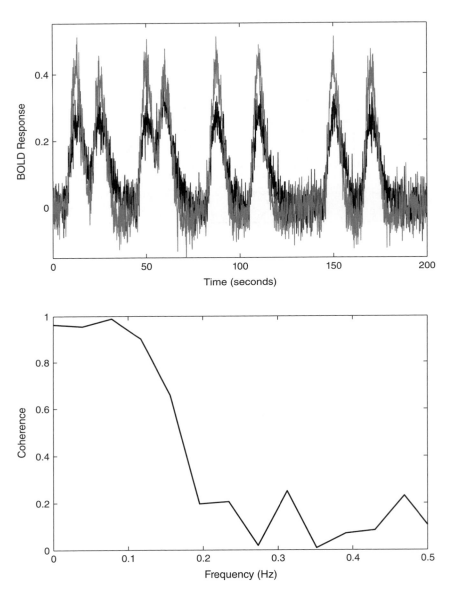

**Figure 8.7**
Two hypothetical BOLD responses and their coherence. The BOLD responses are identical to those used to generate figure 8.6 except that independent zero-mean Gaussian noise has been added at each time point (with standard deviation 0.04).

for all frequencies $f$. If for example, $|H_j(f)| = 0$ for some frequency $f$, then from the identity expressed in equation 8.13, it is clear that $P_{jk}(f) = 0$, and this will be true even if the cross-power spectrum between $N_j(t)$ and $N_k(t)$, $P_{N_j N_k}(f)$, is greater than zero. Coherence is undefined for such frequencies, as one of the power-spectra will also equal zero (see equation 8.13).

Most models of the hrf contain low frequencies but few high frequencies. For example, figure 8.8 shows an hrf defined as the difference of two gamma functions (i.e., see equation 3.7) and its power spectrum. Note that power quickly drops off as frequency increases above about 0.08 Hz. For frequencies above about .15 Hz, power is very small. Equation 8.14 tells us that the cross-power spectrum of $B_j(t)$ and $B_k(t)$ will be small at any frequency for which either hrf has low power. From figure 8.8, we see that hrfs have low power for all high frequencies. Thus, the hrf acts as a low-pass filter. By this we mean that any high-frequency information in the neural activations $N_j(t)$ and $N_k(t)$ will be attenuated by the hrfs and so fail to appear in the observable cross-power spectrum [i.e., in $P_{jk}(f)$]. In other words, high temporal frequencies in the neural activations fail to pass through the "black box" that describes the transformation between neural activation and the BOLD response because of temporal blurring by the hrf. This phenomenon partly explains why the coherence shown in figure 8.6 begins decreasing above 0.3 Hz. For this reason, we expect the coherence $C_{jk}(f)$ to be meaningful only for the low temporal frequencies that are passed by the hrf. In practice, this typically means a range of 0 to around .15 Hz (Sun, Miller, & D'Esposito, 2004).

Coherence can be computed between BOLD responses recorded from any pair of voxels. With 100,000 voxels, this means that potentially $100{,}000 \times 99{,}999 = 9{,}999{,}900{,}000$ possible coherence values could be computed. The exorbitant computing time this would require makes such calculations highly impractical, but even if all these coherence values were computed, Herculean efforts would be required to sift through them all and interpret the results. For these reasons, current applications do not attempt to compute all possible coherence values. Instead, the most common approach is to identify a single region of interest, called the seed, and then to compute the coherence between this region and all other voxels in the brain. In many applications, the seed region will either be an ROI rather than a single voxel, or else some subset of voxels within an ROI. In such cases, the BOLD response used as the seed would typically be constructed by averaging BOLD responses from all selected voxels.

As an illustration of how this method is applied, consider the coherence analysis reported by Sun et al. (2004). In this experiment, subjects performed a bimanual tapping task in an event-related design. In one condition, they were required to alternate tapping with fingers on their right and left hands. Switching between hands like this is facilitated by connections between the hemispheres.

The first step in the coherence analysis is to identify seeds. Sun et al. (2004) used the literature and results from a standard GLM analysis to choose the right and left primary

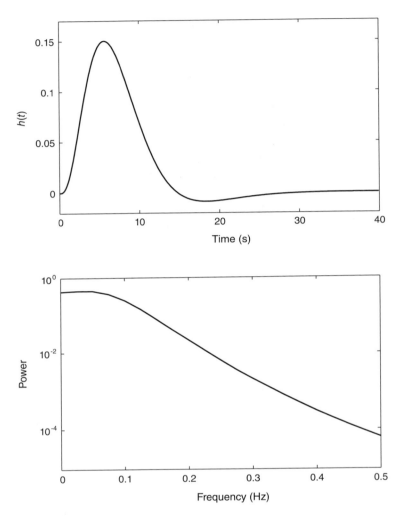

**Figure 8.8**
An hrf (i.e., difference of gamma functions) and its power spectrum.

motor cortices as their seeds. Within each of these regions, they found the 10 voxels with the most significant task-related activation (i.e., the voxels with the 10 largest statistics in the statistical parametric map). Presumably, the BOLD responses from these 10 voxels were then averaged together to produce the seed BOLD response. Next, the average coherence in the bandwidth from 0 to .15 Hz was computed between the seed BOLD response and the BOLD response from every other voxel in the brain.

Figure 8.9 shows a coherence map from one subject in the Sun et al. (2004) experiment that was generated in this method. The $Z$-values denote coordinates in the $Z$-direction, which is parallel to the bore of the magnet. The circle in the left hemisphere of the $Z = 56$ image identifies the location of the seed (left primary motor cortex). Shaded regions denote coherence values between .25 and .80 (higher values are brighter). Note that high coherence was found in expected regions, including (right) primary motor cortex, supplementary motor area, premotor cortex, and posterior parietal cortex.

Hypothesis testing on coherence estimates is also possible. In particular, suppose we want to test whether the coherence between two regions of interest, denoted as regions 1 and 2, is greater than what we might expect from two regions that are not functionally connected in the task we are studying. We begin by selecting two control regions 3 and 4 to serve as two arbitrary reference regions that we expect to be unconnected and not related to the task. Then we wish to test the null hypothesis

$$H_0 : C_{12}(f) = C_{34}(f)$$

against the alternative

$$H_1 : C_{12}(f) > C_{34}(f).$$

Brillinger (1975) showed that if the null hypothesis is true that $C_{12}(f) = C_{34}(f)$ for all frequencies $f$, then when the number of TRs is large, the following statistic is normally distributed:

$$D_{12,34} = \tanh^{-1}[C_{12}(f)] - \tanh^{-1}[C_{34}(f)], \qquad (8.15)$$

where tanh is hyperbolic tangent.[3] Under the null hypothesis, the mean of $D_{12,34} = 0$ and the variance depends on the method used to estimate coherence. For example, if the default MATLAB cohere(B1,B2) command is used,[4] then the variance of $D_{12,34} = \frac{1}{2}$.

3. The hyperbolic tangent of $x$ is defined as

$$\tanh(x) = \frac{e^{2x} - 1}{e^{2x} + 1}.$$

4. In general, the variance of $D_{12,34} = 1/L$, where $L$ is the number of periodograms averaged to compute the components of each coherence. The default in MATLAB is 2.

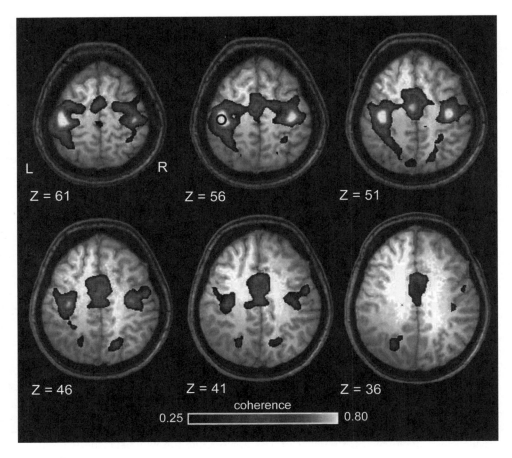

**Figure 8.9**
Coherence values above 0.25 for one subject from the experiment by Sun, Miller, and D'Esposito (2004). Here the coherence was computed between the BOLD response from a seed region in left primary motor cortex (identified by the circle in the $Z = 56$ image) and BOLD responses from all other voxels in the brain. (Reprinted from Sun, Miller, & D'Esposito, "Measuring interregional functional connectivity using coherence and partial coherence analyses of fMRI data," *NeuroImage*, 2004, *21*, 647–658, with permission from Elsevier.)

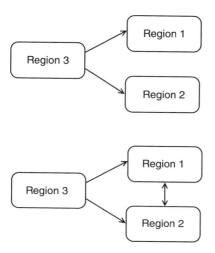

**Figure 8.10**
Two hypothetical neural architectures. In the top panel, regions 1 and 2 are not connected, but they receive a common input from region 3. In the bottom panel, regions 1 and 2 are directly interconnected, and they also receive common input from region 3.

## Partial Coherence

Consider the two alternative connectivity patterns illustrated in figure 8.10. In the architecture shown in the top panel, brain regions 1 and 2 are not connected but they receive a common input from region 3. In the bottom panel, regions 1 and 2 share reciprocal projections and they also receive common input from region 3. In both cases, the BOLD responses recorded from regions 1 and 2 will be correlated and the coherence will be high. As a result, the methods we have considered thus far cannot distinguish between these two possibilities.

In this section we consider a generalized form of coherence that can be used to test between the two figure 8.10 architectures. The generalization is inspired by the notion of partial correlation. In the top panel of figure 8.10, the correlation (and coherence) between the BOLD responses from regions 1 and 2 is due completely to the fact that they are both correlated with the BOLD response from region 3. In other words, if we wanted to predict the activation in region 2, knowledge of activation in region 3 would help, but once this was known, we would gain nothing further by also knowing about activation in region 1. In the bottom panel, however, only some of the correlation between $B_1(t)$ and $B_2(t)$ is due to the fact that both are correlated with $B_3(t)$. So, for example, our prediction of activation in region 2 is again helped by knowledge about the activation in region 3, but now this prediction is further improved by adding additional knowledge about activation in region 1. The partial correlation between BOLD responses $B_1(t)$ and $B_2(t)$ measures the linear correlation between these two BOLD responses that would exist if the influence of region 3 was removed.

Let $\rho_{12}$ denote the Pearson correlation between regions 1 and 2. Then the squared correlation between regions 1 and 2 with region 3 partialled out is defined as (e.g., Cohen, Cohen, West, & Aiken, 2003)

$$\rho_{12\cdot3}^2 = \frac{(\rho_{12} - \rho_{13}\rho_{23})^2}{(1 - \rho_{13}^2)(1 - \rho_{23}^2)}. \tag{8.16}$$

As with standard squared correlation, the squared partial correlation is also bounded below by 0 and above by 1. If the squared partial correlation in equation 8.16 equals 0, then the only possible association between activity in regions 1 and 2 is because of their mutual correlation with region 3. Once the association with region 3 is partialled out, then activity in regions 1 and 2 is uncorrelated. This describes the top panel in figure 8.10, so presumably a partial correlation computed on data collected from this architecture would equal 0. If the squared partial correlation is 1, then activity in region 2 is perfectly predicted from activity in region 1 (and vice versa), even after accounting for activity in region 3.

Partial coherence is modeled after partial correlation, and the equation defining partial coherence has the same form as equation 8.16. However, recall that coherence is analogous to squared correlation. The numerator of equation 8.16 has correlation terms that are not squared. Therefore, to define partial coherence, we need the coherence analogue of correlation, rather than of squared correlation. If coherence is defined as

$$C_{jk}(f) = \frac{[P_{jk}(f)]^2}{P_j(f)P_k(f)},$$

then the appropriate term is

$$Q_{jk}(f) = \sqrt{C_{jk}(f)} = \frac{P_{jk}(f)}{\sqrt{P_j(f)P_k(f)}}. \tag{8.17}$$

Note that, unlike a correlation coefficient, $Q_{jk}(f)$ cannot be negative.[5] This is because the numerator is the cross-power spectrum, which is an amplitude, and amplitudes can never be negative.

Given equation 8.17, we can now define the partial coherence between regions 1 and 2 with region 3 partialled out as

5. Note that $Q_{jk}(f)$ is not equal to the so-called coherency (Rosenberg, Amjad, Breeze, Brillinger, & Halliday, 1989) of $B_j(T)$ and $B_k(T)$. Instead, $Q_{jk}(f)$ is the amplitude of the coherency. The nonstandard term $Q_{jk}(f)$ is introduced here to simplify the exposition [e.g., $Q_{jk}(f)$ is real, whereas coherency is complex].

$$C_{12 \cdot 3}(f) = \frac{[Q_{12}(f) - Q_{13}(f)Q_{23}(f)]^2}{[1 - C_{13}(f)][1 - C_{23}(f)]}. \tag{8.18}$$

Like coherence, partial coherence is also restricted to the interval [0, 1]. And like squared partial correlation, it measures the relative improvement in predicting the BOLD response in region 2 from the BOLD response in region 1 (and vice versa), after we have already accounted for any possible (linear) effects of region 3. Unlike partial correlation, however, the partial coherence measures this ability at each frequency $f$.

Rather than using the BOLD response from some brain region 3 when computing partial coherence, Sun et al. (2004) recommended partialling out a hypothetical BOLD response that is driven purely by the stimulus. The idea here is that different brain regions that are only weakly connected may nevertheless respond strongly to the presentation of a stimulus and that this similar stimulus sensitivity could cause their coherence to be high. If the partial coherence is high after partialling out the effects of a hypothetical region that is driven solely by the stimulus, then we can be confident that the two regions in question are functionally interconnected in some nontrivial way.

The first step in computing this type of partial coherence is to construct a boxcar function that has a value of 1 whenever a stimulus is presented and a value of 0 everywhere else. Next, this boxcar is convolved with a typical hrf to produce a hypothetical BOLD response. Finally, the partial coherence given by equation 8.18 is computed where regions 1 and 2 are the regions of interest, and region 3 is a hypothetical region that generates our constructed BOLD response.

Figure 8.11 shows an example of this type of analysis from Sun et al. (2004) for the two architectures shown in figure 8.10. In both cases, BOLD responses are simulated for regions 1, 2, and 3 by convolving a boxcar function describing stimulus presentations with a canonical hrf. In the top panel, there is no further relationship between regions 1 and 2, but in the bottom panel, these two regions share an additional modulatory input (denoted by M). In the top panel, the partial coherence $C_{12 \cdot 3}(f)$ is low for all frequencies, suggesting that the coherence between regions 1 and 2 is due almost entirely to their common stimulus sensitivity. In the bottom panel, however, partial coherence is high for low frequencies, which suggests that these regions are functionally connected in a more meaningful way (i.e., they are not merely unconnected regions that happen to receive a common input). MATLAB box 8.4 presents code for computing partial coherence with and without the influence modeled in figure 8.11.

## Using the Phase Spectrum to Determine Causality

If the coherence and partial coherence between BOLD responses from regions $i$ and $j$ are large, then we have strong evidence that these two regions are functionally connected in the

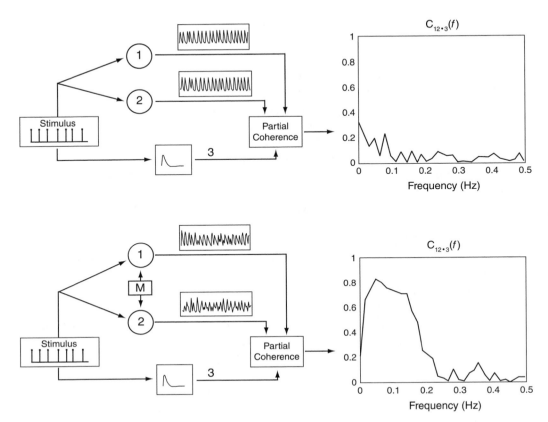

**Figure 8.11**
Partial coherence functions for simulated BOLD responses from the two architectures shown in figure 8.10. (Reprinted from Sun, Miller, & D'Esposito, "Measuring interregional functional connectivity using coherence and partial coherence analyses of fMRI data," *NeuroImage*, 2004, *21*, 647–658, with permission from Elsevier.)

task we are studying. However, we cannot tell from this analysis alone whether region $i$ causes activation in region $j$ or vice versa. Coherence is a measure of correlation, not causation. One way to infer the direction of causality from coherence results is to gather information about which region was activated first.

Coherence analysis focuses on the *amplitude* of the cross-spectral density $S_{jk}(f)$ (see equation 8.7). In this section, we consider the phase or argument of the cross-spectral density because, as we will see, the phase carries information about the temporal ordering of the neural activations that are driving $B_j(t)$ and $B_k(t)$. If activation in region $j$ causes activation in region $i$, then the BOLD response in region $i$ should be similar to the BOLD response in region $j$ (i.e., the coherence should be high), but shifted ahead in time. The phase spectrum of $S_{jk}(f)$ provides an estimate of this temporal shift.

**MATLAB Box 8.4**

Compute partial coherence between two BOLD responses without and with extra influence between them (as in figure 8.11)

```
clear all; close all; clc;                    % Clear all workspaces
ntime=2000; T=200; t=T*[0:ntime-1]/ntime;    % define time
tlag=10;   % lag of n2 relative to n = tlag*T/ntime

n=4; lamda=2; n2=7; lamda2=2; a=.3;    % Create the hrf
hrf=(t.^(n-1)).*exp(-t/lamda)/((lamda^n)*factorial(n-1));

% Create the boxcars
n=zeros(1,ntime); n(26:50)=ones(1,25); n(151:175)=ones(1,25);
n(401:425)=ones(1,25); n(501:525)=ones(1,25); n(776:800)=ones(1,25);
n(1001:1025)=ones(1,25); n(1401:1425)=ones(1,25); n(1601:1625)=ones(1,25);
n2=[zeros(1,tlag),n(1:ntime-tlag)];    % lags behind n
n3=[zeros(1,250),n(1:ntime-250)];    % lags further behind n

% Convolve hrf & boxcar, add noise
B1wo=conv(hrf,n)/10; B2wo=conv(hrf,n2)/10;
B3=B1wo(1:ntime)+.03*randn(1,ntime);
B1wo=B1wo(1:ntime)+.03*randn(1,ntime);
B2wo=B2wo(1:ntime)+.03*randn(1,ntime);
B1=conv(hrf,n+n3)/10; B2=conv(hrf,n2+n3)/10;
B1=B1(1:ntime)+.03*randn(1,ntime); B2=B2(1:ntime)+.03*randn(1,ntime);

% Compute partial coherence when there is no further influence between 1 & 2
[C12wo,freq]=cohere(B1wo,B2wo,[],[]);
[C13wo,freq]=cohere(B1wo,B3,[],[]);
[C23wo,freq]=cohere(B2wo,B3,[],[]);
Q12wo=abs(sqrt(C12wo)); Q13wo=abs(sqrt(C13wo)); Q23wo=abs(sqrt(C23wo));
C12dot3wo=(Q12wo-Q13wo.*Q23wo).^2./((1-C13wo).*(1-C23wo));
freq=freq*ntime/(T*2);
subplot(2,1,1); plot(freq, C12dot3wo); axis([0 0.5 0 1]);

% Compute partial coherence when there is extra influence between 1 & 2
[C12,freq]=cohere(B1,B2,[],[]);
[C13,freq]=cohere(B1,B3,[],[]);
[C23,freq]=cohere(B2,B3,[],[]);
Q12=abs(sqrt(C12)); Q13=abs(sqrt(C13)); Q23=abs(sqrt(C23));
C12dot3=(Q12-Q13.*Q23).^2./((1-C13).*(1-C23));
freq=freq*ntime/(T*2);
subplot(2,1,2); plot(freq, C12dot3); axis([0 0.5 0 1]);
```

To get an intuitive appreciation for what an analysis of the phase spectrum has to offer, consider again figure 8.3, which shows two BOLD responses and their cross-correlation function. The BOLD responses were generated from two neural activations that were identical except that the neural response used to produce $B_k(t)$ lagged 10 seconds behind the neural response used to produce $B_j(t)$. Note that the peak of the cross-correlation function occurs at $-10$ seconds. This is because shifting $B_k(t)$ backward in time by 10 seconds maximizes its correlation with $B_j(t)$. The cross-power spectrum conveys no information about such temporal shifts because shifting the cross-correlation to the right or left does not affect the frequency of sine and cosine waves in its Fourier representation. However, it does affect the phase of these waves. So information about the temporal shift seen in figure 8.3 should be maintained in the phase spectrum of the Fourier transform of the cross-correlation function.

Recall (from equation 8.7) that the cross-spectral density of BOLD responses $B_j(t)$ and $B_k(t)$, denoted by $S_{jk}(f)$, is the Fourier transform of the cross-correlation function $R_{jk}(t)$:

$$S_{jk}(f) = \Im[R_{jk}(t)].$$

$S_{jk}(f)$ is a complex-valued function, because it has both real and imaginary parts. The cross-power spectrum $P_{jk}(f)$ is defined as the amplitude of $S_{jk}(f)$ [i.e., $P_{jk}(f) = |S_{jk}(f)|$; i.e., see equation 8.8]. The phase spectrum of $B_j(t)$ and $B_k(t)$, denoted by $\varphi_{jk}(f)$, is defined as the phase of $S_{jk}(f)$; that is, as

$$\varphi_{jk}(f) = \arg[S_{jk}(f)], \tag{8.19}$$

where arg is defined as in equation 8.6.

To see how the phase spectrum can be used to determine the temporal order of neural events, suppose $B_j(t)$ and $B_k(t)$ are produced from identical neural activations $N_j(t)$ and $N_k(t)$, except that $N_j(t)$ occurs $\tau$ seconds after $N_k(t)$. In other words, suppose

$$N_j(t) = N_k(t - \tau).$$

Proposition 8.2 establishes the key result that makes the phase spectrum useful for determining temporal order.

**Proposition 8.2**    Suppose the neural activation $N_j(t)$ that produces BOLD response $B_j(t)$ is identical to the neural activation $N_k(t)$ that produces BOLD response $B_k(t)$, except that $N_j(t)$ occurs $\tau$ seconds after $N_k(t)$ [i.e., so $N_j(t) = N_k(t - \tau)$]. Denote the phase spectrum between $B_j(t)$ and $B_k(t)$ by $\varphi_{jk}(f)$. Then

$$\tau = -\frac{1}{2\pi}\frac{d\varphi_{ij}(f)}{df}.$$

In other words, the delay between $N_j(t)$ and $N_k(t)$ is proportional to the slope of the phase spectrum, and the constant of proportionality equals $-\frac{1}{2\pi}$.

**Derivation**   Proposition 8.1 showed that the coherence between $B_j(t)$ and $B_k(t)$ equals the coherence between $N_j(t)$ and $N_k(t)$. It is straightforward to show that a similar result holds for the phase spectrum; that is, the phase spectrum of $B_j(t)$ and $B_k(t)$ equals the phase spectrum of $N_j(t)$ and $N_k(t)$ (i.e., repeat the proposition 8.1 derivation with the cross-spectral density substituted for the cross-power spectrum).

Because $N_j(t) = N_k(t - \tau)$, the cross-correlation function between $N_j(t)$ and $N_k(t)$ is equal to

$$R_{N_j N_k}(t) = E[N_j(T + t)N_k(T)]$$

$$= E[N_k(T + t - \tau)N_k(T)]$$

$$= R_{N_k N_k}(t - \tau).$$

Therefore, the cross-spectral density of $N_j(t)$ and $N_k(t)$, denoted by $S_{N_j N_k}(f)$, equals

$$S_{N_j N_k}(f) = \Im[R_{N_j N_k}(t)]$$

$$= \Im[R_{N_k N_k}(t - \tau)]$$

$$= e^{-i2\pi f \tau}\Im[R_{N_k N_k}(t)].$$

The latter equality holds by the shift property of Fourier transforms (e.g., Bracewell, 1965).

The phase spectrum of $N_j(t)$ and $N_k(t)$ is therefore

$$\varphi_{N_j N_k}(f) = \arg[S_{N_j N_k}(f)]$$

$$= \arg\{e^{-i2\pi f \tau}\Im[R_{N_k N_k}(t)]\}$$

$$= \arg(e^{-i2\pi f \tau}) + \arg\{\Im[R_{N_k N_k}(t)]\}$$

$$= \arg(e^{-i2\pi f \tau}).$$

The third equality holds because the argument of a product equals the sum of the arguments in that product (e.g., Churchill, Brown, & Verhey, 1974), and the last equality holds because the Fourier transform of any autocorrelation function is real. Therefore

$$\arg\{\Im[R_{N_k N_k}(t)]\} = 0.$$

Now any complex number $z$ can be written as

$z = x + iy = |z|e^{i\phi}$,

where $|z|$ is the amplitude of $z$ and $\phi$ is the phase. Therefore,

$\varphi_{N_j N_k}(f) = \arg(e^{-i2\pi f\tau}) = -2\pi f\tau$.

As mentioned earlier, the phase spectrum of $B_j(t)$ and $B_k(t)$ equals the phase spectrum of $N_j(t)$ and $N_k(t)$. Therefore,

$\varphi_{jk}(f) = -2\pi f\tau$,

from which the result easily follows.                                              ∎

Figure 8.12 shows an illustration of this method for determining the temporal order of neural activations that comes from Sun, Miller, and D'Esposito (2005). First, two identical neural activations (i.e., spike trains) were generated, except one was delayed 1 second after the other. Next, both spike trains were convolved with the same hrf, and then independent noise was added to each (see figure 8.12A). This process produced the simulated BOLD responses shown in figure 8.12B. Figure 8.12C shows the coherence between the two BOLD responses. As expected, coherence is high for frequencies below 0.15 Hz. Finally, figure 8.12D shows the phase spectrum of the BOLD responses. Note that for frequencies below 0.15 Hz, this plot is approximately linear with a slope of around −6.67 (i.e., for a run of 0.15, the rise is approximately −1). Proposition 8.2 therefore tells us that

$$\hat{\tau} = -\frac{1}{2\pi}(-6.67) = 1.06 \text{ seconds}.$$

As the actual delay was 1 second, this is very close. Rather than judge the slope visually, as we did to obtain our estimate of −6.67, Sun et al. (2005) used linear regression and arrived at −6.25, which produced the estimate $\hat{\tau} = .9954$ seconds.

Although coherence is straightforward to compute using the cohere command in the MATLAB signal processing toolbox, unfortunately the same is not true for phase. MATLAB has a phase command (i.e., angle), but because of the discrete time sampling properties of fMRI data, this command, by itself, is insufficient for the phase analysis described in this section. Estimation of the phase spectrum shown in figure 8.12D used a much more sophisticated algorithm. See Sun et al. (2005) for details.

Among the earliest applications of proposition 8.2 to neuroscience data was reported by Rosenberg et al. (1989), who used it on simultaneous single-unit recordings to determine temporal lag. Its use in fMRI research presents some additional and significant challenges. With single-unit recordings, time is essentially a continuous variable. In fMRI, however, our sampling rate is limited by the TR. With a typical TR of 2.5 seconds, the sampling rate is only 0.4 Hz (i.e., 1/2.5). Using continuous sampling, Rosenberg et al. (1989) estimated one delay to be 29.8 milliseconds. In the figure 8.12 simulation, sampling is nearly con-

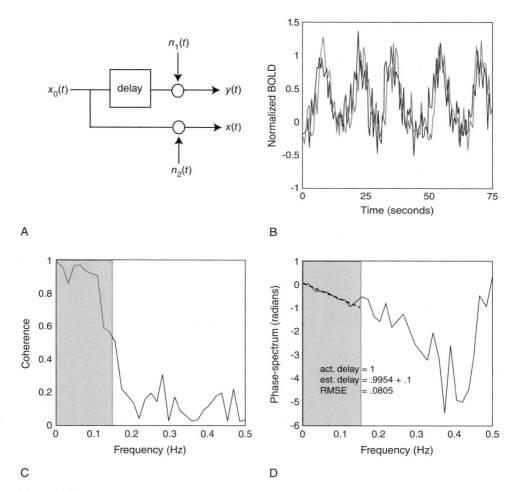

**Figure 8.12**
Coherence (C) and phase spectrum (D) of the BOLD responses shown in (B). The two BOLD responses were generated from the architecture shown in (A). First, two identical neural activations (i.e., spike trains) were generated except one was delayed 1 second after the other. Next, both spike trains were convolved with the same hrf, and then independent noise was added to each. (Reprinted from Sun, Miller, & D'Esposito, "Measuring temporal dynamics of functional networks using phase spectrum of fMRI data," *NeuroImage*, 2005, *28*, 227–237, with permission from Elsevier.)

tinuous, and the delay was 1 second. With many cognitive tasks, it is not difficult to imagine that the delays we would be interested in would typically be much less than 1 second. For example, delays of 50–200 milliseconds might be of interest. If we only sample the relevant BOLD responses every 2.5 seconds, is it reasonable to expect any method to identify a temporal lag between signals of 100 milliseconds?

One key result that provides an important clue about this issue is the Nyquist–Shannon sampling theorem. As we saw in chapter 4, this result specifies that the highest frequency that one could ever hope to measure is half the sampling rate. Thus, if the TR is 2.5 seconds, which means the sampling rate is 0.4 Hz, then the highest temporal frequency that can theoretically be measured in an fMRI experiment is 0.2 Hz. The idea is that we must sample each sine wave at least twice per cycle to determine its frequency. And it should be emphasized that this is the theoretical minimum. Accurate estimation requires significant oversampling of the data.

We have already seen that because the hrf acts as a low-pass filter, coherence and phase spectrum analyses focus on frequencies in the band from 0 to 0.15 Hz. Thus, theoretically, a TR of 2.5 seconds is fast enough. In practice, though, this upper limit of 0.15 Hz may seem uncomfortably close to the theoretical lower Nyquist limit of 0.2 Hz, and we might therefore worry about the quality of our coherence and phase spectrum estimates near 0.15 Hz. This is more of a problem for phase spectrum analysis than for coherence analysis. In coherence analysis, we can use the equation 8.15 statistic to determine whether the coherence between the BOLD responses from a pair of regions is significant for each separate frequency below 0.15 Hz. If we find significance for all frequencies below, say, 0.1 Hz, we would probably conclude that the two regions are functionally connected. In this case, poor coherence estimates between 0.1 and 0.15 Hz would not greatly affect our conclusion. However, in phase spectrum analysis, linear regression is used to estimate the slope of the phase spectrum between 0 and 0.15 Hz. In this case, poor estimates of the phase between 0.1 and 0.15 Hz could greatly affect this single slope estimate. Of course, we could limit the regression to frequencies between 0 and, say, 0.10 Hz. This excludes data near the Nyquist limit, but anytime we exclude data from a regression analysis, we reduce statistical power.

A different potential problem occurs when the delay of interest is short. The decision-making process in phase spectrum analysis includes two stages. First, by determining whether the slope of the phase spectrum (for low frequencies) is positive or negative, we decide which region is causing activation in the other; that is, we decide upon the direction of causality. Second, by determining the exact slope of the phase spectrum, we estimate the temporal lag between regions. If the temporal lag estimate is off by 500 milliseconds, this could catastrophically affect the outcome of the first decision when the true delay is short. In many cognitive tasks, response times are of the order 1 second or less. In such cases, the delay between any two regions that participate in the task will be at most a few hundred milliseconds, and so the direction of causality may be difficult to determine.

One final issue that could limit the usefulness of proposition 8.2 is the strong assumption it makes that the neural activations in the two regions of interest (e.g., regions $j$ and $k$) are identical, except one is shifted ahead in time. Of course, real brain regions are not simple delay devices. Instead, we expect them to actively process the neural activations they receive and to produce their own activations that are some transformation of these inputs (albeit delayed). Unfortunately, I know of no attempts to systematically investigate how violations of this strong temporal-shift assumption affect the initial linearity and slope of the phase spectrum. As a consequence, at this time, the results of applying proposition 8.2 must be interpreted cautiously.

## Conclusions

All of the methods discussed in previous chapters of this book could be classified as exploratory data analysis techniques, as none of them test strong *a priori* predictions derived from a specific model. For example, GLM approaches typically repeat the same analyses on every voxel in the brain in an effort to find *all* task-related voxels, regardless of one's theoretical orientation. In contrast, coherence analysis and also Granger causality, which we consider in the next chapter, are probably best used as confirmatory data analysis tools. One reason for this is sheer numbers. Whereas a complete GLM analysis might require 100,000 or so separate applications (i.e., one for each voxel), as we saw earlier, a coherence analysis could be performed on each pair of voxels, thereby raising the number of possible applications to the staggering figure of $100,000 \times 99,999$, or 9,999,900,000. This enormous number necessitates some careful thought about which subset of voxels or regions to study. A strong theory is critical to this selection process.

# 9 Granger Causality

As we saw in chapter 8, coherence analysis provides a powerful tool for determining whether two brain regions are functionally interconnected in a particular task. It can also be used to assess the direction of causality by estimating the temporal lag between the onsets of two neural activations. In this chapter, we consider an alternative method for assessing causality that has its roots in the economics literature. The method was originally proposed in 1969 by Granger and is now known as Granger causality. The idea is conceptually simple. If event X causes event Y, then knowledge of past values of X should improve our prediction of the current value of Y.

As before, let $B_i(t)$ denote the BOLD response in ROI (or voxel) $i$ at TR $= t$. The first step is to formalize what we mean by prediction. In *linear autoregressive prediction*, we attempt to predict the value of $B_i(t)$ from a linear combination of earlier BOLD responses from this same region. The *order* of the resulting model is the number of previous time points that are used in the prediction. So an autoregressive model of order $p$ for region $i$ would be

$$B_i(t) = a_{i1}B_i(t-1) + a_{i2}B_i(t-2) + \cdots + a_{ip}B_i(t-p) + \varepsilon_i(t), \tag{9.1}$$

where $\varepsilon_i(t)$ is the error term, which in Granger causality is assumed to be normally distributed with mean 0 and variance $\sigma_i^2$.

The error variance, $\sigma_i^2$, is a measure of the accuracy of prediction. To see this, note that we can rewrite equation 9.1 as

$$\varepsilon_i(t) = [B_i(t)] - [a_{i1}B_i(t-1) + a_{i2}B_i(t-2) + \cdots + a_{ip}B_i(t-p)],$$

where the term in the first set of square brackets is the current observed value of the BOLD response, and the terms in the second set of square brackets are the current value of the BOLD response as predicted by the model. Thus, if the model exactly predicts the BOLD response, the error $\varepsilon_i(t)$ will always equal zero, and consequently the error variance will be zero. If the predictions are poor, then the magnitude of the error will be large, and hence the error variance will be large (i.e., because the mean error is always zero).

Figure 9.1 shows examples of this model. To create this figure, a BOLD response was first simulated by convolving a boxcar function with a canonical hrf (i.e., a gamma

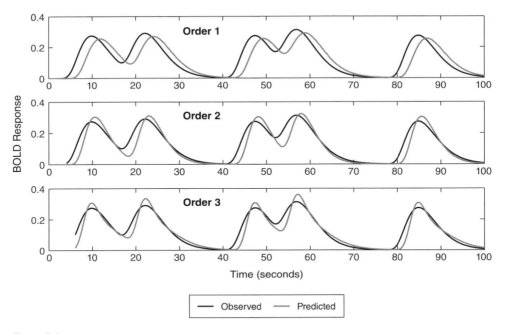

**Figure 9.1**
In each panel, the black curve denotes the same simulated BOLD response. The gray curve is the predicted BOLD response of an autoregressive model of order 1 (top), 2 (middle panel) or 3 (bottom panel).

function). No noise was added in an effort to improve the visual comparison between observed and predicted responses. The simulated BOLD response becomes the observed data. Next, three autoregressive models were created of orders 1, 2, and 3, respectively. Figure 9.1 shows time as a continuous variable, but of course, in any real fMRI experiment, time is discrete because the BOLD response is sampled only every TR seconds. Therefore, the autoregressive models assumed a TR of 2 seconds. In other words, for example, the order 1 model predicts that the BOLD response at time 20 seconds is equal to

$$B_i(20 \text{ seconds}) = a_{i1}B_i(18 \text{ seconds}) + \varepsilon_i(20 \text{ seconds}).$$

Similarly, the order 3 models predicts this same response is equal to

$$B_i(20 \text{ seconds}) = a_{i1}B_i(18 \text{ seconds}) + a_{i2}B_i(16 \text{ seconds})$$

$$+ a_{i3}B_i(14 \text{ seconds}) + \varepsilon_i(20 \text{ seconds}).$$

Fitting these three models to the observed BOLD response requires estimating the unknown values of the $a_{ij}$. As we will see shortly, the equation 9.1 autoregressive model is a special case of the GLM, and as a result, the $a_{ij}$ parameters can be estimated (optimally) via the

**MATLAB Box 9.1**
Create and fit autoregressive models of orders 1, 2, and 3 (as in figure 9.1)

```
clear all; close all; clc;                     % Clear all workspaces
ntime=2000; T=200; t=T*[0:ntime-1]/ntime;      % define time
TR=2;                                          % TR in seconds
TR=TR*ntime/T;

n=4; lamda=2;    % Create the hrf
hrf=(t.^(n-1)).*exp(-t/lamda)/((lamda^n)*factorial(n-1));

% Create the boxcar & BOLD response
n=zeros(1,ntime); n(26:50)=ones(1,25); n(151:175)=ones(1,25);
n(401:425)=ones(1,25); n(501:525)=ones(1,25); n(776:800)=ones(1,25);
n(1001:1025)=ones(1,25); n(1401:1425)=ones(1,25); n(1601:1625)=ones(1,25);
B=conv(hrf,n)/10; B=B(1:ntime);

% Order 1
X=[B(1:ntime-TR)]'; Y=[B(TR+1:ntime)]';
A=(inv(X'*X))*X'*Y; P=X*A;
tt=(TR+1)*T/ntime:T/ntime:T;
subplot(3,1,1); plot(tt,Y,tt,P); axis([0 200 0 .4]);

% Order 2
X=[[B(TR+1:ntime-TR)]' [B(1:ntime-2*TR)]']; Y=[B(2*TR+1:ntime)]';
A=(inv(X'*X))*X'*Y; P=X*A;
tt=(2*TR+1)*T/ntime:T/ntime:T;
subplot(3,1,2); plot(tt,Y,tt,P); axis([0 200 0 .4]);

% Order 3
X=[[B(2*TR+1:ntime-TR)]' [B(TR+1:ntime-2*TR)]' [B(1:ntime-3*TR)]'];
Y=[B(3*TR+1:ntime)]'; A=(inv(X'*X))*X'*Y; P=X*A;
tt=(3*TR+1)*T/ntime:T/ntime:T;
subplot(3,1,3); plot(tt,Y,tt,P); axis([0 200 0 .4]);
```

normal equations (i.e., see equation 5.13). MATLAB code that will produce figure 9.1 is shown in MATLAB box 9.1.

Several features of figure 9.1 are of interest. First, note that even the order 1 model makes reasonably accurate predictions. This is not a general property of all order 1 auto-regressive models. Rather, the figure 9.1 success is because the length of the TR (2 seconds) is much less than the temporal blurring induced by the hrf (i.e., 25–30 seconds). Because of this blurring, the BOLD response at any point in time is not hugely different from the BOLD response 2 seconds earlier. In other words, because the BOLD response varies so slowly in time, it is possible to accurately predict what the BOLD response looks like 2 seconds in the future.

Second, note that the BOLD response predicted by the order 1 model is nearly equal to the observed BOLD response shifted ahead in time by 2 seconds. In fact, the best-fitting value of $a_{i1}$ was 0.922, so the order 1 model was

$$B_i(t) = .922B_i(t-1) + \varepsilon_i(t),$$

where $t-1$ now refers to a time one TR before time $t$. Thus, the order 1 model predicts that the BOLD response at TR $t$ is almost identical to the BOLD response one TR earlier.

Third, note that the predictions of the order 2 model are significantly better than the predictions of the order 1 model. The order 2 predicted response still lags behind the observed response, but by much less, and it is no longer a simple translation of the observed BOLD response. The best-fitting version of the order 2 model was

$$B_i(t) = 1.55B_i(t-1) - .68B_i(t-2) + \varepsilon_i(t),$$

so the contribution of the previous TR is moderated down by the contribution from two TRs in the past [i.e., the weight on $B_i(t-2)$ is negative].

Finally, note that the order 3 model is only slightly more accurate than the order 2 model. Because the order 3 model has one more parameter than the order 2 model, one must question whether this extra parameter significantly improves the fit of the model. We will consider a statistical test that answers this question later in the chapter.

Granger causality uses equation 9.1 to predict the current value of $B_i(t)$ from previous BOLD responses recorded from that same region. A similar model is constructed to predict the current BOLD response in region $j$ [i.e., $B_j(t)$] from previous BOLD responses recorded from region $j$

$$B_j(t) = a_{j1}B_j(t-1) + a_{j2}B_j(t-2) + \cdots + a_{jp}B_j(t-p) + \varepsilon_j(t)$$

$$= \sum_{k=1}^{p} a_{jk}B_j(t-k) + \varepsilon_j(t). \tag{9.2}$$

The fundamental assumption of Granger causality is that if activation in region $i$ causes activation in region $j$, then adding prior BOLD responses from region $i$ to the equation 9.2 model should improve our prediction of $B_j(t)$ (i.e., decrease the error variance). Thus, our next step is to form the more complex model

$$B_j(t) = d_{i1}B_i(t-1) + d_{j1}B_j(t-1) + d_{i2}B_i(t-2) + d_{j2}B_j(t-2) + \cdots$$

$$+ d_{ip}B_i(t-p) + d_{jp}B_j(t-p) + \varepsilon_{j|ij}(t)$$

$$= \sum_{k=1}^{p} [d_{ik}B_i(t-k) + d_{jk}B_j(t-k)] + \varepsilon_{j|ij}(t). \tag{9.3}$$

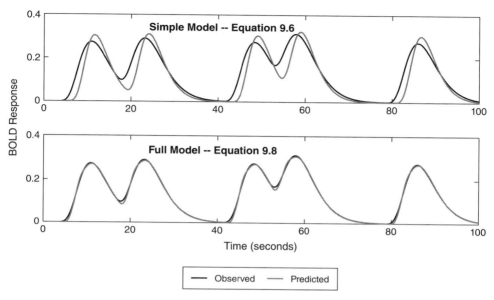

**Figure 9.2**
In each panel, the black curve denotes the same simulated BOLD response. The gray curve is the predicted BOLD response of an autoregressive model of order 2. In the top panel, the model only includes prior observations from the same voxel (i.e., the equation 9.6 model; this panel is the same as the middle panel from figure 9.1). The model in the bottom panel also includes prior observations from a voxel that caused the observed BOLD response (i.e., the equation 9.8 model).

Note that equation 9.3 has twice as many terms as equation 9.2, as there are $p$ previous $B_j$ terms on the right as well as $p$ previous $B_i$ terms. Each has its own regression weight. So $d_{ik}$ denotes the regression weight parameter on the BOLD response from region $i$ that was observed $k$ TRs before the current TR (which is denoted by $t$), and $d_{jk}$ denotes the analogous parameter[1] for the BOLD response from region $j$. The error variance $\varepsilon_{j|ij}(t)$ is again assumed to be normally distributed with mean 0, although now the variance is denoted by $\sigma^2_{j|ij}$, because we assume the accuracy of the equations 9.2 and 9.3 models may differ. The subscript on the error term and on the error variance, $j|ij$, indicates that the error is on predictions of the BOLD response in region $j$ from a model that considers prior BOLD responses from both regions $i$ and $j$.

Figure 9.2 shows an example of the equation 9.3 model and compares its accuracy with the simpler equation 9.2 model. The observed BOLD response, $B_j(t)$, was generated from the neural activation in a hypothetical region $i$ in the following way. First, the BOLD

---

1. Note that we will use the letters $c$ and $d$ to denote regression weights in the more complex models (e.g., equation 9.3) and $a$ to denote regression weights in the simple models (e.g., equation 9.2).

response in region $i$, which is identical to the observed BOLD response shown in figure 9.1, was simulated by convolving a spike train with a canonical hrf (i.e., a gamma function). Next, the neural activation in region $j$ was identical to the activation in region $i$, except delayed by 1 second. This delayed neural activation was then convolved with a different hrf (i.e., difference of gammas) to produce the observed BOLD response in figure 9.2.

The top panel of figure 9.2 shows the best fit of the simple equation 9.2 model of order 2 when the TR is 2 seconds. This panel is essentially the same as the middle panel of figure 9.1. The bottom panel of figure 9.2 shows the best fit of the more complex equation 9.3 model. Note that this fit is virtually perfect, despite the different hrfs used to generate $B_i(t)$ and $B_j(t)$. The best-fitting version of the simple model was

$$B_j(t) = 1.59B_j(t-1) - .75B_j(t-2) + \varepsilon_j(t),$$

whereas the best-fitting version of the complex model was

$$B_j(t) = .56B_i(t-1) + .85B_j(t-1) - .09B_i(t-2) - .38B_j(t-2) + \varepsilon_{j|ij}(t).$$

Note that the greatest weight in this latter model is placed on prior observations from region $j$. Nevertheless, substantial weight is also placed on observations from region $i$, and figure 9.2 makes it clear that these region $i$ contributions substantially improve the fit of the model. MATLAB box 9.2 shows code that could be used to produce figure 9.2 (although different hrfs are not included).

In the figure 9.2 example, it seems clear that adding prior observations from region $i$ improved our ability to predict the current BOLD response in region $j$. In such cases, the conclusion from Granger causality is that activation in region $i$ is causing activation in region $j$. But how can we quantify the amount of this causality? And how can we test statistically whether the improvement in fit seen in figure 9.2 is due to causality rather than to the fact that the more complex model has extra free parameters? We next consider a method of answering the first question, and then later we consider the second question.

## Quantitative Measures of Causality

The key to constructing a quantitative measure of causality is to realize, as mentioned before, that the variance parameter associated with the error term can be interpreted as a measure of goodness-of-fit. The error terms in each model are literally the mispredictions of the model. In the bottom panel of figure 9.2, the fit is almost perfect. Therefore, the error terms are all almost zero, and as a result the variance of these errors will be very small. In contrast, in the top panel of figure 9.2, at some time points the fit is good and at other time points the predicted BOLD response is substantially different than the observed BOLD response. In this case, some errors are small and some are large, and therefore the error variance is large.

**MATLAB Box 9.2**

Compute Granger causality $F_{x \to y}$ (i.e., a measure of how strongly the BOLD response in voxel or region $x$ causes activation in voxel or region $y$). Also produce figure 9.2

```
clear all; close all; clc;                        % Clear all workspaces
ntime=2000; T=200; t=T*[0:ntime-1]/ntime;         % define time
TR=2; TR=TR*ntime/T;                              % TR in seconds
lag=1; lag=lag*ntime/T;                           % ny lag in seconds

n=4; lamda=2;                                     % Create the hrf
hrf=(t.^(n-1)).*exp(-t/lamda)/((lamda^n)*factorial(n-1));

% Create the boxcars & BOLD responses
n=zeros(1,ntime); n(26:50)=ones(1,25); n(151:175)=ones(1,25);
n(401:425)=ones(1,25); n(501:525)=ones(1,25); n(776:800)=ones(1,25);
n(1001:1025)=ones(1,25); n(1401:1425)=ones(1,25); n(1601:1625)=ones(1,25);
Bx=conv(hrf,n)/10; Bx=Bx(1:ntime);
ny=[zeros(1,lag), n(1:ntime-lag)]; By=conv(hrf,ny)/10; By=By(1:ntime);

% Simple Order 2 model
X=[[By(TR+1:ntime-TR)]' [By(1:ntime-2*TR)]']; Y=[By(2*TR+1:ntime)]';
A=(inv(X'*X))*X'*Y; P=X*A;
tt=(2*TR+1)*T/ntime:T/ntime:T;
subplot(2,1,1); plot(tt,Y,tt,P); axis([0 200 0 .4]);
sigsimp=(Y-P)'*(Y-P)                              % sum of squared error

% Full Order 2 model
X=[[By(TR+1:ntime-TR)]' [Bx(TR+1:ntime-TR)]' [By(1:ntime-2*TR)]'
[Bx(1:ntime-2*TR)]'];
Y=[By(2*TR+1:ntime)]';
A=(inv(X'*X))*X'*Y; P=X*A;
tt=(2*TR+1)*T/ntime:T/ntime:T;
subplot(2,1,2); plot(tt,Y,tt,P); axis([0 200 0 .4]);

sigfull=(Y-P)'*(Y-P)                              % sum of squared error
Fij=log(sigsimp/sigfull)                          % Granger causality
```

The critical test for causality is therefore to ask whether $\sigma_{j|ij}^2 < \sigma_j^2$. If it is, then adding previous values of the BOLD response from region $i$ improves our ability to predict the current BOLD response in region $j$. This seems straightforward, but there are two complications—one statistical and one logical.

The statistical complication is that the more complex equation 9.3 model has more free parameters than the simpler equation 9.2 model. In fact, equation 9.2 is a special case of equation 9.3 in which the $d_{ik}$ of equation 9.3 all equal 0 and each $d_{jk} = a_{jk}$. Because of this, equation 9.2 can never fit better than equation 9.3, and the only time the fits will be equal is if equation 9.2 fits the data perfectly. If there is any noise in the data, a perfect fit will occur with probability 0, so in any real application, the predictions of equation 9.3 will be better than the predictions of equation 9.2, and therefore $\sigma_{j|ij}^2 < \sigma_j^2$. Consider the case though where the simpler model is correct but there is noise in the data. In this case, the extra parameters of the more complex model will fit the noise. As a result, $\sigma_{j|ij}^2$ will be smaller than $\sigma_j^2$, but only by a small amount. Thus, to solve this statistical complication, we need to test the null hypothesis that the simpler model is correct (in which case the extra parameters of the more complex model are just fitting noise) against the alternative that the more complex model is capturing some real structure in the data that is missed by the simpler model. In the current case, that real structure is a causal connection between the two regions. We will develop this statistical test in a later section of this chapter.

The logical complication is that regions $i$ and $j$ might be reciprocally connected, so that neither is causing activation in the other. This conclusion (i.e., that neither region causes activation in the other) assumes a definition of causality that includes direction. A more liberal definition might conclude that reciprocally connected regions are each causing activation in the other. In either case, however, if $\sigma_{j|ij}^2 < \sigma_j^2$, we might conclude that region $i$ is functionally connected to region $j$, but we could not know from this information alone whether this connection is unidirectional.

To determine whether the causality is unidirectional (i.e., that activation in region $i$ causes activation in region $j$, but not vice versa) requires constructing and fitting the model analogous to equation 9.3 that attempts to predict activation in region $i$

$$B_i(t) = c_{i1}B_i(t-1) + c_{j1}B_j(t-1) + c_{i2}B_i(t-2) + c_{j2}B_j(t-2) + \cdots$$

$$+ c_{ip}B_i(t-p) + c_{jp}B_j(t-p) + \varepsilon_{i|ij}(t)$$

$$= \sum_{k=1}^{p}[c_{ik}B_i(t-k) + c_{jk}B_j(t-k)] + \varepsilon_{i|ij}(t), \tag{9.4}$$

where $\varepsilon_{i|ij}(t)$ is normally distributed with mean 0 and variance $\sigma_{i|ij}^2$. Now, if activation in region $i$ causes activation in region $j$, but not vice versa, then it should be the case that $\sigma_{j|ij}^2 < \sigma_j^2$; that is, adding previous BOLD responses from region $i$ (significantly) improves our prediction of the region $j$ data, but $\sigma^2_{i|ij} \not< \sigma^2_i$ (adding previous BOLD response from region $j$ does not significantly improve our prediction of the region $i$ data).

In summary, we have four models that must be fit to the data:

$$B_i(t) = \sum_{k=1}^{p} a_{ik} B_i(t-k) + \varepsilon_i(t), \tag{9.5}$$

$$B_j(t) = \sum_{k=1}^{p} a_{jk} B_j(t-k) + \varepsilon_j(t), \tag{9.6}$$

$$B_i(t) = \sum_{k=1}^{p} [c_{ik} B_i(t-k) + c_{jk} B_j(t-k)] + \varepsilon_{i|ij}(t), \tag{9.7}$$

and

$$B_j(t) = \sum_{k=1}^{p} [d_{ik} B_i(t-k) + d_{jk} B_j(t-k)] + \varepsilon_{j|ij}(t). \tag{9.8}$$

Each model has a set of unknown regression weights and an error variance. In addition, because equations 9.7 and 9.8 have terms in common, the error terms associated with these two models will be positively correlated. As we will see, accounting for this correlation will be important in our decisions about causality, so we will also need to estimate this parameter. In particular, let $\mathrm{cov}_{ij}$ denote the covariance between these two errors; that is,

$$\mathrm{cov}_{ij} = \mathrm{cov}[\varepsilon_{i|ij}(t), \ \varepsilon_{j|ij}(t)]$$

$$= E[\varepsilon_{i|ij}(t)\varepsilon_{j|ij}(t)]. \tag{9.9}$$

The latter equality holds because both error terms have mean 0.

The obvious next question is as follows: How can we tell from fitting these four models whether activation in some region $i$ is causing activation in another region $j$? Geweke (1982) proposed a solution to this problem. Specifically, Geweke proposed that a measure of the amount by which activation in region $i$ is causing activation in region $j$ is given by the parameter

$$F_{i \to j} = \ln \left( \frac{\sigma^2_j}{\sigma^2_{j|ij}} \right). \tag{9.10}$$

First, note that equation 9.6 is a special case of equation 9.8, so $\sigma^2_j$ can never be less than $\sigma^2_{j|ij}$. As a result, it is always true that $F_{i \to j} \geq 0$. Second, note that if the activations in regions

$i$ and $j$ are independent, or in other words that region $i$ has no causal influence over region $j$, then adding prior observations of $B_i(t)$ will not improve our prediction of the current value of $B_j(t)$. In this case, $\sigma_j^2 = \sigma_{j|ij}^2$ and $F_{i \to j} = 0$. Finally, we see that the greater the causal influence that $B_i(t)$ has over $B_j(t)$, then the more improvement there will be when prior observations of $B_i(t)$ are added to our model that predicts the current value of $B_j(t)$. As a result, the difference between $\sigma_j^2$ and $\sigma_{j|ij}^2$ will increase with this causal influence and, consequently, so will $F_{i \to j}$.

In figure 9.2, $F_{i \to j} = 3.63$. As a comparison, if independent and normally distributed noise with zero mean and standard deviation equal to .01 is added to the BOLD responses from regions $i$ and $j$, then this measure of causality drops to $F_{i \to j} = 1.26$, and if the standard deviation is increased to .05, then $F_{i \to j}$ drops further to .23. Thus, this measure of Granger causality is sensitive to noise; that is, the presence of noise in $B_i(t)$ reduces our ability to predict current values of $B_j(t)$ from prior values of $B_i(t)$, and this loss of predictive ability is interpreted as a reduced causality. Recall that to produce figure 9.2, different hrfs were used to generate $B_i(t)$ and $B_j(t)$. If the same hrf is used in both regions, then, in the absence of noise, $F_{i \to j}$ rises from 3.63 to 3.76. Thus, unlike coherence analysis, hrf differences across brain regions will reduce their Granger causality. Even so, the existence of independent noise in the two regions will typically reduce Granger causality more than the existence of different hrfs. MATLAB box 9.2 includes code that computes $F_{i \to j}$.

Equation 9.10 measures the amount by which activation in region $i$ is causing activation in region $j$. A similar parameter describes the amount by which activation in region $j$ is causing activation in region $i$:

$$F_{j \to i} = \ln\left(\frac{\sigma_i^2}{\sigma_{i|ij}^2}\right). \tag{9.11}$$

The causal measures $F_{i \to j}$ and $F_{j \to i}$ do not capture the total linear dependence between regions $i$ and $j$ because activation in these two regions could have some instantaneous linear association. For example, they might respond simultaneously to the stimulus presentation but not be functionally connected in any immediate way. As a measure of the instantaneous, undirected influence between regions $i$ and $j$, Geweke (1982) proposed the parameter

$$F_{i \cdot j} = \ln\left(\frac{\sigma_{i|ij}^2 \sigma_{j|ij}^2}{\sigma_{i|ij}^2 \sigma_{j|ij}^2 - \text{cov}_{ij}^2}\right). \tag{9.12}$$

Note that this parameter depends completely on $\text{cov}_{ij}$. If $\text{cov}_{ij} = 0$, then $F_{i \cdot j} = 0$, and if $\text{cov}_{ij} > 0$, then $F_{i \cdot j} > 0$. Recall from equation 9.9 that $\text{cov}_{ij}$ is the covariance between $\varepsilon_{i|ij}(t)$ and $\varepsilon_{j|ij}(t)$; that is, between the current error terms in the full model. Thus, $F_{i \cdot j} > 0$ only if the current BOLD responses in regions $i$ and $j$ are correlated (i.e., linearly related).

Together, equations 9.10–9.12 completely describe the total linear relationship between the two time series $B_i(t)$ and $B_j(t)$. In other words, if we define this total linear relationship as $F_{i,j}$, then

$$F_{i,j} = F_{i \to j} + F_{j \to i} + F_{i \cdot j}.$$ (9.13)

Thus, equation 9.13 specifies that the total linear relationship between regions $i$ and $j$ can be decomposed into the amount by which activation in region $i$ causes activation in region $j$ plus the amount by which activation in region $j$ causes activation in region $i$, plus the instantaneous linear relationship between $i$ and $j$.

### Parameter Estimation

The models used in Granger causality, which are specified by equations 9.5–9.8, are all linear regression models. As a result, the regression coefficients (e.g., the $a_{ik}$, $c_{ik}$, and $d_{ik}$) can all be estimated from the normal equations of the GLM (via equation 5.13). For example, consider the single influence model specified by equation 9.5. Suppose $p = 4$ and we have data available from the first 10 TRs. Then in matrix form the model becomes

$$\begin{bmatrix} B_i(10) \\ B_i(9) \\ B_i(8) \\ B_i(7) \\ B_i(6) \\ B_i(5) \end{bmatrix} = \begin{bmatrix} B_i(9) & B_i(8) & B_i(7) & B_i(6) \\ B_i(8) & B_i(7) & B_i(6) & B_i(5) \\ B_i(7) & B_i(6) & B_i(5) & B_i(4) \\ B_i(6) & B_i(5) & B_i(4) & B_i(3) \\ B_i(5) & B_i(4) & B_i(3) & B_i(2) \\ B_i(4) & B_i(3) & B_i(2) & B_i(1) \end{bmatrix} \begin{bmatrix} a_{i1} \\ a_{i2} \\ a_{i3} \\ a_{i4} \end{bmatrix} + \begin{bmatrix} \varepsilon_i(10) \\ \varepsilon_i(9) \\ \varepsilon_i(8) \\ \varepsilon_i(7) \\ \varepsilon_i(6) \\ \varepsilon_i(5) \end{bmatrix}.$$

In the general case, when the value of $p$ is arbitrary and we collect a total of $n$ TRs of data, the model can be written in matrix form as

$$\begin{bmatrix} B_i(n) \\ B_i(n-1) \\ \vdots \\ B_i(p+1) \end{bmatrix} = \begin{bmatrix} B_i(n-1) & B_i(n-2) & \cdots & B_i(n-p) \\ B_i(n-2) & B_i(n-3) & \cdots & B_i(n-p-1) \\ \vdots & \vdots & \ddots & \vdots \\ B_i(p) & B_i(p-1) & \cdots & B_i(1) \end{bmatrix} \begin{bmatrix} a_{i1} \\ a_{i2} \\ \vdots \\ a_{ip} \end{bmatrix} + \begin{bmatrix} \varepsilon_i(n) \\ \varepsilon_i(n-1) \\ \vdots \\ \varepsilon_i(p+1) \end{bmatrix}.$$ (9.14)

If we now define

$$\underline{y} = \begin{bmatrix} B_i(n) \\ B_i(n-1) \\ \vdots \\ B_i(p+1) \end{bmatrix}, \quad X = \begin{bmatrix} B_i(n-1) & B_i(n-2) & \cdots & B_i(n-p) \\ B_i(n-2) & B_i(n-3) & \cdots & B_i(n-p-1) \\ \vdots & \vdots & \ddots & \vdots \\ B_i(p) & B_i(p-1) & \cdots & B_i(1) \end{bmatrix},$$

$$\beta = \begin{bmatrix} a_{i1} \\ a_{i2} \\ \vdots \\ a_{ip} \end{bmatrix}, \quad \text{and} \quad \varepsilon = \begin{bmatrix} \varepsilon_i(n) \\ \varepsilon_i(n-1) \\ \vdots \\ \varepsilon_i(p+1) \end{bmatrix},$$

then equation 9.14 becomes

$$y = X\beta + \varepsilon,$$

which is the equation that defines the GLM (see chapter 5). As a consequence, minimum variance unbiased estimators of the $a_{ik}$ can be quickly computed by solving the normal equations

$$\hat{\beta} = (X'X)^{-1}X'y. \tag{9.15}$$

A similar approach can be taken to estimate the parameters of the more general models (i.e., the $c_{ik}$, $c_{jk}$, $d_{ik}$, and $d_{jk}$). For example, to estimate the $c_{ik}$ and $c_{jk}$ of equation 9.7, we rewrite the model in matrix form as

$$\begin{bmatrix} B_i(n) \\ B_i(n-1) \\ \vdots \\ B_i(p+1) \end{bmatrix} = \begin{bmatrix} B_i(n-1) & B_j(n-1) & \cdots & B_i(n-p) & B_j(n-p) \\ B_i(n-2) & B_j(n-2) & \cdots & B_i(n-p-1) & B_j(n-p-1) \\ \vdots & \vdots & \ddots & \vdots & \vdots \\ B_i(p) & B_j(p) & \cdots & B_i(1) & B_j(1) \end{bmatrix} \begin{bmatrix} c_{i1} \\ c_{j1} \\ \vdots \\ c_{ip} \\ c_{jp} \end{bmatrix} + \varepsilon_{i|ij}.$$

Thus, as with the single influence model, the vector of parameter values can be estimated using equation 9.15.

As in other applications of the GLM, the variances are estimated via the method of maximum likelihood. First, in each model form the vector of residuals

$$\hat{\varepsilon} = y - X\hat{\beta},$$

which is simply the difference between the observed and predicted BOLD responses. Then the maximum likelihood estimate is

$$\hat{\sigma}^2 = \frac{1}{m}\hat{\varepsilon}'\hat{\varepsilon}, \tag{9.16}$$

where $m$ is the length of the $\hat{\varepsilon}$ vector (i.e., note that $m$ will be less than the number of TRs). The estimate of $\text{cov}_{ij}$ has a similar form

$$\hat{\text{cov}}_{ij} = \frac{1}{m}\hat{\varepsilon}'_{i|ij}\hat{\varepsilon}_{j|ij}. \tag{9.17}$$

The final unknown is $p$, which is the order of the model, or equivalently, the number of previous time points that are included in each model. For any model, increasing $p$ must improve the overall fit because a version of the model with a smaller value of $p$ is always a special case of a version with a larger value of $p$. When $p$ is small, increasing it will add terms to the model that improve the fit because they account for some real temporal correlation. At some point, however, $p$ becomes large enough that $B_i(t)$ and $B_i(t-p)$ are not correlated. In this case, increasing $p$ still improves the fit, but only marginally because the new terms are simply fitting noise. Thus, the strategy for selecting $p$ is to fit the model with different values of $p$, note the improvement in fit each time $p$ is incremented, and then select the largest value of $p$ before this improvement becomes negligible. The trick here, of course, is to define "negligible" rigorously. The standard is to use the Bayesian information criterion (BIC; Schwarz, 1978), which in the current application equals

$$BIC(p) = \ln(\hat{\sigma}^2) + \frac{Dp}{m}\ln(m), \tag{9.18}$$

where $D = 1$ for equations 9.5 and 9.6 and $D = 2$ for equations 9.7 and 9.8. The first term is a measure of absolute fit, and the second term is a penalty for extra parameters. The strategy is to choose the value of $p$ for which $BIC(p)$ is smallest. Increasing $p$ will always decrease the first term and increase the second term. Initially, $BIC(p)$ will tend to decrease when $p$ is incremented because the improvement in fit will tend to be greater than the increased penalty. Eventually, however, increasing $p$ will add term(s) that mostly just fit noise. At this point, the improvement in fit will be less than the penalty paid for the extra parameter(s), and $BIC(p)$ will begin to increase. Thus, choosing the value of $p$ for which $BIC(p)$ is minimum accomplishes our selection strategy.

Once these parameters are all estimated, we can estimate the three causality measures by substituting our variance estimates into equations 9.10–9.12. This process produces

$$\hat{F}_{i \to j} = \ln\left(\frac{\hat{\sigma}_j^2}{\hat{\sigma}_{j|ij}^2}\right), \tag{9.19}$$

$$\hat{F}_{j \to i} = \ln\left(\frac{\hat{\sigma}_i^2}{\hat{\sigma}_{i|ij}^2}\right), \tag{9.20}$$

and

$$\hat{F}_{i.j} = \ln\left(\frac{\hat{\sigma}_{i|ij}^2 \hat{\sigma}_{j|ij}^2}{\hat{\sigma}_{i|ij}^2 \hat{\sigma}_{j|ij}^2 - \hat{cov}_{ij}^2}\right). \tag{9.21}$$

Finally, we can estimate the total linear relationship between regions $i$ and $j$ by

$$\hat{F}_{i,j} = \hat{F}_{i \to j} + \hat{F}_{j \to i} + \hat{F}_{i.j}. \tag{9.22}$$

### Inference

The next step after estimating all the parameters in the various models is statistical inference. For example, we would like a statistical test of whether activation in region $i$ is causing activation in region $j$. In other words, we would like to test the null hypothesis

$$H_0 : F_{i \to j} = 0$$

against the alternative that

$$H_1 : F_{i \to j} > 0.$$

Recall that this is equivalent to asking whether the extra parameters of equation 9.8 are just fitting noise (i.e., the null hypothesis is true) or whether they are accounting for some real causal structure in the data (i.e., the alternative hypothesis is true).

Geweke (1982) showed that if this null hypothesis is true, then the statistic $n\hat{F}_{i \to j}$ has an asymptotic $\chi^2$ distribution with degrees of freedom equal to $p$; that is,

$$n\hat{F}_{i \to j} \sim \chi^2(p), \tag{9.23}$$

where $\sim$ means "is distributed as," and, as usual, $n =$ total number of TRs. Similarly, if $F_{j \to i} = 0$, then

$$n\hat{F}_{j \to i} \sim \chi^2(p), \tag{9.24}$$

and if $F_{i \cdot j} = 0$, then

$$n\hat{F}_{i \cdot j} \sim \chi^2(1). \tag{9.25}$$

Recall from equation 9.13 that the total linear relationship between regions $i$ and $j$, $F_{i,j}$, equals the sum of these three more restricted types of relationship; that is,

$$F_{i,j} = F_{i \to j} + F_{j \to i} + F_{i \cdot j}.$$

Because none of the terms on the right can be negative, note that $F_{i,j} = 0$ if and only if each of $F_{i \to j}$, $F_{j \to i}$, and $F_{i \cdot j}$ equal 0. For this reason, we might begin by testing the null hypothesis

$$H_0 : F_{i,j} = 0 \tag{9.26}$$

against the alternative that

$$H_1 : F_{i,j} > 0.$$

Geweke (1982) showed that this null hypothesis also can be tested via a $\chi^2$ test because

$$n\hat{F}_{i,j} \sim \chi^2(2p+1).$$ (9.27)

If we fail to reject the equation 9.26 null hypothesis, then we have no evidence that the activations in regions $i$ and $j$ are linearly related. As a result, there is no reason to test for a causal relationship between these two areas.

Finally, Geweke (1982) also derived approximate confidence intervals on the equation 9.19 and equation 9.20 estimates of $F_{i \to j}$ and $F_{j \to i}$. In particular, an approximate $100(1 - \alpha)\%$ confidence interval on $F_{i \to j}$ is

$$\left[ \left( \sqrt{\hat{F}_{i \to j} - \frac{p-1}{3n}} - \frac{z_{1-\frac{\alpha}{2}}}{\sqrt{n}} \right)^2 - \frac{2p+1}{3n}, \left( \sqrt{\hat{F}_{i \to j} - \frac{p-1}{3n}} + \frac{z_{1-\frac{\alpha}{2}}}{\sqrt{n}} \right)^2 - \frac{2p+1}{3n} \right],$$ (9.28)

where $z_{1-\frac{\alpha}{2}}$ is the value on a z-distribution (i.e., standard normal with mean 0 and variance 1) for which the area to the left equals $1 - \frac{\alpha}{2}$.

### Conditional Granger Causality

In the previous chapter, we reviewed the concept of partial (or conditional) coherence, which was a measure of the association between two regions after conditioning on or partialling out the effects of a third region or variable. A similar computation is possible with Granger causality. For example, consider the two alternative neural architectures shown in figure 9.3. In the top panel, regions $i$ and $j$ are not directly connected, but they indirectly connect via region $k$. In the bottom panel, regions $i$ and $j$ are still connected via region $k$, but in addition, region $i$ now also projects directly to region $j$.

In these examples, we would like to measure the degree to which activation in region $i$ causes activation in region $j$, but we would like this measure not to be influenced by contributions from region $k$. Let $\sigma^2_{j|ijk}$ denote the variance of an autoregressive model that predicts current activation in region $j$ from prior activation in regions $i$, $j$, and $k$. Then the Granger causality of region $i$ to region $j$, conditioned on region $k$, is (Geweke, 1984)

$$F_{i \to j|k} = \ln \left( \frac{\sigma^2_{j|jk}}{\sigma^2_{j|ijk}} \right).$$ (9.29)

Note that $F_{i \to j|k}$ is greater than 0 only if adding prior activation from region $i$ improves our ability to predict current activation in region $j$ based on prior activation from regions $j$ and $k$. Similarly,

$$F_{j \to i|k} = \ln \left( \frac{\sigma^2_{i|ik}}{\sigma^2_{i|ijk}} \right).$$ (9.30)

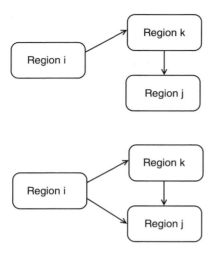

**Figure 9.3**
Two hypothetical neural activations. In the top panel, regions $i$ and $j$ are not directly connected, but their BOLD responses will be correlated because they are indirectly connected via region $k$. In the bottom panel, regions $i$ and $j$ are directly connected, but in addition they are indirectly connected via region $k$.

The conditional instantaneous undirected influence is analogously defined as

$$F_{i \bullet j|k} = \ln \left( \frac{\sigma^2_{i|ijk} \sigma^2_{j|ijk}}{\sigma^2_{i|ijk} \sigma^2_{j|ijk} - \mathrm{cov}^2_{ij|ijk}} \right), \tag{9.31}$$

The covariance term in the denominator is defined as

$$\mathrm{cov}_{ij|ijk} = \mathrm{cov}[\varepsilon_{i|ijk}(t),\ \varepsilon_{j|ijk}(t)],$$

which is the covariance between the error terms in the full region $i$ and $j$ models (i.e., the models that include past activations in regions $i, j$, and $k$). Finally, the total linear relationship between the BOLD responses in regions $i$ and $j$, conditioned on region $k$, is

$$F_{i,j|k} = F_{i \to j|k} + F_{j \to i|k} + F_{i \bullet j|k}. \tag{9.32}$$

Geweke (1984) established a useful identity that defines $F_{i \to j|k}$ in terms of unconditional measures of causality. This result is described in the following proposition.

**Proposition 9.1** The conditional causality measure $F_{i \to j|k}$ is equivalent to

$$F_{i \to j|k} = F_{ik \to j} - F_{k \to j}, \tag{9.33}$$

where

$$F_{ik \to j} = \ln\left(\frac{\sigma_j^2}{\sigma_{j|ijk}^2}\right).$$

**Derivation** From the definitions of the various causality terms, it follows that

$$F_{i \to j|k} = \ln\left(\frac{\sigma_{j|jk}^2}{\sigma_{j|ijk}^2}\right)$$

$$= \ln\left(\frac{\sigma_j^2}{\sigma_{j|ijk}^2}\right) + \ln\left(\frac{\sigma_{j|jk}^2}{\sigma_j^2}\right)$$

$$= \ln\left(\frac{\sigma_j^2}{\sigma_{j|ijk}^2}\right) - \ln\left(\frac{\sigma_j^2}{\sigma_{j|jk}^2}\right)$$

$$= F_{ik \to j} - F_{k \to j},$$

which establishes the proposition.  ∎

Proposition 9.1 indicates that the amount by which activation in region $i$ is causing activation in region $j$ when the influence of region $k$ is partialled out is equal to the amount that $i$ and $k$ together cause activation in $j$ minus the amount by which $k$ alone causes activation in $j$. Thus, we are essentially asking how much our ability to predict $j$ from $k$ is improved if we add $i$ as a predictor.

Figures 9.4 and 9.5 show a numerical example of conditional Granger causality. Figure 9.4 describes results when regions $i$ and $j$ have only an intermediate connection through region $k$ (as in the top panel of figure 9.3), and figure 9.5 describes results when regions $i$ and $j$ are also directly connected (as in the bottom panel of figure 9.3). The solid line curves in all four panels are the BOLD responses from region $j$ over the course of 200 seconds of an event-related design. The dotted line curves show the predicted response in region $j$ from a best-fitting order 2 autoregressive model. In the top graph of each figure, the model predicts the current BOLD response in region $j$ from prior responses in regions $j$ and $k$, whereas the model in the bottom graph of each figure predicts the current BOLD response in region $j$ from prior responses in regions $i$, $j$, and $k$.

To generate these data, a square wave of neural activation was generated in region $i$ to each stimulus event in a jittered, event-related design. The neural activation for region $k$ was identical except the neural response to each stimulus event was delayed, relative to region $i$, by a random number of seconds (geometrically distributed). Similarly, the neural activation in region $k$ was passed on to region $j$, again with a random delay added to each

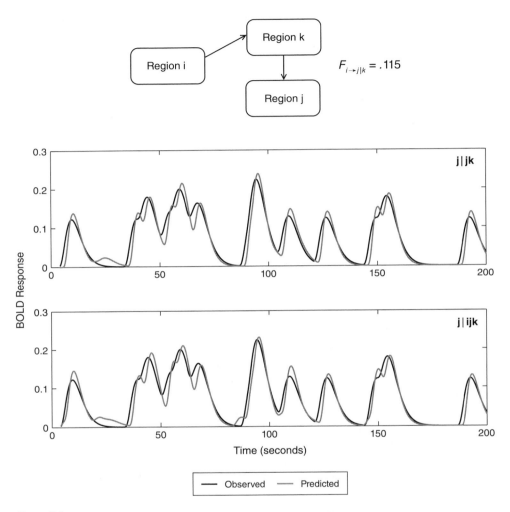

**Figure 9.4**
The two graphs show observed (black curves) and predicted (gray curves) BOLD responses from region $j$ of the network shown in the top panel. The predicted BOLD responses were generated from an order 2 autoregressive model that either included prior BOLD responses from regions $j$ and $k$ (top graph) or from regions $i$, $j$, and $k$ (bottom graph). Also shown is the numerical value of the conditional Granger causality $F_{i \to j|k}$.

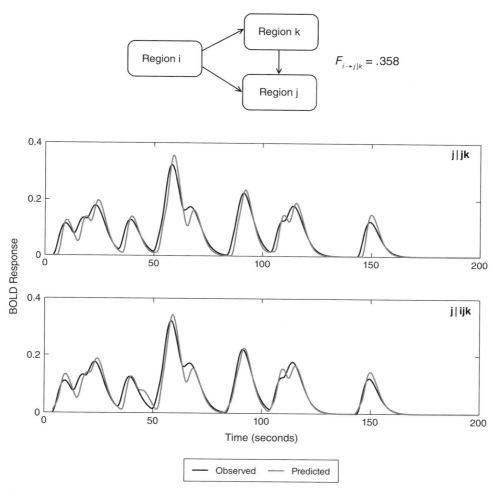

**Figure 9.5**
The two graphs show observed (black curves) and predicted (gray curves) BOLD responses from region $j$ of the network shown in the top panel. The predicted BOLD responses were generated from an order 2 autoregressive model that either included prior BOLD responses from regions $j$ and $k$ (top graph) or from regions $i$, $j$, and $k$ (bottom graph). Also shown is the numerical value of the conditional Granger causality $F_{i \to j|k}$.

**MATLAB Box 9.3**
Compute conditional Granger causality $F_{i \to j|k}$ (i.e., a measure of how strongly the BOLD response in voxel or region $i$ causes activation in voxel or region $j$ when the effects of voxel or region $k$ have been partialled out). Also produce figure 9.4

```
clear all; close all; clc;              % Clear all workspaces
ntime=2000; T=200; t=T*[0:ntime-1]/ntime;  % define time
TR=2; TR=TR*ntime/T;                    % TR in seconds
lag=1; lag=lag*ntime/T;                 % ny lag in seconds

n=4; lamda=2;                           % Create the hrf
hrf=(t.^(n-1)).*exp(-t/lamda)/((lamda^n)*factorial(n-1));

% Create the boxcars & BOLD responses
% ni
ni=zeros(1,ntime); ni(1:10)=1; ni(150:160)=1; ni(400:410)=1; ni(500:510)=1;
ni(800:810)=1;
ni(1000:1010)=1; ni(1400:1410)=1;
Bi=conv(hrf,ni)/10; Bi=Bi(1:ntime);

% nk
lag=30;
nk=zeros(1,ntime); nk(1+5*lag:10+5*lag)=1; nk(150+lag:160+lag)=1;
nk(400+2*lag:410+2*lag)=1; nk(500+lag:510+lag)=1; nk(800+6*lag:810+6*lag)=1;
nk(1000+3*lag:1010+3*lag)=1; nk(1400+lag:1410+lag)=1;
Bk=conv(hrf,nk)/10; Bk=Bk(1:ntime);

% nj with inputs from k only
nj=zeros(1,ntime); nj(1+lag:10+lag)=1; nj(390:400)=1; nj(150+6*lag:160+6*lag)=1;
nj(1200:1210)=1; nj(400+3*lag:410+3*lag)=1; nj(540:550)=1; nj(500+4*lag:510+4*lag)=1;
nj(30:40)=1; nj(800+2*lag:810+2*lag)=1; nj(1490:1500)=1; nj(1000+1*lag:1010+1*lag)=1;
nj(890:900)=1; nj(1400+lag:1410+lag)=1; nj(1860:1870)=1;
Bj=conv(hrf,nj)/10; Bj=Bj(1:ntime);

% nj with inputs from i and k
njik=zeros(1,ntime); njik(1+lag:10+lag)=1; njik(1+4*lag:10+4*lag)=1;
njik(150+6*lag:160+6*lag)=1; njik(150+1*lag:160+1*lag)=1;
njik(400+3*lag:410+3*lag)=1;
njik(400+4*lag:410+4*lag)=1; njik(500+4*lag:510+4*lag)=1;
njik(500+1*lag:510+1*lag)=1;
njik(800+2*lag:810+2*lag)=1; njik(800+1*lag:810+1*lag)=1;
njik(1000+1*lag:1010+1*lag)=1; njik(1000+3*lag:1010+3*lag)=1;
njik(1400+lag:1410+lag)=1;
Bjik=conv(hrf,njik)/10; Bjik=Bjik(1:ntime);
```

**MATLAB Box 9.3**
(continued)

```
% Evaluate (Order 2) model: j given j & k
X=[[Bj(TR+1:ntime-TR)]' [Bk(TR+1:ntime-TR)]' [Bj(1:ntime-2*TR)]'
[Bk(1:ntime-2*TR)]'];
Y=[Bj(2*TR+1:ntime)]';
A=(inv(X'*X))*X'*Y; P=X*A;
tt=(2*TR+1)*T/ntime:T/ntime:T;
subplot(2,1,1); plot(tt,Y,tt,P); axis([0 200 0 .25]);
sigsimp=(Y-P)'*(Y-P);

% Evaluate (Order 2) model: j given i, j & k model
X=[[Bj(TR+1:ntime-TR)]' [Bk(TR+1:ntime-TR)]' [Bi(TR+1:ntime-TR)]' ...
    [Bj(1:ntime-2*TR)]' [Bk(1:ntime-2*TR)]' [Bi(1:ntime-2*TR)]'];
Y=[Bj(2*TR+1:ntime)]';
A=(inv(X'*X))*X'*Y; P=X*A;
tt=(2*TR+1)*T/ntime:T/ntime:T;
subplot(2,1,2); plot(tt,Y,tt,P); axis([0 200 0 .25])
sigfull=(Y-P)'*(Y-P);

% Compute Granger causality
Fij=log(sigsimp/sigfull)
```

square wave. In figure 9.4, a set of random square waves was also added to the region $j$ activation. In figure 9.5, rather than add random square waves, the square waves from region $i$ were passed to region $j$, again with each being delayed by a random number of seconds. Finally, these neural activations (i.e., boxcar functions) were each convolved with a gamma hrf to produce a BOLD response for each region. MATLAB box 9.3 shows the code that produced these figures.

First, note that in both figures, the order 2 prediction of the current BOLD response in region $j$ based on the previous BOLD responses in regions $j$ and $k$ (top graph in both figures) are quite good. In both cases, however, adding previous BOLD responses from region $i$ improves the fit somewhat. The calculated values of conditional Granger causality confirm that this improvement is greater in figure 9.5 than in figure 9.4. In particular, in figure 9.4, $F_{i \rightarrow j|k} = .115$, whereas in figure 9.5, $F_{i \rightarrow j|k} = .358$. This difference indicates that activation in region $i$ has a greater causal influence over activation in region $j$ in figure 9.5 than it does in figure 9.4.

One might ask, though, why the conditional Granger causality in figure 9.4 is greater than zero. After all, region $k$ is simply acting as a relay station for activation in region $i$. In other words, it seems that if we know the activation in region $k$, then adding region $i$ to the model should not improve our prediction of activation in region $j$. In general, this argument is correct. However, recall that random delays were added to each region $i$ square wave as it was successively passed to region $k$ and then to region $j$. Thus, the input to region $j$ from region $k$ was an imperfect copy of activation in region $i$. As a result, adding activation from region $i$ to the model improved our prediction of activation in region $j$ because it added a second noisy version of the same thing.

### Comparing Granger Causality to Coherence Analysis

Granger causality and coherence analysis are both methods for testing whether different brain regions are functionally connected. Thus, it is obvious to ask how these two methods are related. Kayser, Sun, and D'Esposito (2009) reported that the two methods were equally effective at detecting causal connections that were known to exist in a well-studied motor task (e.g., between supplementary motor area and primary motor cortex). Thus, in many applications there might not be good reason to prefer one method over the other. The two methods, however, are not mathematically equivalent, and each has its own strengths and weaknesses.

Coherence analysis measures the nondirected influence between two regions, whereas Granger causality measures the directed influence. Thus, coherence analysis measures correlation, and Granger causality measures causality. For example, if regions $i$ and $j$ are reciprocally connected, it is possible that their mutual effects could cancel at certain frequencies, leaving a coherence of zero (Geweke, 1982). Presumably, this mutual influence would be detected with Granger causality.

Coherence analysis gains the ability to detect directed influences when the phase spectrum is analyzed. Proposition 8.2 showed that the slope of the phase spectrum in coherence analysis is proportional to the temporal lag between the onsets of the two neural regions. Thus, if two regions have a high coherence, then theoretically one could tell which region was driving the other by examining whether the phase spectrum between the two regions had an initial positive or negative slope. Proposition 8.2, however, assumed that the neural activation in the two regions is identical, except one is a delayed version of the other. Of course, in real applications this condition would never be met. Unfortunately, to my knowledge, there has not been a systematic investigation of how violations of this strong assumption affect the initial linearity and slope of the phase spectrum. In contrast, Granger causality makes the much weaker assumption that the activations in the two regions are only linearly related.

On the other hand, coherence analysis has its own unique advantages. In particular, unlike Granger causality, coherence is unaffected by hrf differences across regions. In addition, high-frequency noise does not affect coherence at the low frequencies that are most important in fMRI data analysis (e.g., below .15 Hz). These advantages occur because coherence analysis is done in the frequency domain, whereas Granger causality is computed in the time domain. Granger causality has been extended to the frequency domain (Chen, Bressler, & Ding, 2006; Geweke, 1982), but these extensions have not yet been applied to fMRI data. In summary, if the primary goal is to establish the direction of causality between two ROIs then Granger causality may be the better choice, whereas coherence is superior given the less ambitious goal of simply establishing that there is some sort of functional connection between the ROIs.

# 10 Principal Components Analysis

Thus far, all of the analyses considered in this book have been univariate. This means that we have only examined methods that analyze the data one voxel at a time. For example, in a whole-brain analysis with 100,000 voxels, the GLM methods considered in chapter 5 would be repeated 100,000 times. The obvious problem with this approach is that there are massive correlations between BOLD responses in neighboring voxels. Yet the GLM methods assign completely separate parameters to every voxel, which means that they essentially assume that the data in neighboring voxels have no relationship to each other. Post hoc methods, which are applied after all the GLM parameters have been estimated, try to overcome this obviously incorrect assumption. For example, chapter 6 described post hoc methods for correcting for the multiple comparisons problem that arises from this univariate approach, and chapters 8 and 9 described methods for attempting to recover information about spatial correlations from the many independent GLM tests.

In this and the next chapter, we consider multivariate methods for analyzing fMRI data. In these methods, rather than running the same analysis 100,000 times, as the GLM requires, we run only one (admittedly time-consuming) analysis. The GLM assumes that each voxel generates an independent data set. In an experiment with $n$ TRs, the GLM would consider the $n$ BOLD responses in each voxel to be $n$ samples from the same model and the $n$ BOLD responses from the neighboring voxel to be $n$ samples from a completely independent model. In contrast, the multivariate methods considered in this and the next chapter assume that all BOLD responses collected at each TR form a single (multivariate) observation. Thus, with 100,000 voxels, the multivariate methods consider a single observation to be a $100,000 \times 1$ vector and the complete set of data collected in the entire experiment to form $n$ samples from one model.

This chapter considers *principal components analysis* (PCA), which is a popular method from multivariate statistics. In the next chapter, we consider the related method of *independent component analysis* (ICA). ICA is arguably the much preferred method for analyzing fMRI data, but ICA is easier to understand if one already has a basic understanding of PCA, and some ICA applications begin with a preliminary PCA to eliminate as much noise from the data as possible. For these reasons, we take time in this chapter to briefly consider PCA. Our main focus will be on PCA as a method for eliminating noise from fMRI data. Because ICA seems the preferable method for analyzing fMRI data, this chapter is considerably shorter than the next.

The theoretical basis of PCA depends critically on the mathematical concepts of *eigenvectors* and *eigenvalues*. These concepts from matrix algebra are reviewed in appendix A. Readers not familiar with eigenvectors and eigenvalues should review that material before continuing with this chapter.

## Principal Components Analysis

Suppose we have two tests—one that measures spatial ability and one that measures mathematical ability—and that we are interested in determining whether people have unique spatial and mathematical cognitive abilities or whether there is one underlying cognitive skill that mediates performance in both tasks. To answer this question, we administer both tests to a large collection of students. Let $x_i$ and $y_i$ denote the scores of student $i$ on the spatial and mathematical tests, respectively. Across all students who take these tests, suppose the pair of scores $(x_i, y_i)$ has a bivariate normal distribution with mean $(\mu_x, \mu_y)$ and variance-covariance matrix

$$\Sigma = \begin{bmatrix} \sigma_x^2 & \mathrm{cov}_{xy} \\ \mathrm{cov}_{xy} & \sigma_y^2 \end{bmatrix}. \tag{10.1}$$

For a review of multivariate normal distributions, see appendix B.

Figure 10.1 illustrates a hypothetical idealized example of such data. The ellipse represents the contour within which 95% of the samples would fall (called a contour of equal likelihood). Note that the scores on the two tests are positively correlated, as large values of $x_i$ (i.e., high spatial scores) tend to co-occur with large values of $y_i$ (i.e., high mathematical scores). If the two tests were measuring exactly the same ability, however, then there should be a single number that measures this ability in each subject, and furthermore, all differences among students on the pair of tests should reduce to their differences on this single number. Thus, our mathematical question is as follows: What is the optimal method of reducing these $(x_i, y_i)$ pairs to a single number, and how much information is lost by this dimensionality reduction?

In the case of linear transformations, the optimal solution is known to depend on the diagonal representation of the variance-covariance matrix:

$$\Sigma = VDV' = \begin{bmatrix} \underline{v}_1 & \underline{v}_2 \end{bmatrix} \begin{bmatrix} d_1 & 0 \\ 0 & d_2 \end{bmatrix} \begin{bmatrix} \underline{v}_1' \\ \underline{v}_2' \end{bmatrix}, \tag{10.2}$$

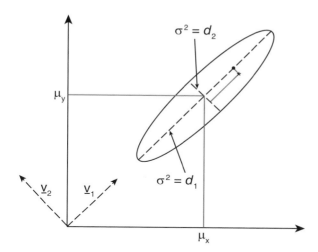

**Figure 10.1**
Contour of equal likelihood of a bivariate normal distribution with positive correlation and approximately equal $x$ and $y$ variances. The dotted line vectors, $\underline{v}_1$ and $\underline{v}_2$, are the eigenvectors of the variance-covariance matrix, and $d_1$ and $d_2$ are the eigenvalues. Note that the eigenvalues specify the variances in the directions specified by the eigenvectors.

where $d_1$ and $d_2$ are the eigenvalues of $\Sigma$, and $\underline{v}_1$ and $\underline{v}_2$ are the associated eigenvectors. Variance-covariance matrices are always positive semidefinite, so $d_1$ and $d_2$ must both be greater than or equal to zero. The eigenvectors $\underline{v}_1$ and $\underline{v}_2$ are shown in figure 10.1. Note that they are parallel to the major and minor axes of the ellipse that describes the distribution of scores. This is not a coincidence. Regardless of the number of dimensions, the contours of equal likelihood of a multivariate normal distribution are always (hyper) ellipsoids, and the eigenvectors of the distribution's variance-covariance matrix are always parallel to the ellipsoid's axes. Furthermore, note that the eigenvectors in figure 10.1 are also orthogonal (i.e., at a right angle). This is also always true, no matter the dimensionality, because the axes of all ellipsoids are always orthogonal. These properties of the eigenvectors of the variance-covariance matrix are the first key result that makes PCA possible. The second key property is that the eigenvalues turn out to equal the variances along the directions specified by the associated eigenvectors. Thus, in figure 10.1, $d_1$ is the variance along the major axis of the ellipse (corresponding with the eigenvector $\underline{v}_1$), and $d_2$ is the variance along the minor axis (corresponding with the eigenvector $\underline{v}_2$).

Because the major axis of an ellipsoid specifies the direction of greatest width across the ellipsoid, it follows that the eigenvector of the variance-covariance matrix that is associated with the largest eigenvalue specifies the direction in one's data along which there is greatest variability (i.e., assuming the data have a multivariate normal distribution).

Furthermore, the eigenvector associated with the second largest eigenvalue specifies the independent direction along which there is the second most variability, and so on. We can also use the eigenvalues to quantify these relations. Specifically, with $n$-dimensional data, the percentage of variance due to variation in the direction specified by the i$^{th}$ eigenvector equals

$$\frac{d_i}{d_1 + d_2 + \cdots + d_n}.$$

Thus, if we were to reduce the $(x_i, y_i)$ scores described by the figure 10.1 ellipse to a single number, it makes sense that we should choose to describe each pair of scores relative to their position along the ellipse's major diagonal. For example, if we do this, then the data point denoted by the star in figure 10.1 would be recoded as the point denoted by the filled circle. The loss of information by recoding in this way equals the amount by which the positions of these two points differ. PCA provides an optimal method for reducing dimensionality in the sense that it minimizes the sum of squared information losses. In the figure 10.1 example, we might therefore conclude that the spatial and mathematical tests are measuring a single underlying cognitive ability if $d_1/(d_1 + d_2)$ is sufficiently large (e.g., greater than .95).

The mathematical basis for PCA is summarized in the following proposition.

**Proposition 10.1**    Suppose an $n$-dimensional random vector $\underline{x}$ has a multivariate normal distribution with mean vector $\underline{\mu}$ and variance-covariance matrix $\Sigma$. Let $\underline{v}_1, \underline{v}_2, \ldots, \underline{v}_n$ denote the $n$ eigenvectors of $\Sigma$ and let $d_1, d_2, \ldots, d_n$ denote the $n$ corresponding eigenvalues, where the ordering is such that $d_1 > d_2 > \cdots > d_n$. Then the direction along which the data have greatest variance is $\underline{v}_1$ (with variance $d_1$), the independent direction along which the data have second greatest variance is $\underline{v}_2$ (with variance $d_2$), and in general the independent direction along which the data have the i$^{th}$ greatest variance is $\underline{v}_i$ (with variance $d_i$).

Note that PCA does not require the estimation of any free parameters. In this sense, then, it is qualitatively different from other multivariate statistical techniques, such as factor analysis or ICA. Thus, PCA is not a model that must be fit to the data. Instead, it is simply a rigid rotation of the data to a new set of coordinate axes (i.e., the eigenvectors of the variance-covariance matrix).

### PCA with fMRI Data

PCA is a multivariate statistical technique because it operates simultaneously on all the data collected in an fMRI experiment. To apply PCA to fMRI data, we must therefore first collect all fMRI data into one matrix. To do this, we will form the data matrix Y that has a row for every TR and a column for every voxel. In particular, suppose there are $n$ TRs and

$N$ voxels. Let $y_{ij}$ denote the BOLD response on the $i^{th}$ TR in voxel $j$. Then the matrix Y is defined as

$$Y = \begin{bmatrix} y_{11} & y_{12} & \cdots & y_{1N} \\ y_{21} & y_{22} & \cdots & y_{2N} \\ \vdots & \vdots & \ddots & \vdots \\ y_{n1} & y_{n2} & \cdots & y_{nN} \end{bmatrix}. \tag{10.3}$$

To apply PCA, we must first compute the variance of the BOLD responses collected from each voxel and the covariance between the responses from each pair of voxels. These values will then be collected in an $N \times N$ variance-covariance matrix. The first step is to construct a mean-centered version of the data matrix Y, denoted by $Y_C$, by computing the mean in each voxel (i.e., in each column of Y) and then subtracting this value from all BOLD responses collected in that voxel. Following this operation, the mean in each voxel across TRs will be zero. Denote the mean of all BOLD responses in the $j^{th}$ voxel by $\bar{y}_{.j}$ (i.e., before mean centering). Then the matrix $Y_C$ is defined as

$$Y_C = \begin{bmatrix} y_{11} - \bar{y}_{.1} & y_{12} - \bar{y}_{.2} & \cdots & y_{1N} - \bar{y}_{.N} \\ y_{21} - \bar{y}_{.1} & y_{22} - \bar{y}_{.2} & \cdots & y_{2N} - \bar{y}_{.N} \\ \vdots & \vdots & \ddots & \vdots \\ y_{n1} - \bar{y}_{.1} & y_{n2} - \bar{y}_{.2} & \cdots & y_{nN} - \bar{y}_{.N} \end{bmatrix}. \tag{10.4}$$

The centered data matrix $Y_C$ can be computed via matrix operations if we first define the mean vector

$$\bar{\underline{y}} = \begin{bmatrix} \bar{y}_{.1} \\ \bar{y}_{.2} \\ \vdots \\ \bar{y}_{.N} \end{bmatrix}, \tag{10.5}$$

and the $n \times 1$ vector of ones by

$$\underline{1}_n = \begin{bmatrix} 1 \\ 1 \\ \vdots \\ 1 \end{bmatrix}. \tag{10.6}$$

Then

$$Y_C = Y - \underline{1}_n \bar{\underline{y}}'. \tag{10.7}$$

Given the matrix $Y_C$, the variance-covariance matrix is estimated by

$$\hat{\Sigma} = \frac{1}{n-1} Y_C' Y_C. \tag{10.8}$$

PCA depends on the eigenvectors and eigenvalues of $\hat{\Sigma}$. Note that $\hat{\Sigma}$ is $N \times N$ but $Y_C$ is $n \times N$. If the PCA is applied to the whole brain, then a reasonable value of $N$ might be 100,000. In contrast, $n$ is the number of TRs in the scanning session. For a 30-minute session and a 2-second TR, then $n = 900$. So for a whole-brain analysis, we should expect that $N$ will be much larger than $n$. Now a well-known theorem in matrix algebra states that for any matrix $Y_C$,

$$\text{rank}(Y_C' Y_C) = \text{rank}(Y_C Y_C') = \text{rank}(Y_C') = \text{rank}(Y_C).$$

Because the number of nonzero eigenvalues of a matrix is equal to its rank (see appendix A), we see that, although $\hat{\Sigma}$ is $N \times N$ (e.g., $100,000 \times 100,000$), it can have at most $n$ (e.g., 900) nonzero eigenvalues.

Consider first the eigenvector with the largest eigenvalue. This is called the principal component of the variance-covariance matrix $\hat{\Sigma}$. If we rank order and then number the eigenvalues from largest to smallest, then $\underline{v}_1$ is the principal component. This is the direction along which there is greatest variation across TRs. In other words, if we project the data vector from the $i^{th}$ TR onto $\underline{v}_1$, then the result will be

$$\overline{y} + a_i \underline{v}_1, \tag{10.9}$$

for some constant $a_i$ that will be different for each TR. Because $\underline{v}_1$ is the principal component, the variance of the $a_i$ (i.e., $d_1$) is greater than if we project the data onto any other vector.

Note that $\underline{v}_1$ is an $N \times 1$ vector that specifies a numerical value in each voxel. As equation 10.9 shows, variation along this direction means multiplying all these values by a constant (i.e., by $a_i$). Because $\underline{v}_1$ is the principal component, the variability in the $a_i$ weights across TRs will be greater than for any other direction in the data. Thus, the activation pattern specified by $\underline{v}_1$ will change more across TRs than in any other components. Of course, we expect that voxels corresponding with a distributed neural network that is mediating the responses to stimulus events will modulate up in the TRs after stimulus presentation and down during rest periods. As a result, we expect the weights (i.e., the $a_i$) to fluctuate dramatically across TRs. In contrast, noise should not change much across TRs, so the weights associated with components that are driven by noise should show little variability across TRs. This logic suggests that the task-related components should have large eigenvalues, whereas noise-related components should have small eigenvalues.

Note that any voxel with a zero value in its component map (i.e., in $\underline{v}_i$) will not change as a result of the equation 10.9 multiplications, whereas voxels with large absolute values will change a lot across TRs. For example, suppose the principal component corresponds with a distributed neural network that is mediating the responses to stimuli that are presented on random TRs in our experiment. Voxels from brain regions that play a critical role in this network should show an increased BOLD response shortly after each stimulus presentation and a decreased response after rest TRs. Thus, the BOLD responses in important voxels will vary significantly across TRs, so voxels playing the most important roles in the principal component will have large absolute values in $\underline{v}_1$. These are the voxels that should be emphasized in visual presentations of $\underline{v}_1$. One way to do this is to convert the entries in $\underline{v}_1$ to $z$-scores and then threshold these values at something like $|2|$. A graphic can then be created that color codes all voxels with entries in $\underline{v}_1$ that exceed this threshold.

As we will see in the next chapter, the goals of ICA are essentially the same as the goals of PCA; namely, to identify functionally separate neural networks that each contribute to the observed BOLD response. Although the two approaches make very different assumptions, they produce results in exactly the same form; that is, each component identified by PCA and by ICA is in the form of a spatial map along with numerical weights specifying how strongly the component is activated on each TR. Furthermore, the interpretation of the components and weights produced by PCA and ICA are also essentially the same. Because of these similarities, and because ICA is generally considered more effective than PCA at identifying true task-related networks, we hold off on a more thorough discussion of how to interpret PCA or ICA results until the next chapter.

## Using PCA to Eliminate Noise

With fMRI data, one of the most useful applications of PCA is to eliminate noise. fMRI data are noisy and of very high dimension. For example, as mentioned above, with 100,000 voxels, one could theoretically estimate a $100,000 \times 100,000$ variance-covariance matrix. Applying PCA to this matrix would yield $n$ components; that is, as many components as there are TRs in the experiment. PCA assumes an underlying multivariate normal distribution, so these $n$ components would denote the axes of the $n$-dimensional hyper-ellipsoid that defines a contour of equal likelihood of this underlying distribution. No one would expect these $n$ components to all be signals (i.e., meaningful). In the next chapter, we will see that there is good reason to expect that signals will not be normally distributed. If so, then the principal components of this PCA will misestimate the true signals. On the other hand, it is widely accepted that noise will be normally distributed. Thus, the eigenvectors corresponding with the smallest eigenvalues will most likely estimate independent noise. The following algorithm describes a method for eliminating this noise from the data.

### Algorithm for Eliminating Noise from fMRI Data

*Step 1*  Compute the diagonal representation of the sample variance-covariance matrix: $\hat{\Sigma} = VDV'$.

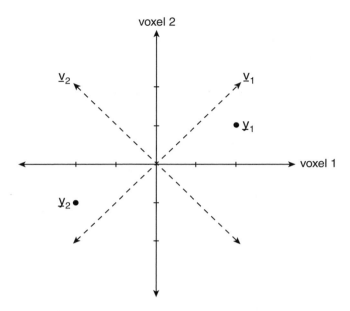

**Figure 10.2**
Hypothetical fMRI data from an experiment with only two voxels and two TRs. The points $\underline{y}_1$ and $\underline{y}_2$ denote the BOLD responses on TRs 1 and 2, respectively.

*Step 2*   Compute the coordinates of the centered data in eigenvector space by forming the matrix $W_C = Y_C V$. Note that $W_C$ and $Y_C$ are both $n \times N$, and V is $N \times N$. The matrix $W_C$ has the same structure as the data matrix $Y_C$; that is, $W_C$ has a row for each TR and a column for each voxel. The difference in the two matrices is in the coordinate system used to describe the data. The matrix $Y_C$ uses a coordinate system in which there is an axis or dimension for each voxel. In contrast, $W_C$ uses a system in which the axes correspond with the eigenvectors of $\hat{\Sigma}$.

For example, consider the simple case illustrated in figure 10.2 in which we only have two voxels and two TRs. Note that the observed BOLD responses at the two TRs are $\underline{y}_1 = [2 \ 1]$ and $\underline{y}_2 = [-2 \ -1]$.

These data have already been centered (i.e., the mean of the voxel 1 coordinates is 0, as is the mean of the voxel 2 coordinates). Suppose that the eigenvectors of the variance-covariance matrix are

$$\underline{v}_1 = \frac{1}{\sqrt{2}}\begin{bmatrix} 1 \\ 1 \end{bmatrix} \quad \text{and} \quad \underline{v}_2 = \frac{1}{\sqrt{2}}\begin{bmatrix} -1 \\ 1 \end{bmatrix}.$$

Then

$$\underline{w}_1 = [\underline{y}_1 \underline{v}_1 \quad \underline{y}_1 \underline{v}_2] = \frac{1}{\sqrt{2}}[3 \quad -1] \quad \text{and} \quad \underline{w}_2 = [\underline{y}_2 \underline{v}_1 \quad \underline{y}_2 \underline{v}_2] = \frac{1}{\sqrt{2}}[-3 \quad 1].$$

So the coordinates of $\underline{y}_1$ when the axes are the eigenvectors of $\hat{\Sigma}$ are $(3/\sqrt{2}, -1/\sqrt{2})$. Note in figure 10.2 that this makes sense because $\underline{y}_1$ falls to the right of the $\underline{v}_2$ axis (hence the first coordinate is positive) and below the $\underline{v}_1$ axis (so the second coordinate is negative).

*Step 3* Reduce dimensionality. This is done by starting at the right and setting as many columns of the $W_C$ matrix to zero as desired. If $r$ nonzero columns remain, call the resulting matrix $W_r$. Remember that each column of V contains an eigenvector of $\hat{\Sigma}$, and that these are ordered from left to right by the magnitude of the corresponding eigenvalues. Thus, the left column of V is associated with the largest eigenvalue and the right column is associated with the smallest.

In our numerical example,

$$W_C = \frac{1}{\sqrt{2}}\begin{bmatrix} 3 & -1 \\ -3 & 1 \end{bmatrix}.$$

We can make our data one-dimensional by setting the second column of $W_C$ to all zeros:

$$W_1 = \frac{1}{\sqrt{2}}\begin{bmatrix} 3 & 0 \\ -3 & 0 \end{bmatrix}.$$

*Step 4* Convert back to voxel coordinates. After step 3, the data are one-dimensional (in this example), but they are still expressed in the eigenvector coordinate system. To convert them back to the voxel coordinate system, we must post-multiply $W_r$ by $V'$, which is the inverse[1] of V, and then add the mean back in (which had been removed by the centering operation). We call the resulting matrix $Y_r$:

$$Y_r = W_r V' + \underline{1}_n \bar{y}', \tag{10.10}$$

where, as before, $\bar{y}$ is the column vector of all such means, and $\underline{1}'_n$ is a $1 \times n$ row vector of all ones.

In our numerical example,

$$Y_1 = \begin{bmatrix} \dfrac{3}{\sqrt{2}} & 0 \\ -\dfrac{3}{\sqrt{2}} & 0 \end{bmatrix}\begin{bmatrix} \dfrac{1}{\sqrt{2}} & \dfrac{1}{\sqrt{2}} \\ -\dfrac{1}{\sqrt{2}} & \dfrac{1}{\sqrt{2}} \end{bmatrix} = \begin{bmatrix} 1.5 & 1.5 \\ -1.5 & -1.5 \end{bmatrix}.$$

---

1. The matrix V is orthogonal, which means that $VV' = V'V = I$. As a result, $V^{-1} = V'$.

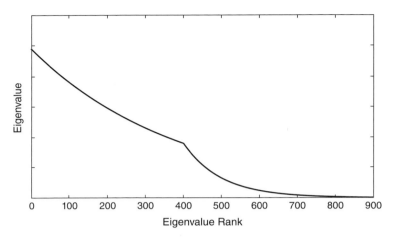

**Figure 10.3**
Idealized ranking of eigenvalues from an fMRI experiment. The obvious kink suggests there may be around 400 components and 500 noise sources.

Thus, the new coordinates of the first data point are (1.5, 1.5) and the second data point becomes (−1.5, −1.5). Note that both of these points fall on the line defined by the first eigenvector of $\hat{\Sigma}$.                                                                                           ∎

An obvious problem when applying this method is to decide how many dimensions to eliminate. Unfortunately, there is no objectively correct solution to this problem. In practice, a combination of several guidelines can be used. The motivating principle here is that the data are a mixture of signal and noise. Ideally, signal and noise would differ in some qualitative manner. For example, perhaps the distribution of signal and noise are different. As we will see in the next chapter, this in fact is a core assumption of ICA. In PCA, however, signal and noise are both assumed to be normally distributed, so distributional differences cannot be used to separate signal from noise. Instead, our only hope rests on the assumption that, relative to signal, any single noise source will only account for a small percentage of variance in the data. Thus, ideally we should separate eigenvectors with large eigenvalues from eigenvectors with small eigenvalues. In practice, of course, this is not so easy to do. In most cases, there will be no obvious gap between the small and large eigenvalues.

A more subtle application of this same method is to order the eigenvalues from largest to smallest and then to look for a change in the rate by which the eigenvalues are decreasing. This is often done visually by plotting the eigenvalues against their rank and looking for a kink. An idealized example of such a plot is shown in figure 10.3 for a scanning session with 900 TRs. Note the obvious kink at 400. The behavior of the eigenvalues is qualitatively different to the left and right of the kink. If we accept that signal and noise are

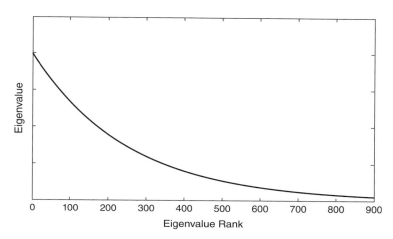

**Figure 10.4**
A hypothetical ranking of eigenvalues from an fMRI experiment that provides no statistical basis for deciding the number of true components.

qualitatively different and that signals account for more variance in the data than noise sources, then it makes sense in this case to conclude that the first 400 eigenvalues come from signal-related eigenvectors and the next 500 come from noise-related eigenvectors. Thus, in this case, the standard decision would be to retain at least 400 dimensions.

In practice, unfortunately, a kink is rarely obvious. Instead, the eigenvalues often tend to decrease at a roughly constant rate, as in the example illustrated in figure 10.4. In this case, PCA, by itself, offers no statistical basis for deciding how many dimensions to eliminate. So some extra theoretical assumptions must be made. For example, one might decide that with fMRI data, there cannot possibly be more than a couple of hundred signals of interest, or perhaps that at least 10% of the total variance in the data must be due to noise. The key here is to be conservative. In most cases, it will be much better to leave some noise in the data than to throw away signal.

For example, a conservative methodology might be to use the following decision rule. First find the smallest value of $K$ such that

$$\frac{\sum_{i=0}^{K} d_{n-i}}{\sum_{j=1}^{n} d_j} > .10.$$

Next eliminate eigenvectors $\underline{v}_n, \underline{v}_{n-1}, \ldots \underline{v}_{n-K+1}$. This rule eliminates the dimensions or eigenvectors with the smallest eigenvalues that collectively account for less than 10% of the variance in the data.

**Conclusions**

PCA orthogonally (i.e., rigidly) rotates data to a new coordinate system. It does this by finding the direction in one's data along which there is maximal variance and then rotating so that this direction becomes a coordinate axis. PCA has no free parameters. It simply allows one to look at data from a different perspective. This can be a useful process, but with fMRI data, at least, not too much should be expected from a PCA analysis. One problem is that the PCA rotation is guaranteed to be optimal only if the data have an underlying multivariate normal distribution, and in the next chapter we will encounter some powerful arguments that this assumption is invalid with fMRI data. On the other hand, PCA is widely regarded as an effective method for reducing noise. Arguably, this may be the most effective use of PCA in fMRI data analysis.

# 11 Independent Component Analysis

Independent component analysis (ICA) has goals similar to those of PCA. Both methods are multivariate techniques that try to decompose the observed BOLD response into a set of independent components. But ICA is considerably more powerful than PCA and depends on more realistic assumptions about the nature of the underlying components. Also, unlike the GLM analyses considered in chapter 5, ICA does not require an identical response to each repeated presentation of a stimulus. This property means that ICA offers the potential to study phenomena such as learning and habituation.

ICA differs from PCA in a number of ways. As described in chapter 10, PCA is a straightforward orthogonal rotation of the data to a new coordinate system that requires no model fitting process. This is because PCA has no free parameters to estimate from the data. PCA simply allows the user to view his or her data from a different perspective. In contrast, ICA is a true model, in the sense that it has many free parameters that must be estimated from the data. Mathematically and statistically, ICA is more like factor analysis than it is like PCA.

ICA and PCA also assume different types of structure in the data. The only assumption of PCA is that the data have a multivariate normal distribution. This is a strong assumption, however, because the components in a multivariate normal distribution are necessarily orthogonal, or equivalently, uncorrelated (i.e., see chapter 10 and appendix B), and also statistically independent. ICA has two key fundamental assumptions. First, ICA assumes components are statistically independent, although it does not require that they are also orthogonal. Second, in contrast with PCA, ICA assumes that components are non-normally distributed. As we will see, this is a critical assumption in the sense that ICA is guaranteed to fail on data constructed from normally distributed components.

## The Cocktail-Party Problem

A good way to gain an intuitive understanding of ICA is through its most widely known application, namely, the cocktail-party problem. Imagine you are hosting a cocktail party where some important matters will be discussed. You want a record of the conversations but you do not want to be distracted by having to take notes. Instead, you place micro-phones around the room with the idea that later you will listen to the recordings and tran-scribe the conversations. To make the discussion concrete, suppose that four people join the conversations and there are four microphones around the room. The problem is that after the party, when you listen to the recordings, they each are unintelligible because dur-ing much of the time, two or more people are speaking simultaneously. To make matters worse, there may also be background noise that makes it difficult to understand even single speakers.

ICA provides an extremely effective method for separating the voices of the different speakers. The conceptual idea is simple. Speech signals produced by different people should be independent of each other. Knowledge that one speaker increases the loudness of his or her voice does not allow us to predict the loudness of other speakers at that same point in time. Therefore, we should look at all the combined data and try to pull out four separate waveforms that are all mutually independent. This signal extraction is done on a purely statistical basis with absolutely no regard to the linguistic content of the separate signals. In fact, it turns out that this process is highly effective. For example, in the case of the cocktail-party problem, it is well known that the waveforms identified via ICA will closely match the speech signals of the four speakers. In other words, ICA can usually solve the cocktail-party problem.

In this application, ICA will identify four signals—the speech signals produced by each of the four speakers. For each signal, the model has four free parameters that must be esti-mated from the data. These are weights that are essentially equivalent to the amplitude of that speaker's voice at each of the four microphones. ICA assumes that the input to each microphone will be a weighted sum of each of the four voices. The parameters fix those weights.

### Applying ICA to fMRI Data

The application of ICA to the cocktail-party problem is an example of *temporal ICA* be-cause the signals that are extracted are temporal waveforms. The weights, on the other hand, carry spatial information because each weight is associated with a particular micro-phone that has a fixed spatial location. When applied to fMRI, however, both temporal and *spatial ICA* are used, although applications of spatial ICA are more common. Spatial ICA reverses the logic of temporal ICA. In spatial ICA, the signals or components are spatial maps, and the weights carry temporal information.

A spatial ICA analogue of the cocktail-party problem might assume that instead of four speakers, there are four functionally independent neural networks that are simultaneously active during some fMRI experiment. For example, one network might mediate the pro-cessing of task-relevant stimulus information, one might mediate processing of any feed-back provided during the course of the experiment, one might monitor the auditory stimulation provided by the scanning environment, and one could be the so-called default network, which can be seen when subjects lie quietly in the scanner with no task to perform (e.g., Buckner, Andrews-Hanna, & Schacter, 2008). Note that each network defines a spatial pattern of activation across all voxels in the brain. When the network is active, voxels in brain regions that are part of the network will be active, and voxels that are not part of the network will be inactive. On any TR, spatial ICA assumes that the observable BOLD response is a mixture of the activation patterns associated with each of these networks plus (perhaps) some noise. As the TRs change, the amount that each network is activated could change. For example, the network that processes the stimulus should become more active on TRs during and immediately after stimulus presentation and become less active during rest periods. Thus, on every TR, spatial ICA will estimate a weight for each neural network that measures how active that network is on that TR. Thus, in this example, ICA estimates four weights (one for every network) on every TR.

In spatial ICA, the spatial pattern of activation associated with each neural network is the analogue of the temporal waveform associated with each speaker in the cocktail-party example. These are the signals or components that ICA tries to identify. The spatial ICA analogue of the microphone weights are the network weights on each TR that measure the network's activation on that TR. So in spatial ICA, the components are spatial maps, and the weights describe the modulation of the components over time.

Applications of temporal ICA to fMRI data are conceptually more similar to the GLM applications we considered in chapter 5. In temporal ICA, the components are temporal waveforms, and a weight is estimated for every voxel. For example, a task-related component might look much like the predicted BOLD response that the correlation GLM generates by convolving an hrf with a boxcar function (e.g., McKeown, Hansen, & Sejnowski, 2003). In addition, the weight in each voxel is conceptually similar to the $\theta$ parameter (e.g., see equation 5.8) that is estimated when the GLM is fit to the data from that voxel. One important difference though is that the ICA is applied to all voxels simultaneously, whereas the GLM is applied independently to the data from each single voxel. Other differences are considered at the end of this chapter.

Although applications of temporal ICA to fMRI are not uncommon (e.g., Biswal & Ulmer, 1999; Calhoun, Adali, Pearlson, & Pekar, 2001; Hu et al., 2005; McKeown et al., 2003), fMRI is especially well suited to spatial ICA because the spatial dimension is typically much larger than the temporal dimension. In other words, most fMRI data sets have many more voxels than TRs. As we will see, ICA algorithms treat the weights as free parameters. These are adjusted in an iterative process with the goal of making the components as signal-like (e.g., independent) as possible. In spatial ICA there is a weight for each TR, whereas in temporal ICA there is a weight for each voxel. Thus, from the perspective of the ICA algorithms, there are fewer unknowns to estimate in spatial ICA than in temporal ICA. Largely for this reason, fMRI applications of spatial ICA have flourished (McKeown et al., 1998). As a result, our mathematical description will focus on spatial

ICA. A description of temporal ICA would largely be the same, except every instance of "voxel" would be replaced by "TR" and vice versa. We will consider temporal ICA again near the end of the chapter when we compare ICA to standard GLM approaches.

### Spatial ICA

This section describes the formal structure of spatial ICA. To begin, denote the $k^{th}$ component identified by ICA by the vector

$$\underline{c}_k = \begin{bmatrix} c_{k1} \\ c_{k2} \\ \vdots \\ c_{kN} \end{bmatrix}.$$

The term $c_{kj}$ denotes the activation in voxel $j$ for component $k$. Denote the weight on component $k$ at TR $i$ by $m_{ik}$. ICA assumes that the observed BOLD response on each TR is a weighted sum of each of these components. Specifically, denote the BOLD response in all $N$ voxels at the $i^{th}$ TR by the vector

$$\underline{y}_{TR(i)} = \begin{bmatrix} y_{i1} \\ y_{i2} \\ \vdots \\ y_{iN} \end{bmatrix}.$$

In its standard form, ICA extracts as many components as there are TRs. Then, with $n$ TRs, ICA assumes

$$\underline{y}_{TR(i)} = m_{i1}\underline{c}_1 + m_{i2}\underline{c}_2 + \cdots + m_{in}\underline{c}_n. \tag{11.1}$$

So the weights specify the contribution of each component at every TR. Neural networks that mediate the processing of the stimulus should be active during TRs immediately following stimulus presentation, and their activation should gradually decrease with each successive TR for which the stimulus is not presented. Thus, if component $k$ mediates stimulus processing, then its associated weights should be correlated with the TR vector that specifies when the stimulus is presented. As we will see in more detail later in this chapter, it is through such correlations that stimulus-related components are identified.

Equation 11.1 is a simple linear equation, but note that we know nothing on the right-hand side. The left side is our observed data at the $i^{th}$ TR, but on the right side we know neither the weights nor the components. All of these must somehow be determined from the data. Without adding some constraints to this problem, there are obviously an infinite number of solutions. ICA constrains the components to be statistically independent and non-normal, but even in this case some ambiguity remains. In particular, it is impossible to determine the variance of each component uniquely. For example, suppose the variance of the elements in component $j$ is $\sigma_j^2$. Then if we multiply each entry in $\underline{c}_j$ by $1/\sigma_j$, the variance has been changed to 1. But if we now multiply each weight $m_{jk}$ by $\sigma_j$ to create a new weight, the model is mathematically identical to our original model. For this reason, without loss of generality, ICA assumes that all component variances equal 1.

Equation 11.1 specifies how the components are mixed together on TR $i$. Of course, there are analogous equations for the other TRs. Collecting all these together into one matrix equation produces

$$
\begin{bmatrix}
y_{11} & y_{12} & \cdots & y_{1N} \\
y_{21} & y_{22} & \cdots & y_{2N} \\
\vdots & \vdots & \ddots & \vdots \\
y_{n1} & y_{n2} & \cdots & y_{nN}
\end{bmatrix}
=
\begin{bmatrix}
m_{11} & m_{12} & \cdots & m_{1n} \\
m_{21} & m_{22} & \cdots & m_{2n} \\
\vdots & \vdots & \ddots & \vdots \\
m_{n1} & m_{n2} & \cdots & m_{nn}
\end{bmatrix}
\begin{bmatrix}
\underline{c}_1' \\
\underline{c}_2' \\
\vdots \\
\underline{c}_n'
\end{bmatrix},
\tag{11.2}
$$

or

$$Y = MC.$$

As in chapter 10, the $n \times N$ matrix Y includes all data from all $N$ voxels at each of the $n$ TRs of the experiment (i.e., Y has a row for each TR and a column for each voxel). C is an $n \times N$ matrix containing a component in each of its $n$ rows. Finally, the $n \times n$ matrix M is called the mixing matrix because it contains the weights that determine the mixture proportions of the components on each TR.

When M is square, it will also be nonsingular, and thus $M^{-1}$ will exist. Denote this inverse by $U = M^{-1}$. Then note that

$$C = UY.
\tag{11.3}$$

The matrix U is often called the unmixing matrix. Equation 11.3 is the form actually used to find the components. There are a variety of ICA algorithms (e.g., Hyvärinen, Karhunen, & Oja, 2001), but they all attempt to find entries in the U matrix that make the rows of C as component-like as possible. Some of these try to maximize the statistical independence of the rows of C in order to find components, whereas others try to maximize the non-normality of these rows. As we will see, however, these two goals are very similar and tend to produce the same solutions. To see why this is true, we need to better understand the criteria that are used to assess independence and non-normality, and we also need to better understand why components or signals should be non-normally distributed. The next two sections address these issues.

### Assessing Statistical Independence

If we grant that separate components should be statistically independent, then a critical problem to solve is to find a method via which we can judge whether the entries in two rows of C are statistically independent. In probability and statistics, two random variables

$X$ and $Y$ are said to be statistically independent if and only if their joint probability density function, $f_{X,Y}(x, y)$, equals the product of the two marginal distributions, $f_X(x)$ and $f_Y(y)$, for all values of $x$ and $y$; that is, if and only if

$$f_{X,Y}(x, y) = f_X(x) f_Y(y), \quad \text{for all } x \text{ and } y. \tag{11.4}$$

In the context of ICA, this is not a useful criterion for establishing independence for two reasons. First, it requires estimating probability density functions, which is a statistically challenging task that has no known optimal solution. Second, independence is satisfied only if the equation 11.4 equality holds for all values of $x$ and $y$. Therefore, we would have to check an infinite number of equalities if equation 11.4 was our test of independence. An ideal method would require that we check only a single equality to verify independence and would use parameters or functions of parameters that are straightforward to estimate. Unfortunately, such an ideal method does not exist, and as a result, many alternative options have been proposed. We will review some of the most important of these in the next major section.

An obvious candidate to solve this problem might seem to be the correlation coefficient, which is easy to estimate, and a test based on the correlation coefficient would require checking only one equality. It is true that statistically independent random variables are necessarily uncorrelated. The problem though is that uncorrelated random variables are not necessarily independent (e.g., Ashby & Townsend, 1986). The Pearson correlation coefficient only measures the strength of the linear relationship between two variables. Statistical independence requires no relationship of any kind. Two random variables could be strongly related in a nonlinear way, yet still be uncorrelated. For example, suppose a scatterplot of $X$ and $Y$ samples is U shaped. In this case, knowledge of $X$ allows one to predict the value of $Y$, so $X$ and $Y$ are not independent, but the best-fitting regression line has a slope of 0, and therefore $X$ and $Y$ are uncorrelated.

The correlation coefficient is insufficient for assessing independence because it depends only on first-order (e.g., mean) and second-order (e.g., variance) statistics, whereas statistical independence depends on statistics of all orders. The *order* of a statistic is equal to the highest power in the expected value that defines that statistic. The mean of $X$ is defined as $\mu = E(X)$. Because the exponent on $X$ is 1, the mean is a first-order statistic. The variance is defined as $\sigma^2 = E(X - \mu)^2$, so the variance is a second-order statistic. Many higher-order statistics depend on the central moments of the distribution. The $r^{th}$ central moment of $X$, which is a statistic of order $r$, is defined as $E(X - \mu)^r$. For example, kurtosis, which is a fourth-order statistic, depends on the second and fourth moments, whereas skewness (a third-order statistic) depends on the second and third moments.

Statistical independence (i.e., equation 11.4) depends on statistics of all orders, so no method that tries to minimize or maximize some function of first- and second-order statistics (such as the correlation coefficient) could ever successfully identify statistical independence—at least not without some extra assumptions (e.g., normality). For this reason, all of the ICA methods discussed below incorporate higher-order statistics at some point in their algorithms. For example, one of the earliest ICA algorithms was based on estimating the first four moments of the component distributions (Comon, 1994).

## The Importance of Non-normality in ICA

As previously mentioned, a second fundamental assumption of ICA is that signals or components have non-normal distributions. More specifically, ICA assumes that the distribution of the elements in each component has a higher peak and higher tails than the normal distribution. Such distributions are said to be leptokurtic or super-Gaussian. One example is the Laplace distribution. Figure 11.1 shows normal and Laplace distributions each of which has mean 0 and variance 1. Note that the Laplace has much higher likelihood around zero and it also has slightly higher tails.

To understand why ICA assumes that components have super-Gaussian distributions, consider a stimulus-related component in some cognitive task. Suppose this component includes the neural network that mediates the perceptual and cognitive processing of the stimulus. Even if this network depends on many brain areas, the vast majority of voxels in the whole brain will fall in areas not in this network. These voxels will not respond to the stimulus, so most voxels in the component will have activation values near zero. The Laplace distribution provides a good model of this because of its high likelihood around zero. In contrast, the normal distribution predicts too few voxels with activations near zero. The other problem with the normal distribution is that it has very low tails. Thus, it predicts that few voxels in each component will have extreme activation values. But all voxels in our hypothetical neural network should have extreme values, so the tails of the component distribution should be higher than in a normal distribution.

From the central limit theorem, we know that normal distributions arise from processes in which many independent factors are added together. This seems like a good model of noise because we think of noise as arising from many small independent sources, rather than from a single source. But we do not typically think of signals in this way. So an ideal model might assume that some components arise from super-Gaussian distributed signals, and the other components represent normally distributed noise. In fact, this is exactly the assumptions of the noisy ICA model, which we will consider later in this chapter.

## Preparing Data for ICA

Almost all ICA algorithms include some data-preparation steps. The most common of these are to mean-center and then whiten the data. Mean centering resets the mean (across TRs) in each voxel to 0, and whitening converts the variance-covariance matrix to the identity, so that all variances equal 1 and all covariances equal 0. The whitening process is especially relevant to the non-normality assumption.

We encountered mean centering in several previous chapters. In this step, for every voxel, we compute the mean BOLD response across all TRs and then subtract this same value from the BOLD response at every TR (see equations 10.4–10.7 for details). All ICA

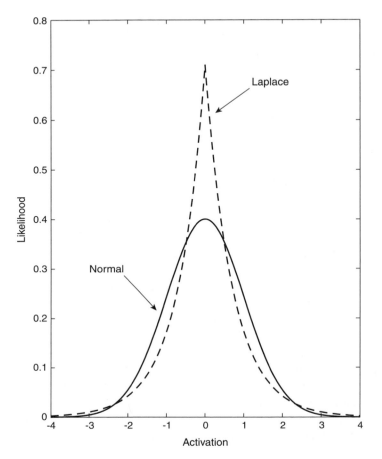

**Figure 11.1**
Probability density functions of Laplace and normal distributions. The mean of both distributions is zero, and in both cases the variance is 1.

algorithms assume mean-centered data, so in the remainder of this chapter we assume that the data matrix Y has already been centered.

Whitening data means to apply a linear transformation so that the variance-covariance matrix equals the identity; in other words, so that all variances equal 1 and all covariances equal 0. To whiten the data, we need to find a matrix P so that the transformation

$$Y_w = PY, \tag{11.5}$$

causes $\hat{\Sigma}_w = I$. There are several known solutions to this problem. One is to choose

$$P = D^{-1/2}V', \tag{11.6}$$

where D is the diagonal matrix of eigenvalues of $\hat{\Sigma}_Y$, and V is the orthogonal matrix with columns equal to the corresponding eigenvectors[1] of $\hat{\Sigma}_Y$ (i.e., see appendix A). A computationally simpler alternative is to use $P = A^{-1}$, where A is the lower triangular Cholesky matrix that results from the Cholesky factorization of $\hat{\Sigma}_Y$ (e.g., see proposition 1.8, Ashby, 1992).

Whitening is theoretically important because after this step, all the eigenvalues of the variance-covariance matrix are 1, and thus the data have equal variance in all directions. As a result, a PCA on whitened data is useless. All a PCA would do is tell us that any direction in the data is just as important as any other direction. Thus, if the components were normally distributed, whitening would throw all useful information about them away. Whitening therefore makes sense only if the components are non-normally distributed.

But why do ICA algorithms take the time to whiten the data? It turns out that whitening the data reduces by more than half the number of parameters in the unmixing matrix that must be estimated. The fewer parameters to estimate, the faster the algorithm will run. Of course, it takes time to whiten the data, but as it happens the time saved in the parameter estimation process when ICA is run on whitened data more than compensates for the extra time required to whiten the data. So the main reason to whiten data is to make the ICA programs run faster.

To see that whitening reduces the number of free parameters in the unmixing matrix, note from equations 11.2 and 11.5 that

$$Y_W = PY = PMC.$$

Therefore, we could define a new mixing matrix for the whitened data as

$$M_W = PM$$

(i.e., because now $Y_W = M_W C$). Because $Y_W$ is whitened, its variance-covariance matrix equals the identity. Therefore

$$I = \hat{\Sigma}_W = \frac{1}{n-1} Y_W Y_W'$$

$$= \frac{1}{n-1}(M_W C)(M_W C)' = M_W \left( \frac{1}{n-1} CC' \right) M_W' = M_W \hat{\Sigma}_C M_W'$$

$$= M_W M_W'. \tag{11.7}$$

---

1. To see that this works, note that

$$\hat{\Sigma}_W = P\hat{\Sigma}_Y P' = (D^{-1/2}V')\hat{\Sigma}_Y(D^{-1/2}V')' = (D^{-1/2}V')(VDV')(VD^{-1/2})$$

$$= (D^{-1/2}V')(VD^{1/2}D^{1/2}V')(VD^{-1/2}) = D^{-1/2}(V'V)D^{1/2}D^{1/2}(V'V)D^{-1/2}$$

$$= (D^{-1/2}D^{1/2})(D^{1/2}D^{-1/2}) = I.$$

Note that this derivation assumes that $\hat{\Sigma}_C = I$. This is true in all forms of ICA. $\hat{\Sigma}_C$ must be diagonal (i.e., all covariances equal zero) because ICA assumes all components are independent (and independent components are necessarily uncorrelated), and as mentioned above, the component variances cannot be estimated uniquely in ICA, so without loss of generality, it is standard to set them all to one. Equation 11.7 shows that $M_W$ is an orthogonal matrix (i.e., a matrix B is orthogonal if and only if $BB' = B'B = I$). This greatly simplifies the parameter estimation process because as with any orthogonal matrix, $M_W^{-1} = M_W'$. Therefore,

$$C = U_W X_W$$

$$= M_W^{-1} X_W$$

$$= M_W' X_W.$$

As a result, the unmixing matrix $U_W$ is also orthogonal. An $n \times n$ orthogonal matrix has only $n(n-1)/2$ free parameters, whereas the original, unconstrained unmixing matrix U has $n^2$ free parameters. In addition, however, note that after parameter estimation is complete, the mixing matrix $M_W$ can be computed quickly by simply transposing the unmixing matrix (rather than inverting it).

Mean centering and whitening the data does throw away information, but it only throws away information about means, variances, and covariances. None of these statistics carry any information about nonnormality. To see this note that the transformations we used to mean center and whiten are all linear. Because linear transformations of normally distributed variables are still normally distributed, mean centering and whitening do not affect the normality or non-normality of the data. This is really all the ICA algorithms care about, so mean centering and whitening only throws away information that ICA algorithms never use anyway.

## ICA Algorithms

The goal of any ICA algorithm is to estimate the parameters of the unmixing matrix U (or $U_W$) and the components. Many such algorithms have been proposed. This section provides a brief overview of the most widely used of these. The goal is to give the reader a theoretical understanding of how these algorithms work. For computational details, the original sources should be consulted.

### Minimizing Mutual Information

A number of algorithms are based on results from information theory. One reason for this is that information theory provides a nonparametric measure of statistical independence that requires checking only one equality. Information theory was developed by Claude

Shannon in an attempt to quantify the effects on communication of transmitting signals across unreliable media (Shannon & Weaver, 1949). A key role in this approach is played by the mathematical concept of *information*, which is also sometimes called *uncertainty* or *entropy*. The basic idea is to quantify the amount of information that is gained when one witnesses the occurrence of some event. For example, suppose we watch someone toss a coin in the air. Before the toss, we know the probability of a heads or a tails occurring are both $\frac{1}{2}$. Now suppose we watch the toss and a heads comes up. How much information have we gained during this process? Shannon essentially decided to arbitrarily call the amount of information gained during this experiment 1 bit. Given that we gained 1 bit of information from this experience, he then worked out how to compute the number of bits of information that would be gained from observing the outcome of any experiment.

**Mathematical Definitions**    Readers not interested in the mathematical details should skip to the next section (i.e., "Conceptual Treatment"). Shannon's solution was to define the information, uncertainty, or entropy in a continuous random variable $X$ as

$$H(X) = E[-\log f(x)] = -\int f(x) \log f(x) \, dx, \tag{11.8}$$

where $E$ denotes expected value, and $f(x)$ is the probability density function of $X$. If $X$ is a discrete random variable, then the integral is replaced by a sum

$$H(X) = -\sum_{x} P(X = x) \log P(X = x). \tag{11.9}$$

If the log has base 2, then $H(X)$ is measured in bits of information. For example, consider our coin-tossing experiment. In this case, we could define a random variable $X$ that equals 0 if the coin toss produces a heads and 1 if it produces a tails. Then

$$H(X) = -[P(X = 0) \log_2 P(X = 0) + P(X = 1) \log_2 P(X = 1)]$$

$$= -[\tfrac{1}{2} \log_2 \tfrac{1}{2} + \tfrac{1}{2} \log_2 \tfrac{1}{2}]$$

$$= -[\tfrac{1}{2}(-1) + \tfrac{1}{2}(-1)]$$

$$= 1 \text{ bit}.$$

So this definition does say that the amount of information gained from observing the results of one coin toss is 1 bit.

Equation 11.8 is readily extended to random vectors. In particular, when $X$ and $Y$ are both random variables, then the *joint information* in the vector $(X, Y)'$ equals

$$H(X, Y) = -\iint f(x, y) \log f(x, y) \, dx \, dy. \tag{11.10}$$

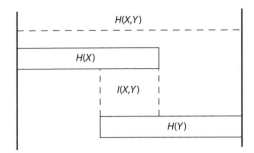

**Figure 11.2**
Schematic illustrating the relationships among the information-theoretic constructs of joint information [$H(X,Y)$], mutual information [$I(X,Y)$], and marginal information [$H(X)$ and $H(Y)$].

Now the *mutual information* contained simultaneously in $X$ and $Y$ is defined as

$$I(X,Y) = H(X) + H(Y) - H(X,Y). \tag{11.11}$$

**Conceptual Treatment**    Figure 11.2 illustrates the relationships among the most important information-theoretic measures. For two random variables $X$ and $Y$, $H(X)$ and $H(Y)$ denote the number of bits of information gained by observing the outcome of a random sample drawn from the $X$ and $Y$ populations, respectively. The joint information $H(X,Y)$ is the amount of information gained by observing both samples simultaneously, and the mutual information $I(X,Y)$, defined by equation 11.11, is a measure of how much information one gains about $Y$ by observing a sample from the $X$ population, or vice versa. Information theory plays a critical role in ICA because of the following well-known theorem.

**Proposition 11.1**    Two random variables $X$ and $Y$ are statistically independent if and only if $I(X,Y) = 0$.

**Proof**    See, for example, Papoulis and Pillai (2002).

Proposition 11.1 provides a straightforward solution to the conceptual problem of assessing the statistical independence of a pair of random variables. In particular, only a single calculation is required. If the mutual information between $X$ and $Y$ is 0, then the random variables are independent. If the mutual information is any nonzero value, then they are statistically dependent.

One ICA approach then is to find the entries in the unmixing matrix U that minimize the mutual information between the rows of C. Although this method requires that we check only a single equality, it is more difficult than it might seem because of the statistical challenges of estimating mutual information. This is not unexpected. As mentioned earlier, statistical independence depends on all higher-order statistics. This fact, coupled with proposition 11.1, therefore guarantees that mutual information must also depend on all higher-order statistics. For example, Comon (1994) proposed an algorithm that minimizes mutual information, and this algorithm estimates mutual information with a statistic that requires estimating the first four moments of the component distributions. One significant weakness of such methods is that the standard error of higher moments is huge. Enormous, noise-free samples are needed to estimate third and fourth moments accurately. If even a few outliers enter the data set, such estimates can change dramatically (e.g., Ratcliff, 1979). For this reason, ICA algorithms based on direct estimation of higher moments have not become popular.

## Methods That Maximize Non-normality

Some ICA algorithms work by trying to find entries in the unmixing matrix U that make the rows of C as super-Gaussian as possible. There are two popular ways that this is done. One tries to maximize kurtosis, which is a measure of the "peakedness" of the probability density function. Kurtosis, which is a function of the fourth and second moments, equals zero in a normal distribution. Leptokurtic or super-Gaussian distributions, like the Laplace, have positive kurtosis. Distributions with negative kurtosis, which are said to be platykurtic, tend to be flatter than the normal distribution. Kurtosis-based ICA algorithms find entries in W that maximize the kurtosis of each row of C (e.g., Hyvärinen & Oja, 1997). However, because kurtosis is a fourth-order statistic, kurtosis estimators are extremely sensitive to outliers. For this reason, ICA algorithms that use other methods of detecting non-normality have been proposed. One such approach uses information theory.

The normal distribution has zero kurtosis, but it also has other special properties. For example, consider the class of all continuous random variables with some specific mean and variance that are defined over the whole real line. There are an infinite number of possible distributions in this class, but of all these, the normal distribution has the greatest information. If $X$ is normally distributed with mean $\mu$ and variance $\sigma^2$, then the information in $X$ can be shown to equal

$$H(X) = \tfrac{1}{2}[1 + \ln(2\pi\sigma^2)].$$
(11.12)

Thus, all other continuous distributions with this same mean and variance have information less than this value. A similar result holds for multivariate distributions. Consider the class of all continuous random vectors with some specific variance-covariance matrix and that are defined on each dimension over the entire real line. Then among all such distributions, the multivariate normal has the greatest joint information.

These results led to the creation of a new construct called *negentropy*, which is defined as

$$J(X) = \tfrac{1}{2}[1 + \ln(2\pi\sigma^2)] - H(X),$$
(11.13)

for any random variable $X$ with variance $\sigma^2$. The first term on the right is the information in a normal distribution. Because $H(X)$ cannot be greater than this value, negentropy can never be negative. Note that negentropy equals zero only if $X$ is normally distributed, so the larger the value of $J(X)$, the more non-normal the distribution of $X$.

So an alternative ICA algorithm is to find the entries in U that maximize the sum of the negentropies in each row of C (Hyvärinen, 1999). Special care must be taken in this process to avoid the possibility that different rows of C converge to the same non-normal solution. This is not a problem if the data are prewhitened. As we saw in a previous section, whitening the data matrix means that the mixing matrix is orthogonal. In other words,

$$U = M^{-1} = M',$$

which implies that

$$U^{-1} = (M^{-1})^{-1} = M,$$

and thus the unmixing matrix is also orthogonal. After whitening, the data matrix Y is also orthogonal, and the product of two orthogonal matrices is orthogonal. Therefore, the component matrix

$$C = UY$$

is itself orthogonal, so

$$CC' = I.$$

If we denote the $i^{th}$ row of C by $\underline{c}_i'$ then the orthogonality of C means that

$$\underline{c}_i' \underline{c}_i = 0,$$

or in other words, that the different components in C must be uncorrelated. If they are uncorrelated, then they cannot be identical. Thus, prewhitening the data matrix guarantees that maximizing the negentropies of the rows of C will produce a set of unique components.

As the reader might anticipate, negentropy is not inherently easier to estimate than mutual information. For example, one estimator uses the third moment and kurtosis (Hyvärinen et al., 2001) and therefore suffers from the same weaknesses as the other methods that we have discussed that also use these statistics. Hyvärinen (1999) proposed an alternative method that replaces the third and fourth moments with the expected value of certain non-polynomial functions that have estimators with better statistical properties. The resulting algorithm, called FastICA, has become quite popular.

We have now seen two ICA algorithms with the different goals of minimizing mutual information and maximizing negentropy that nevertheless both use concepts from information theory. This might cause one to wonder exactly how these two methods are related. As it happens, they are so closely related that minimizing mutual information almost always leads to essentially the same solution as maximizing negentropy. The key to seeing this is to understand how the ICA parameter estimation process affects the joint information of the component matrix C. The data matrix Y remains the same throughout the parameter estimation process, so its joint information is constant. It turns out that the effect of the linear transformation C = UY is to increase the joint information in C by the log of the determinant of the unmixing matrix U; that is,

Information(C) = Information(Y) + log|U|.                                    (11.14)

Thus, although the joint information of Y is unaffected by parameter estimation, the joint information of C changes when the determinant of U changes. If the data are prewhitened, however, then U is orthogonal and |U| = 1 (the determinant of any orthogonal matrix is either +1 or −1). Therefore, if we prewhiten the data, then

Information(C) = Information(Y),

and so the joint information of C does not change during the process of estimating the entries in U. Note from figure 11.2 that for any value of joint information, mutual information is minimized when each marginal information is as small as possible. Equation 11.13 makes it clear that negentropy is maximized when the marginal information is minimized. Thus, minimizing mutual information is essentially the same as maximizing negentropy.[2]

## Maximum Likelihood Approaches
Still another popular method for estimating the entries in the unmixing matrix U is to use the method of maximum likelihood (Gaeta & Lacoume, 1990; Pham & Garrat, 1997). The goal of this method is to find the matrix U that maximizes the likelihood of observing the data that we actually collected in our fMRI experiment, given, of course, that the ICA model is correct.

The derivation of this likelihood depends on several critical assumptions that are made by all versions of ICA. First, of course, is the fundamental assumption of ICA that separate components are statistically independent. Second, because the data have already been centered (i.e., so the mean in all voxels is zero) and whitened, ICA assumes that the distributions of all components have identical form. Third, ICA assumes that for each component, the component values in each voxel are independent samples from the same component distribution. Given these three conditions, it can be shown that the joint likelihood of the data given a particular unmixing matrix U equals (e.g., see Hyvärinen et al., 2001; or Stone, 2004)

---

2. Under these conditions, they are mathematically equivalent (i.e., when the mixing matrix is orthogonal). In practice, however, because the algorithms for minimizing mutual information and maximizing negentropy are different, it is possible that they will yield different solutions.

$$L(Y|U) = |U|^n \prod_{i=1}^{n} \prod_{k=1}^{n} f(c_{ik}), \tag{11.15}$$

where $f(c_{ik})$ is the component probability density function, and as before, $n$ is the number of TRs. So the method of maximum likelihood finds the matrix U that maximizes the right side of equation 11.15. Computationally, it is often easier to maximize the log of this likelihood:

$$\log[L(Y|U)] = n\log(|U|) + \sum_{i=1}^{n} \sum_{k=1}^{n} \log[f(c_{ik})]. \tag{11.16}$$

Because the log is a strictly increasing function, the matrix U that maximizes the right side of equation 11.16 will also maximize the right side of equation 11.15.

An important point to note is that the right side of equation 11.16 can be maximized only if we specify the form of the component distributions [i.e., the $f(c_{ik})$]. For example, one might assume that the components all have Laplace distributions. It turns out that this specification does not need to be precise. Similar solutions are obtained for a reasonably broad class of choices for the $f(c_{ik})$ (e.g., Hyvärinen et al., 2001). However these distributions are identified, it is vital that we assume they are super-Gaussian. When this is done, maximum likelihood algorithms tend to produce solutions that are nearly identical to the ones obtained by the other ICA methods we have considered. Thus, whereas the other methods we have discussed estimate higher-order moments or some other nonlinear functions, maximum likelihood approaches overcome the need for higher-order statistical information by specifying this information *a priori*, in the form of a parametric guess about the component distributions.

## Infomax

**Overview**    Another ICA estimation technique, which is closely related to maximum likelihood, is provided by the infomax principle (Bell & Sejnowski, 1995). Infomax specifies a learning algorithm for a neural network that maximizes the joint information in the outputs—hence the name infomax. The neural network is illustrated in figure 11.3. When used to perform ICA, the entire set of BOLD responses is input to the network, one voxel at a time. The $i^{th}$ set of these inputs is the BOLD responses from the $i^{th}$ voxel at every TR of the experiment. The inputs are multiplied by a set of constants that form the unmixing matrix U, and these are summed to produce the components. So as before, $c_{ij}$ is the value of component $j$ in voxel $i$. Next, the component values are passed through a nonlinear squashing function to produce the outputs $g(c_{ij})$. A common choice for $g$ is the logistic function

$$g(c_{ij}) = \frac{1}{1 + e^{-c_{ij}}}. \tag{11.17}$$

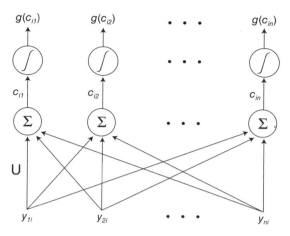

**Figure 11.3**
The infomax neural network. The learning algorithm finds connection weights (elements of the matrix U) that maximize the joint information of the outputs [i.e., the $g(c_{ij})$].

This is the function displayed in figure 11.3. After the data from each voxel propagate through the network, infomax uses a gradient ascent learning algorithm to modify the connection weights (i.e., the entries in U) before the data from the next voxel are input. The goal of this learning algorithm is to maximize the joint information in the $g(c_{ij})$.

As mentioned before, of all distributions defined over the entire real line, the one with the greatest information (i.e., for a given mean and variance) is the normal distribution. But of course, any fixed set of data will have a largest and smallest value, and thus real data are always bounded. If we take all possible distributions defined over a fixed interval, then it turns out that the distribution with the greatest information is the uniform distribution. So by maximizing the joint information in the outputs, infomax is trying to make the outputs as uniformly distributed as possible.

Note that equation 11.11 implies that the joint information satisfies

$$H(X,Y) = H(X) + H(Y) - I(X,Y).$$ (11.18)

Thus, the joint information is increased if the marginal information is increased or if the mutual information is decreased. Infomax maximizes joint information, so it will tend to reduce mutual information. But it will not necessarily drive mutual information to its absolute minimum value. The exception occurs when the squashing function $g$ exactly equals the cumulative distribution function of the component distributions (Bell & Sejnowski, 1995). In this case, infomax not only maximizes the joint information of the outputs, but it also simultaneously minimizes their mutual information—or, in other words, it maximizes the statistical independence of the network outputs. Now a fundamental result of probability theory says that if two random variables are statistically independent, then any order-preserving transformation of those random variables is also independent. Figure 11.3 makes it clear that the relationship between the component values and the network outputs is order preserving. Thus, maximizing the statistical independence of the network outputs is equivalent to maximizing the statistical independence of the components. For this reason, infomax can successfully implement ICA.

In fact, shortly after infomax was proposed, it was shown to be equivalent to maximum likelihood ICA, under this same condition that the squashing function is equal to the cumulative distribution function of the component distributions (Cardoso, 1997; Pearlmutter & Parra, 1997). Thus, if we believe that component distributions are super-Gaussian, then if we use infomax for ICA, it is critical to use a squashing function that is the cumulative distribution function of a super-Gaussian distribution. The logistic function in equation 11.17, which is a popular infomax choice, is the cumulative distribution function of a logistic distribution. Figure 11.4 compares the logistic and normal distributions. Note that the logistic is super-Gaussian, but not as much as the Laplace (i.e., compare figures 11.1 and 11.4).

The nonlinear squashing function is critical to the infomax algorithm. As mentioned earlier, statistical independence depends on all higher-order moments. The nonlinearity of the squashing function provides access to this higher-order statistical information. Without the nonlinearity, maximizing the joint information in the outputs is equivalent to maximizing the determinant of the unmixing matrix U (e.g., Bell & Sejnowski, 1995). Because the determinant is the product of the eigenvalues (e.g., see appendix A), this would be equivalent to maximizing the eigenvalues of U and therefore maximizing the variance along each of the principal components. This method then would not be able to discover independent components. It would merely spread the data out in the original dimensions as far as possible.

**The Infomax Learning Algorithm**    The learning algorithm used by infomax describes how to update the weights in the network after inputting the data from each successive voxel. Readers not interested in the technical details of this learning algorithm should skip ahead to the next section. Ideally, the Infomax updating scheme would guarantee that the unmixing matrix converges to the ICA solution. To appreciate the infomax solution to this problem, we need some new notation. Equation 11.1 specifies how each row of Y is related to the mixing weights and the components. Note that the columns of Y each contain the BOLD responses from one voxel over every TR of the experiment. Denote the $i^{th}$ column by

$$\underline{y}_{v(i)} = \begin{bmatrix} y_{1i} \\ y_{2i} \\ \vdots \\ y_{ni} \end{bmatrix}.$$

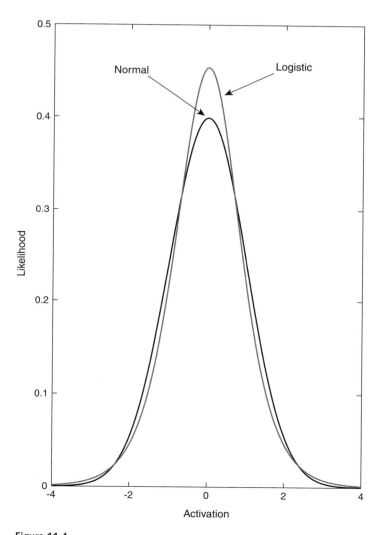

**Figure 11.4**
Normal and logistic probability density functions. Note that the logistic distribution is slightly super-Gaussian (i.e., compare with the Laplace distribution in figure 11.1).

Similarly, whereas the $i^{th}$ row of the component matrix C defines the value of the component $i$ in each voxel, the $i^{th}$ column defines all the component values in voxel $i$. Denote this column by

$$\underline{c}_{V(i)} = \begin{bmatrix} c_{1i} \\ c_{2i} \\ \vdots \\ c_{ni} \end{bmatrix}.$$

The learning algorithm used by infomax depends on the first two derivatives of the squashing function $g$. Remember that $g$ is the cumulative distribution function of the component distribution, so the first derivative of $g$ is the component probability density function, which we denote by $f(c_{ij})$. In other words,

$$\frac{dg(c_{ij})}{dc_{ij}} = f(c_{ij}).$$

We denote the second derivative by

$$\frac{df(c_{ij})}{dc_{ij}} = \dot{f}(c_{ij}).$$

The infomax learning algorithm depends on the ratio of these two derivatives, which we denote by

$$b(c_{ij}) = \frac{\dot{f}(c_{ij})}{f(c_{ij})}. \tag{11.19}$$

Finally, define the vector of all possible $b(c_{ij})$ as

$$\underline{b}(\underline{c}_{V(i)}) = \begin{bmatrix} b(c_{i1}) \\ b(c_{i2}) \\ \vdots \\ b(c_{in}) \end{bmatrix}.$$

Given these definitions, we can now describe the learning algorithm. Following the presentation of the data from voxel $i$, the unmixing matrix U is updated by

$$U_{new} = U_{old} + \eta \left[ (U')^{-1} + \frac{1}{n} \sum_{i=1}^{n} \underline{b}(\underline{c}_{V(i)}) \underline{y}_{V(i)}' \right], \tag{11.20}$$

where $\eta$ is the learning rate (typically around 0.01). For a derivation of equation 11.20, see Bell and Sejnowski (1995) or Stone (2004).

Amari, Cichocki, and Yang (1996) proposed post-multiplying the second term on the right by U'U, which converts equation 11.20 into

$$U_{new} = U_{old} + \eta \left[ I + \frac{1}{n} \sum_{i=1}^{n} \underline{b}(\underline{c}_{V(i)})(\underline{y}_{V(i)}U)' \right] U$$

$$= U_{old} + \eta \left[ I + \frac{1}{n} \sum_{i=1}^{n} \underline{b}(\underline{c}_{V(i)})\underline{c}_{V(i)}' \right] U. \qquad (11.21)$$

This form of the learning rule avoids computing the matrix inverse required in equation 11.20 and converges more quickly to the optimal solution. In the case where a logistic squashing function is used, it is straightforward to show[3] that $b(c_{ij})$ reduces to:

$$b(c_{ij}) = 1 - 2g(c_{ij}). \qquad (11.22)$$

Bell and Sejnowski (1995) computed this term for seven different possible choices for the squashing function (i.e., see their table 1).

To apply the equation 11.21 learning rule, the first step is to set up the figure 11.3 neural network and define an initial unmixing matrix U (e.g., set U to the identity or generate random samples to fill U). Next, data from the different voxels are input to the network, and U is updated according to equation 11.21. After all the voxels have been input, the process is repeated until the changes in U become negligible (e.g., after the root mean square change over all elements of U is less than $10^{-6}$; McKeown et al., 1998). During this process, it is common to gradually reduce the learning rate $\eta$.

## Interpreting ICA Results

The results of an ICA should be largely the same, regardless of which method is used to estimate the components and the mixing parameters. With any method, two principle problems remain to be solved after the estimation process is complete. First, unlike PCA, ICA provides no direct information about which components are most important. This is because of the indeterminacy in the variance of each component. As we saw earlier, it is

---

3. If $g(c) = (1 + e^{-c})^{-1}$, then $f(c) = e^{-c}(1 + e^{-c})^{-2} = g(c)[1 - g(c)]$. Therefore, by the product rule,

$$\dot{f}(c) = f(c)[1 - g(c)] - f(c)g(c) = g(c)[1 - g(c)]^2 - [g(c)]^2[1 - g(c)] = g(c)[1 - g(c)]\{[1 - g(c)] - g(c)\}$$

$$= g(c)[1 - g(c)][1 - 2g(c)].$$

Combining these two results produces

$$b(c) = \frac{\dot{f}(c)}{f(c)} = \frac{g(c)[1 - g(c)][1 - 2g(c)]}{g(c)[1 - g(c)]} = 1 - 2g(c).$$

mathematically impossible to estimate the variance of a component uniquely. As a result, all component variances are set to 1. This means that ICA does not partition the total variance in a data set into a set of independent sources. As a result, ICA can identify components and weights, but it cannot directly determine the relative importance of these components.[4]

The second problem in interpreting ICA results is to assign interpretations to the various components. Theoretically, any independent source of variation will be identified as a separate component. This includes neural networks that mediate the perceptual and cognitive processing of the stimulus, but it also includes artifacts due to head movements, respiration, and even the subject's heartbeat. A typical ICA will identify as many components as there are TRs in the experiment. Somehow we must sift through these several hundred components to find the few that are related to the task we are studying. This section describes standard methods of solving these two problems.

### Determining the Relative Importance of Each Component

The relative importance of a component can be determined by examining how different the data would look if that component were lost or eliminated. Eliminating an unimportant component would not alter the data in any meaningful way, but eliminating a critical component would fundamentally change the look of the data. There are several ways to do this, but perhaps the simplest is to set each component successively to the zero vector, $\underline{0}' = [0 \ 0 \ \ldots \ 0]$, reconstruct the data matrix Y, and then compare the new data matrix that results from this operation with the original matrix.

For example, we can compute what the data would look like if the first component were eliminated by forming the product

$$
Y_{\text{without } \underline{c}_1} = \begin{bmatrix} m_{11} & m_{12} & \cdots & m_{1n} \\ m_{21} & m_{22} & \cdots & m_{2n} \\ \vdots & \vdots & \ddots & \vdots \\ m_{n1} & m_{n2} & \cdots & m_{nn} \end{bmatrix} \begin{bmatrix} \underline{0}' \\ \underline{c}_2{}' \\ \vdots \\ \underline{c}_n{}' \end{bmatrix}.
$$

Note that this is identical to equation 11.2 except we have set all component 1 values to 0. Next, we need to compare the original data matrix Y to $Y_{\text{without } \underline{c}_1}$. A straightforward method of doing this is to compute the sum of squared differences between the entries in the two matrices:

---

4. This has nothing to do with whether or not we choose to whiten the data before running our ICA. Instead, it is a consequence of the inherent ambiguity in the ICA model $Y = MC$. The problem is that nothing on the right side of this equality is known beforehand. As a result, there are an infinite number of solutions. Assuming the separate components are independent and non-normally distributed helps hugely. In particular, these extra constraints guarantee that the components can be identified uniquely. However, they are not enough to determine the relative importance of each component.

$$SSD(\underline{c}_1) = \sum_{j=1}^{N} \sum_{i=1}^{n} [Y(i,j) - Y_{\text{without } \underline{c}_1}(i,j)]^2. \tag{11.23}$$

The larger this value, the more important the component.

This process is then repeated for every component. Rank ordering the resulting $SSD(\underline{c}_i)$ rank orders the relative importance of all of the components. Furthermore, because the components are independent, the percentage of variance accounted for by the $i^{th}$ component equals

$$\frac{SSD(\underline{c}_i)}{\sum_{k=1}^{n} SSD(\underline{c}_k)}.$$

## Assigning Meaning to Components

Once the most important components have been identified, the next step is to figure out what they mean. This is a much trickier step because there is no known algorithm that is guaranteed to work for every component. The accepted approach, however, is to determine the meaning of a component by examining its weights. The basic idea is that we expect a component to be most active shortly after the event to which it is responding. The weights associated with a component specify the relative contribution of that component at each TR in the experiment. Thus, a zero weight means that the component made no contribution, whereas a large weight means the component was very active at that TR. For example, a component associated with head movements should have a large value when the subject moves his or her head and should be near zero on all other TRs. Because head movements should be rare, we would expect only a few large weights during the whole experiment.

An example from a real ICA is shown in figure 11.5. This experiment used a simple event-related design in which the stimuli were arrows that pointed either to the left or to the right, and the subject's task was to press a response key on the side to which the arrow was pointing. The top panel of figure 11.5 shows a component map that was thresholded at ±2.9 to aid visual interpretation. Remember that a component map specifies a numerical value in each voxel. These values will have mean 0 (because the data matrix Y was mean centered) and variance 1. So to threshold at ±2.9, all component values less than 2.9 and greater than −2.9 are set to 0. The idea here is that voxels with extreme values are most important because when multiplied by the weights, they will change most across TRs (e.g., a voxel with a component value of 0 has a predicted value of 0 for all TRs).

It is important to note, though, that this thresholding process cannot be used to determine statistical significance. This means that we are not justified in saying that the voxels that exceed the threshold are the ones making a statistically significant contribution to the component map. This is because the components were selected to have non-normal distributions, and therefore, even though the component values have mean 0 and variance 1, they

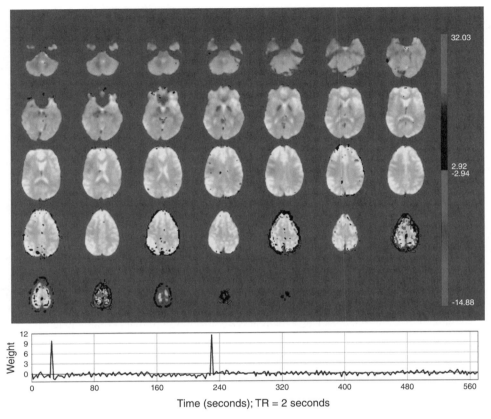

**Figure 11.5**
A component map (top panel) and its associated weights (bottom panel). Voxels in the component map are thresholded at ±2.9. It is highly likely that this component is driven by two discrete head movements.

do not follow a z-distribution. As a result, the true *p*-value associated with any particular threshold is unknown. We will discuss a possible solution to this problem in the next section (i.e., "The Noisy ICA Model"). For now, though, it must suffice to keep in mind that the thresholding evident in figure 11.5 (and in figure 11.6) has no statistical interpretation and is only done to aid visual inspection of the component maps.

The bottom panel of figure 11.5 shows the component weights. Note that these hover around 0, except for two TRs, when they take on values greater than 9. In this experiment, many more than two left and right arrows were displayed, so it is not likely that this component is task related. Figure 11.5 describes about 10 minutes of data, so the component displayed there was much too infrequent to be related to the subject's respiration or heart rate. An obvious candidate is head movement. The component map supports this hypothesis because almost all voxels that exceed threshold are around the edges of the brain.

We can use a similar approach to find task-related components. A component that identifies the neural network that is processing a stimulus will be most active shortly after stimulus presentation. As the time since stimulus presentation increases, we expect activation in such components to decrease consistently. So to determine if a particular component is task-related, we could create an $n \times 1$ vector with a 1 at each TR when the stimulus is presented and a 0 everywhere else, and then correlate this TR vector with the vector of weights associated with the component. Better yet would be to correlate the weight vector with a vector containing the predicted BOLD response at each TR that is created using the methods of chapter 5. For example, we could use the TR vector to create a boxcar model of predicted neural activation and then convolve this boxcar with a canonical hrf, such as a gamma function (e.g., as in figure 5.2).

This approach was used to identify the component shown in figure 11.6. The solid curve in the bottom panel of figure 11.6 gives the component weights at each TR of the experiment. The dotted curve is the predicted BOLD response to the right-pointing arrow. This curve was generated by creating a boxcar function with a value of 1 during times when the right-pointing arrow was displayed and zero at all other times. The boxcar was then convolved with a gamma hrf to produce the dotted curve. There are obvious discrepancies between the dotted and solid curves in figure 11.6. Nevertheless, the two curves have a reasonably high correlation (around $r = 0.78$). Furthermore, the component map shows lots of left-hemisphere activation, which is consistent with the subject allocating visual attention to the right and pressing a response key with the right hand.

If physiologic data are collected, one would also expect to find components that are correlated with the subject's respiration rate and heart rate. Many components will have no obvious interpretation. Typically, no attempt is made to identify all components. Instead the emphasis is on finding task-related components.

## The Noisy ICA Model

The standard ICA model assumes no noise. All components are assumed to have the non-normal distribution that is expected from true signals. This seems like an unrealistic assumption—and it causes statistical problems. Without a noise model, slight differences in BOLD responses must be interpreted as real effects, and there is no underlying statistical theory that would allow significance testing. The noisy ICA model solves these problems (also called probabilistic ICA) (e.g., Beckmann & Smith, 2004; Hyvärinen et al., 2001).

Whereas the standard noise-free ICA model assumes that the data from voxel $i$ can be expressed as

$$\underline{y}_{V(i)} = M\underline{c}_{V(i)},$$

the noisy ICA model assumes

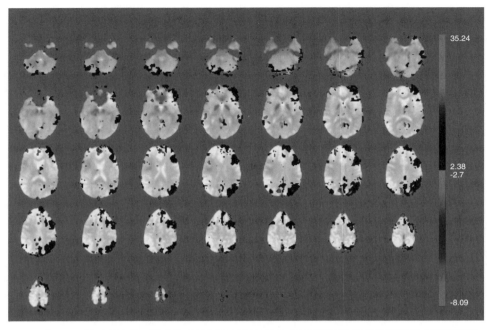

**Figure 11.6**
A component map (top panel) and its associated weights (solid curve, bottom panel). The component map is thresholded at 2.38 and −2.7. The dotted curve in the bottom panel is the predicted BOLD response to the right-pointing arrow.

$$\underline{y}_{V(i)} = M\underline{c}_{V(i)} + \underline{\varepsilon}_{V(i)}, \tag{11.24}$$

where $\underline{\varepsilon}_{V(i)}$ is a multivariate normal random vector with mean $\underline{0}$ and variance-covariance matrix $\Sigma_i$. The component and noise vectors are assumed to be independent. Estimating the components and weights in noisy ICA is a two-step process. The first problem is to estimate the unmixing matrix $U = M^{-1}$. In standard ICA, this is really the only problem because once $U$ is known, the components can be computed from $C = UY$. In the noisy model, however, this process is more complicated because when we premultiply both sides of equation 11.24 by $U$, rather than recover the components, we recover a noise-corrupted version of the components:

$$U\underline{y}_{V(i)} = \underline{c}_{V(i)} + U\underline{\varepsilon}_{V(i)}. \tag{11.25}$$

So the second problem in noisy ICA is to obtain an optimal estimate of the components once the unmixing matrix has been estimated.

Although there has been less work on the noisy ICA model than on standard ICA, various methods for estimating the unmixing matrix in the presence of noise have been proposed (for a review, see Hyvärinen et al., 2001). In general, standard methods do not need much modification. To see this note that $U\underline{\varepsilon}_{V(i)}$ in equation 11.25 is a multivariate normal random vector, because it is a linear transformation of the multivariate normal vector $\underline{\varepsilon}_{V(i)}$. Therefore, for example, because kurtosis is 0 in normal distributions, standard ICA methods that select entries in U that maximize the kurtosis of $U\underline{y}_{V(i)}$ will necessarily maximize the kurtosis of $\underline{c}_{V(i)}$ (because the kurtosis of $U\underline{\varepsilon}_{V(i)}$ will be 0). Thus, methods that find estimates of U that maximize kurtosis should produce the same estimates of U regardless of whether noise has been added to the data. Similar arguments hold for most other ICA methods (i.e., because they all depend on higher-order statistics).

The second problem—removing the effects of noise on the component estimates—is more challenging. One complication occurs because it is impossible to determine the noise variances exactly (Davies, 2004). The solutions that have been proposed for this problem depend on the assumptions that are made about the noise variance-covariance matrix $\Sigma_i$. In the general case, when few constraints are placed on the form of $\Sigma_i$, maximum likelihood estimators have been developed, although these tend to be computationally complex (Attias, 1998). When restrictive assumptions are made about the form of $\Sigma_i$, then the problem simplifies. For example, the noisy ICA module used by FSL (called MELODIC 3.0) assumes $\Sigma_i = \sigma^2 I$. In this case, correcting the component estimates for noise is fairly straightforward (Beckmann & Smith, 2004).

One advantage of the noisy ICA model is that it provides a theoretical basis for statistical inference. For example, FSL models the intensity values in each component map as samples from a mixture of normal distributions (e.g., Beckmann & Smith, 2004). Let $f_i(c)$ denote the probability density function of the intensity values in the $i^{th}$ component map, and denote the probability density function of a normal distribution with mean $\mu_j$ and standard deviation $\sigma_j$ by $N(\mu_j, \sigma_j)$. Then FSL assumes

$$f_i(c) = \sum_{j=1}^{K} \theta_j N(\mu_j, \sigma_j), \qquad (11.26)$$

where the $\theta_j$ are constants that sum to 1. The number of terms in this sum, $K$, is an unknown parameter that is estimated from the data. In addition, all of the $\mu_j$ and $\sigma_j$ are also parameters that require estimation. If there are no restrictions on any of these parameters (including $K$), then this is a weak assumption because almost any probability density function can be approximated to a high degree of accuracy by some version of equation 11.26 (e.g., Bishop, 1995).

The idea behind this model is that if a component is due simply to noise, then the best fit of equation 11.26 will be with $K = 1$ (i.e., a purely normal distribution). Higher values of $K$

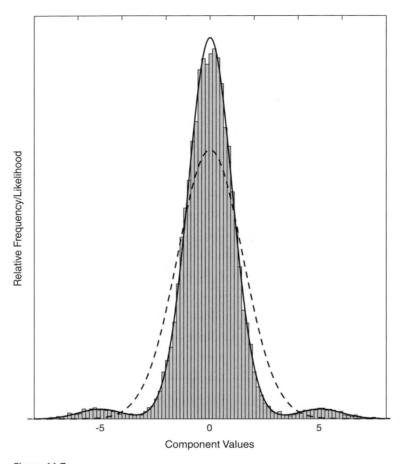

**Figure 11.7**
The gray bars depict the relative frequency histogram of hypothetical component values. The solid line curve is the best-fitting mixture of three normal probability density functions. The dotted line curve is the best-fitting normal distribution. Note that this mixture of normals is super-Gaussian.

are therefore assumed to model signal. An example of this approach is shown in Figure 11.7. The gray bars depict the relative frequency histogram of a hypothetical set of activation values from a component map. The solid curve is the best-fitting mixture of normal distributions. In this case, an almost perfect fit is obtained with a mixture of three normals (so $K = 3$). The dotted line curve shows the best-fitting single normal distribution. Note that the high tails in the histogram cause the (pure) normal distribution to underpredict both the mode and the tails. Thus, the mixture of normals is super-Gaussian (e.g., compare figures 11.7 and 11.1) and so would be appropriate as a model of the component distributions in standard ICA approaches.

The mixture of normals model can be used to separate voxels in this component map that are part of the neural network that is driving the component (i.e., signal) from voxels that are responding merely to noise. The key is to realize that the noise is normally distributed. Thus, one of the normal distributions in the sum on the right side of equation 11.26 should model noise, whereas the other distributions should model signal. According to the noisy ICA model, the mean of the noise distribution is zero, so the distribution with the estimated mean nearest zero could be assumed to model noise. In most cases, this will also be the dominant normal distribution in the mixture; that is, the one with the largest value of $\theta_j$. This is because most voxels in any component should be responding to noise, and only a small percentage should show signal-related activity.

The top panel in figure 11.8 shows this dominant (i.e., central) component of the figure 11.7 mixture model. If this distribution models the noise, then we can use a standard $z$-table to set upper and lower thresholds to control the type I error rate at any desired value (e.g., $\alpha$ in figure 11.8). These thresholds can then be used on all the data, as in the bottom panel of figure 11.8, to identify signal-related voxels. Specifically, any voxel in the component with a value that is more extreme than these thresholds is assumed to be signal related.

### Other Issues

In equation 11.2 we assumed there were as many components as TRs (i.e., $n$). Because of this assumption, the mixing matrix M is square, and so $U = M^{-1}$ is defined if M is nonsingular. With $n$ separate components, M must be nonsingular if these components are truly independent. Most of the methods we reviewed work by estimating the entries in U and then solving for M by inverting the final estimate of U. So a critical assumption of these methods is that the number of components equals the number of TRs. If it is known that there are fewer components than TRs, then M will not be square and so $M^{-1}$ will not be defined. This greatly complicates the ICA process (e.g., Hyvärinen et al., 2001), so this situation is usually avoided. In other words, it is common to estimate the full model with $n$ components, even if one believes that there are fewer than $n$ true components. If there are less than $n$ components, but the full model is used, the ICA algorithms will still work (noise will fill in for the missing components), but some of the estimated components should account for only a small percentage of variance in the data (i.e., using equation 11.23). On the other hand, some ICA algorithms allow the user to specify the number of components beforehand. One example is the FastICA algorithm that maximizes negentropy, which we considered earlier in this chapter. The main advantage of specifying a number of components less than the maximum value of $n$ is speed. In FastICA, the components are estimated successively, so specifying a smaller number of components will decrease computing time.

Another common practice with ICA is to first run a PCA and then use these results to reduce the amount of noise in the data (i.e., see chapter 10). This should be done conservatively to avoid the error of eliminating true components during the noise reduction process.

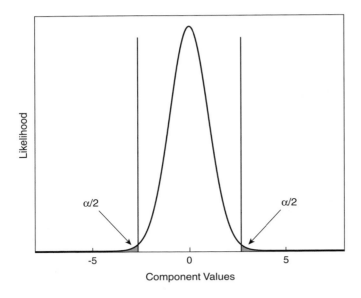

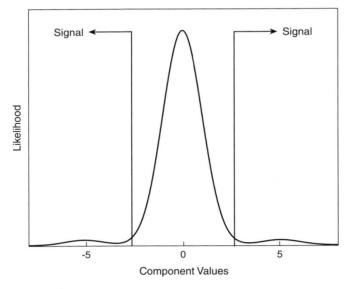

**Figure 11.8**
FSL method for separating signal and noise in component maps. The top panel shows the dominant normal distribution from fitting the mixture of normals model to the relative frequency histograms shown in figure 11.7. Upper
and lower thresholds are set so that the type I error rate equals some specified value of $\alpha$. These thresholds are then
used on the full mixture model (bottom panel) to separate signal and noise.

It is important to realize, however, that in general, reducing the dimensionality of the data matrix Y can cause mathematical complications. To see this, recall from equation 11.2 that the fundamental ICA model assumes

$$\underset{n \times N}{Y} = \underset{n \times n}{M} \underset{n \times N}{C}.$$                                                (11.27)

The number of voxels ($N$) is almost always much greater than the number of TRs ($n$), so without PCA preprocessing, Y will typically be full row rank. As a result, the sample variance-covariance matrix of Y will have rank $n$ and will therefore have $n$ nonzero eigenvalues. Using PCA to eliminate noise will reduce the rank of Y to some value less than $n$. This will also reduce the number of independent components and the rank of M to a value less than $n$. If M is not full rank, then its inverse U will not exist, so eliminating noise from Y will cause some ICA algorithms to fail. For this reason, if PCA is used for noise reduction, then the ICA should use an algorithm such as FastICA, where it can be specified beforehand that there are a reduced number of components (i.e., some number less than $n$). FastICA will still succeed in this reduced rank case because it estimates components successively, rather than simultaneously.

It is also important to realize that the question of whether PCA should be used to reduce dimensionality before running ICA is controversial. A large part of this controversy is due to reports that even very conservative uses of PCA to reduce dimensionality can adversely affect the ability of an ensuing ICA to detect task-related components (Green, Nandy, & Cordes, 2002). For example, in the Green et al. (2002) study, adverse effects were found even when PCA was used to eliminate components that only accounted for a total of .01% of the variance in the observed data.

### Comparing ICA and GLM Approaches

Table 11.1 compares spatial and temporal ICA with the two GLM approaches that we considered in chapter 5. Remember that in the correlation version of the GLM, we construct a predicted BOLD response by convolving a boxcar function with a canonical hrf and then use the GLM to correlate this predicted signal with the observed BOLD response in each voxel. The FBR GLM defines a separate GLM parameter for each successive BOLD response following presentation of an experimental event.

The first difference among these methods is that ICA is applied simultaneously to the whole brain, whereas the GLM approaches are applied separately to data from each single voxel. In statistical parlance, this means ICA is a multivariate statistical technique, whereas the GLM approaches are univariate. The obvious advantage of ICA in this regard is that it can identify entire brain networks that all work together to accomplish the task under study. In contrast, all the GLM approaches can accomplish is to make a set of separate decisions about whether each voxel does or does not show task-related activation. Nothing in either GLM analysis can tell us if task-related voxels in two different brain regions are part of the

**Table 11.1**
A comparison of ICA and two standard GLM approaches

|  | Spatial ICA | Temporal ICA | Correlation GLM | FBR GLM |
|---|---|---|---|---|
| Applied to | Whole brain | Whole brain | Single voxel | Single voxel |
| Statistical model | Nonparametric | Nonparametric | Parametric | Nonparametric |
| Components | Spatial maps | Temporal waveforms | Temporal waveforms | Temporal waveforms |
| Weights | Vary across time but not space | Vary across space but not time | Vary across space but not time | Vary across space but not time |
| Parameters | Weights and components unknown | Weights and components unknown | Weights unknown, components known | Weights known, components unknown |

same or different neural networks. To answer this question, additional methods, such as coherence analysis (chapter 8) or Granger causality (chapter 9), are needed.

ICA makes no parametric assumptions about the hrf or the nature of the BOLD response. In this sense, it is like the FBR GLM. In contrast, the correlation GLM makes strong parametric assumptions about task-induced neural activation (typically, that it follows a boxcar function) and about the form of the hrf (e.g., gamma). Poor choices in these models will reduce correlations with task-related BOLD activation and therefore reduce statistical power.

ICA also differs from both GLM approaches in the nature of the components. In spatial ICA, the components are spatial maps, whereas in temporal ICA and in both GLM approaches, the components are temporal waveforms. In univariate approaches like the GLM, the data are a time series from a single voxel, and therefore temporal waveforms are the only possible components. In the correlation GLM, the components are computed by convolving an hrf with a boxcar function. This convolution is computed before data analysis begins, and thus the components are assumed to be known *a priori*. In contrast, the weights are unknown (i.e., the $\theta_i$ parameters; see chapter 5), and they define the parameters that are estimated from the data. This situation is reversed in the FBR GLM. Now the components are unknown and are estimated from the data, whereas the weights are assumed to be known (i.e., the ones and zeroes in the design matrix; see chapter 5). ICA differs in this sense from both methods because both forms of ICA assume that neither the components nor the weights are known beforehand and therefore that both must be estimated from the data. The less that is known and the more that must be estimated from the data, the more challenging the statistical problem. This is the primary reason that ICA is a more difficult statistical challenge than the GLM.

A final important difference between ICA and GLM approaches is that the weights are assumed to remain constant in the GLM, whereas they are free to vary with time in spatial

ICA. The normal equations in the GLM work by averaging across similar events. Such averaging makes sense only if all samples that are averaged are from the same population. In statistics, this assumption is called stationarity. Stationarity is a critical restriction. In the FBR GLM it means that there can be no learning or habituation during the experimental session. The correlation GLM has some limited ability to deal with changes to the BOLD response within a session (e.g., by using the subject's response times to define the durations of each boxcar), but the correlation GLM requires that these changes are known exactly beforehand. In contrast, spatial ICA allows the weights to differ on every TR and thus does not assume stationarity. Thus, if learning or habituation effects are expected, ICA might be a better choice than the GLM.

### Conclusions

ICA is a multivariate statistical technique that has great potential for use with fMRI data. It has some significant advantages over standard GLM-based approaches. First, because it operates on all data simultaneously, it largely avoids the intractable multiple comparisons problem that plagues GLM analyses. Second, it identifies networks of event-related voxels, rather than single voxels, so it simultaneously addresses questions of functional connectivity. In addition, ICA is not constrained by the stationarity assumptions of the GLM, which makes it useful for studying learning or habituation. In contrast, such effects reduce power of GLM-based analyses. On the other hand, ICA does have weaknesses. First, it is time and resource consuming to run. Second, it is a purely exploratory data-analytic technique, in the sense that it provides no straightforward method of testing specific *a priori* hypotheses about any of the components. Finally, it provides no foolproof method of identifying task-related components. In many cases, an ICA analysis might identify several hundred components, only a few of which are likely related to the task under study. Finding these few components of interest among the hundreds identified can be a difficult challenge.

Currently, GLM approaches to analyzing fMRI data are much more common than ICA approaches. The GLM dates back at least to the publication of R. A. Fisher's 1935 book, *The Design of Experiments,* and since the 1960s or so, ANOVA and regression have been required courses in virtually all doctoral programs in psychology. Not surprisingly, the GLM was among the first statistical techniques applied to neuroimaging data (e.g., Friston et al., 1991, 1995b). In contrast, although ICA dates back to the early 1980s (for a review, see Hyvärinen et al., 2001), it did not become popular until the mid-1990s (e.g., with Bell & Sejnowski, 1995; Comon, 1994), and it was not introduced as a method for analyzing fMRI data until 1998 (McKeown et al., 1998). It seems likely, therefore, that the relatively infrequent use of ICA is due as much to its unfamiliarity as to its computational and statistical drawbacks. As ICA inevitably becomes more widely known, its use as a standard method of analyzing fMRI data is also likely to increase.

# 12 Other Methods

fMRI data analysis is a rapidly evolving research area. New methods are developed every year. This book surveyed the most widely used current methods, but other methods are also in use. This chapter briefly introduces some of these. The goal is not to describe the methods in the level of detail used in previous chapters. Instead, the goal is to give a brief intuitive description of these methods and direct interested readers to appropriate references that provide more detail.

## Pattern Classification Techniques

One of the most exciting recent developments in fMRI data analysis is the application of machine learning classification methods to BOLD response data (Haynes & Rees, 2006; Norman, Polyn, Detre, & Haxby, 2006; Pereira, Mitchell, & Botvinick, 2009). The basic idea is that if some brain region is responding differently to two different event types, then it should be possible to find a classification scheme that can look at the responses of all voxels in that region and correctly identify which event triggered the response.

As a concrete example, consider a slow-event related design with a TR of 2 seconds where on each trial the subject is shown a picture of either a shoe or a chair (similar to Haxby et al., 2001). Suppose we focus on 2000 object-sensitive voxels in the ventral temporal cortex. Our question of interest is whether these 2000 voxels respond differently to pictures of shoes than they do to pictures of chairs. After each stimulus presentation, a typical application would sum the BOLD response in each voxel over a series of TRs that is likely to include the peak response (e.g., TRs 4, 6, and 8 seconds after stimulus onset). Finally, these sums from trial $i$ would be loaded into a $2000 \times 1$ vector, which we denote $\underline{B}_i$.

Now imagine a 2000-dimensional space with a coordinate axis for each of the 2000 voxels. Each vector $\underline{B}_i$ specifies a numerical value on each of these dimensions, and therefore we could plot each $\underline{B}_i$ as a single point in this high-dimensional space. The idea is that the $\underline{B}_i$ from trials when a shoe is presented should cluster in a different part of the space from the $\underline{B}_i$ from trials when a chair is presented if this brain region responds differently to these two stimulus classes. On the other hand, if this region does not discriminate between shoes and chairs, then the points should all fall in the same region.

Of course, it would be impossible to decide whether the points fall in the same or different regions by visual inspection. Instead, machine learning classification techniques are used. A standard application might proceed as follows. First, all available $\underline{B}_i$ are divided arbitrarily into two sets. One of these is called the training set, and the other is called the testing set. For example, data from even-numbered trials could form the training set, and data from odd-numbered trials could form the testing set. Next, a machine learning pattern classifier is chosen. Popular choices include the support vector machine and the naïve Bayes classifier (e.g., Bishop, 2006). The third step is to estimate the parameters of this classifier by using the data in the training set. This estimation process uses both the spatial coordinates of each point in the training set and the identity of the stimulus that was presented when that data point was collected. For example, a simple classifier might use these data to find the (hyper)plane that best separates the chair $\underline{B}_i$ from the shoe $\underline{B}_i$ in the training set. The final step is to test the classifier by examining its ability to identify the stimulus label (i.e., shoe vs. chair) of the $\underline{B}_i$ in the testing set. An important restriction is that during this testing process, all parameters are left fixed at their final training values. If the classifier correctly classifies more $\underline{B}_i$ in the testing set than would be expected by chance, then we conclude that this brain region is responding differentially to the two stimulus classes.

Pattern classification methods are multivariate techniques because they simultaneously consider all voxels in the search region. Note that a standard GLM approach to this same problem would identify any single voxels within this region that respond differentially to the two stimulus classes. If none of the GLM contrasts for any voxel within this ROI reach significance, then a tempting conclusion might be that the region does not differentially respond to the stimuli. Note though that this does not follow logically. A failure of the GLM to find any significant voxels in the region means at best that no single voxel shows a strong differential response to the two stimulus classes, but it cannot rule out the possibility that stimulus discrimination is encoded by small to moderate differences distributed across many voxels in the region. Pattern classifiers are designed to answer this more subtle question. For example, Haxby et al. (2001) reported that the ability of a pattern classifier to discriminate between stimulus categories was almost unaffected by removing those voxels that showed the strongest differential response to the two categories.

### Partial Least Squares

Partial least squares is a multivariate technique that generalizes PCA (see chapter 10). It is also closely related to canonical correlation and structural equation modeling. The first application to neuroimaging was by McIntosh, Bookstein, Haxby, and Grady (1996). For more recent treatments, see McIntosh, Chau, and Protzner (2004), McIntosh and Lobaugh (2004), and Rayens and Andersen (2006).

Recall from chapter 10 that PCA is based on the eigenvectors and eigenvalues of the sample variance-covariance matrix of the BOLD responses (see equation 10.8):

$$\hat{\Sigma} = \frac{1}{n-1} Y_C' Y_C, \tag{12.1}$$

where $Y_C$ is the matrix of mean-centered data, and $n$ is the number of TRs. Thus, PCA takes no account of the design matrix of the GLM. As such, it is a purely exploratory data analysis tool, because the components that result need have no relation to the components that we expect based on our knowledge of the task under study. In contrast, partial least squares is based on the singular-value decomposition of $X'Y_C$ (Höskuldsson, 1988), where X is the design matrix of the GLM. Pre-multiplying the data matrix by $X'$ essentially computes the correlation between each column of the design matrix and the data in each voxel in the brain (or ROI), and singular-value decomposition can be thought of as a generalization of eigenvector, eigenvalue decomposition (e.g., Poole, 2006). Thus, unlike PCA or ICA, partial least squares focuses on components that are directly related to the experimental design (e.g., the TR vector that describes event occurrences).

A primary advantage of partial least squares then is that it simplifies the process of finding task-relevant components. With PCA, for example, there is no reason to expect that the principal component or any of the components with large eigenvalues will be task relevant. In fact, the neural network mediating the task may be related to a number of PCA components, which would make it especially difficult to identify. With partial least squares, however, the components are constrained to that part of the covariance structure of the data that can be ascribed to task manipulations. Thus, in theory, all partial least squares components are task relevant.

## Dynamic Causal Modeling

Dynamic causal modeling is a sophisticated confirmatory data analysis technique that allows the user to test highly specific assumptions about functional connectivity (Friston, Harrison, & Penny, 2003; Lee, Friston, & Horwitz, 2006; Marreiros, Kiebel, & Friston, 2008; Stephan et al., 2007, 2010). To begin, the user must specify a number of brain regions that are presumed to interact in the same functional network. A dynamic causal model is then constructed that models instantaneous changes in neural activation within this network via a series of nonlinear (i.e., bilinear) differential equations. The resulting activations are then converted to predicted BOLD responses via a version of the balloon model (see chapter 3). The most important free parameters are the connection strengths among the different brain regions. These are estimated by fitting the model to observed fMRI data from an experiment that is assumed to activate the neural network under study. Alternative versions of the model can be constructed that assume different neural architectures, and these can be compared in their ability to account for the BOLD data. Dynamic causal modeling can also be used to investigate how variables manipulated during the experiment affect the network under study. For example, Friston et al. (2003) used this approach to conclude that attention to visual motion potentiates backward projections from inferior frontal gyrus to superior parietal cortex and from superior parietal cortex to motion-sensitive neurons in V5.

Dynamic causal modeling represents an exciting attempt to bring biologically plausible models to fMRI data analysis. Although the bilinear models of neural activation that underlie dynamic causal modeling would not be considered biologically detailed by current computational neuroscience standards, they nevertheless represent a significant improvement on this dimension over any other current method of analyzing fMRI data. For example, they directly model neural activation (unlike, e.g., Granger causality or coherence analysis), they model networks of interacting brain regions (also unlike Granger causality or coherence analysis), and they are dynamic (unlike, e.g., structural equation modeling). For these reasons, the popularity of dynamic causal modeling is likely to increase.

### Bayesian Approaches

This book has focused on traditional null hypothesis testing approaches to fMRI data analysis. A less common but potentially more powerful approach is to use Bayesian methods (Friston et al., 2002; Friston & Penny, 2003; Genovese, 2000; Woolrich, Behrens, Beckmann, Jenkinson, & Smith, 2004; Woolrich et al., 2009). In traditional null-hypothesis testing of the sort discussed in chapter 5, for example, one computes the probability of obtaining the observed data or something more extreme given that there is no effect of the task (i.e., this is the well-known $p$-value that forms the basis of null-hypothesis testing). However, there will almost always be at least some small effect, so this probability is guaranteed to keep decreasing as we collect more scans or run more subjects. The Bayesian approach acknowledges that there is likely to be some effect, so the goal instead is to estimate the probability distribution of the effect given the observed data. Because there is no null hypothesis in Bayesian approaches, there are no false-positive decisions. The analogue of an activation map would be to identify for purposes of visual presentation those voxels where activation is above some predetermined threshold. It turns out that this thresholding process produces results similar to methods that control false discovery rate (see chapter 7; Friston & Penny, 2003).

The Bayesian approach requires knowledge of the prior distribution of activation and of all other parameters specified by the model. In most applications, these prior distributions are unknown, so either an arbitrary assumption is made or a noninformative prior is chosen that attempts to take a neutral position. For example, in the case of a probability, a noninformative prior might assume a uniform distribution over the range [0,1]. For proponents of null hypothesis testing, this inherent subjectivity has always been the theoretical weak point of Bayesian methods. In response, Friston proposed using empirical Bayesian methods, in which the prior distributions are estimated from the available data (Friston et al., 2002; Friston & Penny, 2003). The idea is that the application of the GLM in fMRI analysis can proceed in a hierarchical fashion. We saw an example of this in chapter 7 where we first applied the GLM to the data of each individual subject, and then we used these results to create a higher-level group GLM. With hierarchical models, the empirical Bayesian approach uses the data at the higher level to estimate the distribution of parameters in the lower-level model. This multilevel parameter estimation process is accomplished iteratively using the expectation-maximization (EM) algorithm (Dempster, Laird, & Rubin, 1977). By estimating priors empirically, much of the subjectivity of Bayesian approaches is eliminated. For example, the variance in effect size across all voxels can be used as an estimate of the variance of the prior effect size distribution when the GLM is applied to a single voxel (Friston & Penny, 2003).

A second criticism of Bayesian methods is that they typically require considerably more computation to implement than standard null hypothesis testing methods. This is because some complex multiple integrals must often be evaluated numerically. Fast computers and sophisticated numerical algorithms have reduced this concern, but even so, Bayesian methods are slower and more complex to implement than the methods used in null hypothesis testing.

The discovery of better methods for modeling prior distributions and faster and more efficient numerical algorithms is slowly increasing the popularity of Bayesian approaches in fMRI data analysis. For example, Bayesian methods now play prominent roles in both the SPM and FSL software packages (e.g., Friston et al., 2007; Woolrich et al., 2009).

# Appendix A: Matrix Algebra Tutorial

## Matrices and Their Basic Operations

A *matrix* is a two-dimensional ordered array of numbers. It can have any number of rows and columns, and it can contain any type of numbers (e.g., positive, negative, real, imaginary). The only requirement is that there are no missing values. The *order* of a matrix is its number of rows and columns. For example, the matrix

$$A = \begin{bmatrix} 2 & 3 & -1 \\ 0 & \frac{1}{2} & 4 \end{bmatrix}$$

is of order 2 × 3 because it has 2 rows and 3 columns. To enter this matrix into MATLAB, at the command line (denoted by >>) type

A = [2 3 −1; 0 .5 4]

Hitting the return key produces

```
              A =
2.0000    3.0000    −1.0000
0         0.5000     4.0000
```

By convention, matrices are typically identified by capital letters, and the order is sometimes expressed below this letter. For example, the 2 × 3 matrix A might be written as $A_{2 \times 3}$. A matrix in which the number of rows equals the number of columns is said to be *square* (i.e., the order is $n \times n$, for some value of $n$). A square matrix in which all entries not on the main diagonal equal 0 is called a *diagonal* matrix. For example,

$$D = \begin{bmatrix} 1 & 0 & 0 \\ 0 & -12 & 0 \\ 0 & 0 & \frac{1}{3} \end{bmatrix}$$

is a 3 × 3 diagonal matrix.

A matrix with one row or one column is called a *vector*. A column vector has a single column, and a row vector has a single row. Vectors are traditionally identified by lowercase underlined letters. So, for example, a $3 \times 1$ column vector might be written as

$$\underline{v} = \begin{bmatrix} 2 \\ -7 \\ 1 \end{bmatrix}.$$

Finally, within matrix algebra, single numbers are referred to as *scalars*.

A variety of mathematical operations can be performed on matrices and vectors. Although addition and multiplication are included in this list, not all pairs of matrices can be added or multiplied. In other words, certain conditions must be met before matrix addition or multiplication is defined. These conditions are different for addition and multiplication. Pairs of matrices that satisfy these conditions are said to be *conformable* for that operation.

Two matrices A and B are conformable for addition if and only if they have the same order. Matrices of different orders cannot be added. If A and B have the same order, then the sum $C = A + B$ is defined as the matrix containing the term-by-term sums of the entries in A and B. Thus, if A and B are both $2 \times 2$, then

$$A + B = \begin{bmatrix} a_{11} & a_{12} \\ a_{21} & a_{22} \end{bmatrix} + \begin{bmatrix} b_{11} & b_{12} \\ b_{21} & b_{22} \end{bmatrix} = \begin{bmatrix} a_{11} + b_{11} & a_{12} + b_{12} \\ a_{21} + b_{21} & a_{22} + b_{22} \end{bmatrix} = C.$$

In MATLAB, the command $A + B$ will compute the sum, provided it exists. Note that matrix addition is commutative; that is, if $A + B = C$, then A and B are also conformable for the sum $B + A$, and $B + A = A + B = C$.

Suppose A is of order $n \times m$ and B is of order $p \times q$. Then A and B are conformable for the product AB if and only if $m = p$; that is, if and only if the number of columns of the pre-multiplier equals the number of rows of the post-multiplier. If this condition is met, then the product $C = AB$ is of order $n \times q$. So C has the same number of rows as the pre-multiplier and the same number of columns as the post-multiplier. If the product $C = AB$ exists, then the entry in row $i$ and column $j$ equals the sum of the term-by-term multiplication of the entries in row $i$ of the pre-multiplier and column $j$ of the post-multiplier. For example, if A is $3 \times 2$ and B is $2 \times 2$, then the product is of order $3 \times 2$ and is defined as

$$\underset{3\times2}{A}\ \underset{2\times2}{B} = \begin{bmatrix} a_{11} & a_{12} \\ a_{21} & a_{22} \\ a_{31} & a_{32} \end{bmatrix}_{3\times2} \begin{bmatrix} b_{11} & b_{12} \\ b_{21} & b_{22} \end{bmatrix}_{2\times2} = \begin{bmatrix} a_{11}b_{11} + a_{12}b_{21} & a_{11}b_{12} + a_{12}b_{22} \\ a_{21}b_{11} + a_{22}b_{21} & a_{21}b_{12} + a_{22}b_{22} \\ a_{31}b_{11} + a_{32}b_{21} & a_{31}b_{12} + a_{32}b_{22} \end{bmatrix}_{3\times2} = \underset{3\times2}{C}.$$

As numerical examples, note that

$$\begin{bmatrix} 2 & 3 \\ 4 & -1 \end{bmatrix} \begin{bmatrix} 1 & -1 \\ 2 & 0 \end{bmatrix} = \begin{bmatrix} 8 & -2 \\ 2 & -4 \end{bmatrix} \tag{A.1}$$

and

$$[2 \quad 1]\begin{bmatrix} 3 & 0 \\ 4 & 1 \end{bmatrix} = [10 \quad 1].$$

To perform the equation A.1 multiplication in MATLAB, one first defines the two matrices

```
>> A = [2 3;4 −1];
>> B = [1 −1;2 0];
```

The semicolon at the end of each line suppresses printing. Next type

```
>> A*B
```

Hitting the return key produces the result

```
          ans =
8      −2
2      −4
```

Unlike addition, matrix multiplication is not commutative. In fact, if A is $n \times m$ and B is $m \times p$, then the product AB is defined (and is of order $n \times p$), but note that BA is not defined unless $p = n$. Even in this case, however, AB will generally not equal BA. Because of this, great care must be taken about the order in which one writes the various terms in each product.

Any matrix can be multiplied by a scalar in an operation known as scalar multiplication. The scalar simply multiplies each entry in the matrix. For example,

$$5\begin{bmatrix} 1 & 2 \\ 3 & 0 \end{bmatrix} = \begin{bmatrix} 5 & 10 \\ 15 & 0 \end{bmatrix}.$$

This scalar multiplication is done in MATLAB via the following commands:

```
>> A = [1 2;3 0];
                >> 5*A
```

Another useful operation is matrix transposition. The *transpose* of a matrix A, denoted by $A'$, is created by switching the rows and columns of A. Specifically, the $i^{th}$ row of A becomes the $i^{th}$ column of $A'$ (for all $i$). So if A is $n \times m$, then $A'$ is $m \times n$. For example,

$$\begin{bmatrix} 2 & 1 & -3 \\ 0 & 4 & 1 \end{bmatrix}' = \begin{bmatrix} 2 & 0 \\ 1 & 4 \\ -3 & 1 \end{bmatrix}.$$

MATLAB will produce the transpose of any matrix A simply by typing

$$>> A'$$

One useful rule regarding transposes is that the transpose of a product equals the product of the transposes in reverse order. So, for example,

$$\left( \underset{n\times m}{A} \; \underset{m\times p}{B} \right)' = \underset{p\times m}{B'} \; \underset{m\times n}{A'} .$$

Note that if the product AB is defined, then B'A' must also be defined.

By convention, the transpose is also used to denote a row vector. Standard notation is to interpret a vector $\underline{v}$ as a column vector. If so, then to denote a row vector one would write $\underline{v}'$.

Matrix algebra is especially useful for simplifying and solving systems of simultaneous linear equations, as, for example, one finds in the GLM. To see how this is done, consider the equations

$$x - y + 2z = 2$$

$$3x + y - z = 4$$

$$5x + 2y - z = 9$$

Note that these equations can be rewritten in matrix form as

$$\begin{bmatrix} 1 & -1 & 2 \\ 3 & 1 & -1 \\ 5 & 2 & -1 \end{bmatrix} \begin{bmatrix} x \\ y \\ z \end{bmatrix} = \begin{bmatrix} 2 \\ 4 \\ 9 \end{bmatrix},$$

which we can rewrite in shorthand form as

$$A\underline{x} = \underline{b} \tag{A.2}$$

where

$$A = \begin{bmatrix} 1 & -1 & 2 \\ 3 & 1 & -1 \\ 5 & 2 & -1 \end{bmatrix}, \quad \underline{x} = \begin{bmatrix} x \\ y \\ z \end{bmatrix}, \quad \text{and} \quad \underline{b} = \begin{bmatrix} 2 \\ 4 \\ 9 \end{bmatrix}.$$

If equation A.2 was a univariate (i.e., scalar) algebraic equation, we would easily solve for $\underline{x}$ by dividing both sides by A. This does not work with matrix equations, though, because matrix division is not defined. However, note that dividing both sides of the scalar equation

$ax = b$

by $a$ is the same as multiplying both sides by the inverse of $a$:

$a^{-1}ax = a^{-1}b$,   which implies that $x = a^{-1}b$.

Fortunately, the inverse of a matrix is defined, at least under certain special conditions.

The value 1/2 is the multiplicative inverse of 2 because their product is the identity element 1, and 1 is the multiplicative identity because

$1 \times x = x \times 1 = x$,

for any value of $x$. So to define a matrix inverse, we must first define an identity matrix. More specifically, we seek a matrix I such that

$$IA = AI = A. \tag{A.3}$$

Note that the only way that both products IA and AI are defined and equal to each other is if A and I are both square and of the same order (i.e., $n \times n$). For any value of $n$, it can be shown that the only matrix I that satisfies equation A.3 is the $n \times n$ matrix

$$I = \begin{bmatrix} 1 & 0 & \cdots & 0 \\ 0 & 1 & \cdots & 0 \\ \vdots & \vdots & \ddots & \vdots \\ 0 & 0 & \cdots & 1 \end{bmatrix},$$

which is a diagonal matrix (nonzero values only appear on the main diagonal) with every entry on the main diagonal equal to 1. To see that I satisfies equation A.3, note, for example, that

$$\begin{bmatrix} 1 & 0 & 0 \\ 0 & 1 & 0 \\ 0 & 0 & 1 \end{bmatrix} \begin{bmatrix} 1 & -1 & 2 \\ 3 & 1 & -1 \\ 5 & 2 & -1 \end{bmatrix} = \begin{bmatrix} 1 & -1 & 2 \\ 3 & 1 & -1 \\ 5 & 2 & -1 \end{bmatrix} \begin{bmatrix} 1 & 0 & 0 \\ 0 & 1 & 0 \\ 0 & 0 & 1 \end{bmatrix} = \begin{bmatrix} 1 & -1 & 2 \\ 3 & 1 & -1 \\ 5 & 2 & -1 \end{bmatrix}.$$

In MATLAB, the $n \times n$ identity matrix is constructed via the command eye($n$). For example, to construct a 3 × 3 identity matrix, type the command

>> I = eye(3)

Hitting the return key produces

I =

| 1 | 0 | 0 |
| 0 | 1 | 0 |
| 0 | 0 | 1 |

The identity matrix can be used to find the inverse of a matrix. If A is $n \times n$, then we seek another $n \times n$ matrix, which we denote $A^{-1}$, for which

$$A^{-1}A = AA^{-1} = I. \tag{A.4}$$

If A is the $2 \times 2$ matrix

$$A = \begin{bmatrix} a_{11} & a_{12} \\ a_{21} & a_{22} \end{bmatrix},$$

then it turns out that

$$A^{-1} = \frac{1}{a_{11}a_{22} - a_{12}a_{21}} \begin{bmatrix} a_{22} & -a_{12} \\ -a_{21} & a_{11} \end{bmatrix}. \tag{A.5}$$

We can verify that this works, for example, by computing

$$A^{-1}A = \frac{1}{a_{11}a_{22} - a_{12}a_{21}} \begin{bmatrix} a_{22} & -a_{12} \\ -a_{21} & a_{11} \end{bmatrix} \begin{bmatrix} a_{11} & a_{12} \\ a_{21} & a_{22} \end{bmatrix}$$

$$= \frac{1}{a_{11}a_{22} - a_{12}a_{21}} \begin{bmatrix} a_{11}a_{22} - a_{12}a_{21} & 0 \\ 0 & a_{11}a_{22} - a_{12}a_{21} \end{bmatrix}.$$

$$= I$$

MATLAB computes the inverse of a matrix A, if it exists, via the command inv(A). For example, to compute the inverse of the matrix

$$A = \begin{bmatrix} 7 & 9 \\ 3 & 4 \end{bmatrix}$$

Type

>> A = [7 9;3 4];
>> inv(A)

This produces the result

$$ans =$$

  4.0000     −9.0000
 −3.0000      7.0000

Note that the inverse defined by equation A.5 exists only if the denominator of the scalar multiple is nonzero; that is, only if

$a_{11}a_{22} - a_{12}a_{21} \neq 0.$

This value is so important that it is given its own name, the *determinant*, which is written as |A|. Specifically, the determinant of a 2 × 2 matrix A is defined as

$$|A| = \begin{vmatrix} a_{11} & a_{12} \\ a_{21} & a_{22} \end{vmatrix} = a_{11}a_{22} - a_{12}a_{21}.$$

It turns out that every square matrix has a determinant, and every square matrix has an inverse if and only if its determinant is nonzero. For matrices 3 × 3 or larger, computing a determinant or inverse can be time consuming and tedious. With MATLAB, however, these computations are trivial. For any square matrix A, det(A) returns the determinant and inv(A) returns the inverse (if it exists). For example, the determinant of the 3 × 3 matrix A from equation A.2 is

$$|A| = \begin{vmatrix} 1 & -1 & 2 \\ 3 & 1 & -1 \\ 5 & 2 & -1 \end{vmatrix} = 5.$$

Therefore A has an inverse.

The following commands compute this determinant in MATLAB:

```
>> A = [1 −1 2;3 1 −1; 5 2 −1];
>> det(A)
```

which produces

ans =
5

The inverse of this matrix is computed from

```
>> inv(A)
```

which produces

$$
\begin{array}{ccc}
& \text{ans} = & \\
.2 & .6 & -.2 \\
-.44 & -2.2 & 1.4 \\
.2 & -1.4 & .8
\end{array}
$$

In summary, any matrix A has an inverse if and only if two conditions are met. First, A must be square, and second, the determinant of A must be nonzero. A matrix with an inverse is said to be *nonsingular*, whereas a square matrix without an inverse is *singular*. So a matrix A is nonsingular if and only if $|A| \neq 0$. Another important property of the inverse is that if it does exist, then it is unique. In other words, for a matrix A satisfying these two conditions there exists only one matrix $A^{-1}$ for which

$$A^{-1}A = AA^{-1} = I.$$

### Rank

A set of vectors is said to be *linearly independent* if and only if it is impossible to write any one of them as a weighted linear combination of the others. A set of vectors that are not linearly independent are said to be *linearly dependent*. For example,

$$\begin{bmatrix} 1 \\ 2 \\ 3 \end{bmatrix}, \quad \begin{bmatrix} 1 \\ 1 \\ 1 \end{bmatrix}, \quad \text{and} \quad \begin{bmatrix} 3 \\ 4 \\ 5 \end{bmatrix}$$

are linearly dependent because

$$\begin{bmatrix} 3 \\ 4 \\ 5 \end{bmatrix} = \begin{bmatrix} 1 \\ 2 \\ 3 \end{bmatrix} + 2\begin{bmatrix} 1 \\ 1 \\ 1 \end{bmatrix}.$$

As another example,

$$\begin{bmatrix} 1 \\ 2 \end{bmatrix} \quad \text{and} \quad \begin{bmatrix} 2 \\ 3 \end{bmatrix}$$

are linearly independent because neither one is a scalar multiple of the other.

Every matrix can be considered either as a collection of row vectors or column vectors. A well-known result in matrix algebra is that the number of linearly independent columns in any matrix must equal the number of linearly independent rows. For example, consider the matrix

$$A = \begin{bmatrix} 1 & 2 \\ 3 & 1 \\ -1 & 3 \\ 2 & -1 \end{bmatrix}. \tag{A.6}$$

As column 2 is not a scalar multiple of column 1, there are two linearly independent columns in this matrix. Therefore, there must also be two linearly independent rows. The first two rows are linearly independent because the second row is not a scalar multiple of the first. Row 3, however, equals

$$\begin{bmatrix} -1 \\ 3 \end{bmatrix} = 2\begin{bmatrix} 1 \\ 2 \end{bmatrix} - \begin{bmatrix} 3 \\ 1 \end{bmatrix},$$

so row 3 is not linearly independent of rows 1 and 2. Similarly, note that row 4 equals row 2 minus row 1. Therefore, there are also two linearly independent rows in this matrix.

The *rank* of a matrix equals the number of linearly independent rows or columns. So for example, the rank of A in the equation A.6 matrix is 2. Rank is a useful construct that has a number of important applications. For example, as we will see, the number of solutions of any set of simultaneous linear equations can be determined by comparing the ranks of two appropriate matrices. Computing the rank of any matrix in MATLAB is simple. For example, the rank of the equation A.6 matrix is computed via

$>> A = [1\ 2;3\ 1;-1\ 3;2\ -1];$

$>> \text{rank}(A)$

which produces

ans =

2

Computing the rank of a matrix by hand can be difficult. The following properties of rank, however, can simplify this process.

*Property 1    The rank of a matrix equals 0 if and only if every entry in the matrix is 0.*

*Property 2    If A is of order n × m, then rank(A) ≤ min(n,m).*    This result follows because the number of linearly independent rows equals the number of linearly independent columns. So for example, if a matrix has fewer rows than columns (i.e., so $n < m$), then at most there are $n$ linearly independent rows, and therefore also at most $n$ linearly independent columns. A corollary to this result says that the maximum rank of an $n \times n$ square matrix is $n$. In this case, note that all rows and all columns are linearly independent. An $n \times n$ square matrix with rank $n$ is said to be *full rank.*

*Property 3    If rank(A) = r, then there must exist an r × r submatrix of full rank.*    A submatrix is created by striking out any number of rows or columns. For example, the rank of the matrix

$$A = \begin{bmatrix} 1 & 1 & 0 & 0 \\ 4 & 7 & 3 & 0 \\ 0 & 1 & 1 & 0 \\ 0 & 0 & 0 & 1 \end{bmatrix}$$

is no greater than 3 because column 2 is the sum of columns 1 and 3. A 3 × 3 submatrix of full rank can be created by striking out row 2 and column 2. Note that this process leaves the 3 × 3 identity matrix, which is full rank. Therefore, this matrix has rank 3.

*Property 4*   *Suppose A is n × n. Then rank(A) = n if and only if |A| ≠ 0.*   This is a very important property. Note that it provides another way to determine whether a matrix is nonsingular (i.e., has an inverse).

In summary, if A is a square $n \times n$ matrix, then the following statements are all equivalent.

1. rank(A) = $n$.

2. $|A| \neq 0$.

3. A is nonsingular (i.e., $A^{-1}$ exists).

Similarly, the following statements are also equivalent.

1. rank(A) < $n$.

2. $|A| = 0$.

3. A is singular.

## Solving Linear Equations

Any set of simultaneous linear equations must have 0, 1, or an infinite number of solutions. Examples of these three possibilities are shown in figure A.1. For example, the equations

$$x + y = 0$$

$$x + y = 2$$

have zero solutions because if $x + y$ equals 0, it cannot also equal 2. Graphically, these equations describe parallel lines with slope $-1$ and y-intercepts 0 and 2 (see the top panel of figure A.1). A solution to these equations would be a point $(x, y)$ that falls on both lines and therefore simultaneously satisfies both equations. Of course, parallel lines share no points in common, so these equations have no solution.

Simultaneous equations with no solutions are said to be *inconsistent*. If at least one solution exists, then the equations are *consistent*. With linear equations, there are only two possibilities if the equations are consistent. They either have one solution or they have an infinite number of solutions.

The middle panel of figure A.1 shows an example of equations with one solution:

$$x - y = 0$$

$$x + y = 2.$$

Solving these equations produces $x = 1$ and $y = 1$, and figure A.1 shows that this is the point where the two lines intersect. In contrast, the equations

$$x + y = 2$$

$$2x + 2y = 4$$

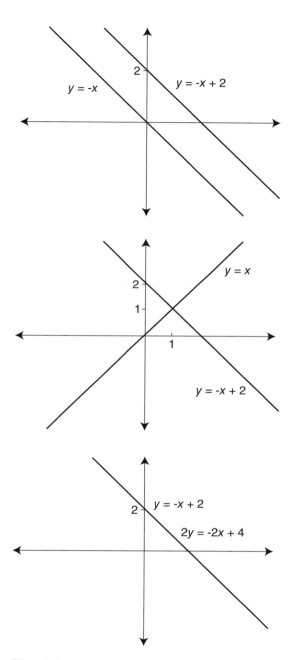

**Figure A.1**
Three possible outcomes when trying to solve a set of simultaneous linear equations. Either there are 0 solutions (top), one solution (middle), or an infinite number of solutions (bottom).

have an infinite number of solutions because they both describe the same line. Therefore, any point on this line is a solution of both equations.

When faced with a set of simultaneous linear equations therefore, our first question is to ask whether they are consistent. If not, then nothing more can be done. If they are consistent, then the next question is to ask whether they have one solution or an infinite number. The question of consistency can be answered by comparing the ranks of two different matrices. Specifically, the equations

$$A\underline{x} = \underline{b}$$

are consistent if and only if

$$\text{rank}(A) = \text{rank}(A \vdots \underline{b}), \qquad\qquad\qquad\qquad\qquad\qquad (A.7)$$

where $A \vdots \underline{b}$ is the matrix $A$ augmented with the vector $\underline{b}$. For example, if $A$ is $n \times n$, then $\underline{x}$ and $\underline{b}$ must both be $n \times 1$. The matrix $A \vdots \underline{b}$, which is of order $n \times n + 1$, contains $A$ in its first $n$ columns and $\underline{b}$ in column $n + 1$.

If $A$ is $n \times n$, then $\text{rank}(A) \leq n$, and adding another column to $A$ cannot decrease its rank. Therefore, note that equation A.7 holds if $\underline{b}$ is linearly dependent on the columns of $A$ and it is violated if $\underline{b}$ is linearly independent of the columns of $A$. Furthermore, note that by rank property no. 2, $\text{rank}(A \vdots \underline{b}) \leq n$ (because this augmented matrix has only $n$ rows). So if $A$ is full rank [i.e., $\text{rank}(A) = n$], then because adding $\underline{b}$ cannot reduce the rank of $A \vdots \underline{b}$, equation A.7 must hold. In other words, the equations $A\underline{x} = \underline{b}$ are always consistent if $A$ is full rank. This means that if $\underline{x}$ and $\underline{b}$ are $n \times 1$, then the only conditions under which the equations $A\underline{x} = \underline{b}$ are not consistent is if $\text{rank}(A) < n$.

To illustrate these results, consider our earlier examples. First, rewriting

$$x + y = 0 \quad \text{and} \quad x + y = 2$$

in matrix form produces

$$\begin{bmatrix} 1 & 1 \\ 1 & 1 \end{bmatrix} \begin{bmatrix} x \\ y \end{bmatrix} = \begin{bmatrix} 0 \\ 2 \end{bmatrix}.$$

Note that

$$\text{rank}(A) = \text{rank} \begin{bmatrix} 1 & 1 \\ 1 & 1 \end{bmatrix} = 1 \quad \text{and} \quad \text{rank}(A \vdots \underline{b}) = \text{rank} \begin{bmatrix} 1 & 1 & 0 \\ 1 & 1 & 2 \end{bmatrix} = 2,$$

so these equations are not consistent. As another example, consider the equations

$$x + y = 2 \quad \text{and} \quad 2x + 2y = 4.$$

In matrix form these become

$$\begin{bmatrix} 1 & 1 \\ 2 & 2 \end{bmatrix} \begin{bmatrix} x \\ y \end{bmatrix} = \begin{bmatrix} 2 \\ 4 \end{bmatrix}.$$

Because

$$\text{rank} \begin{bmatrix} 1 & 1 \\ 2 & 2 \end{bmatrix} = \text{rank} \begin{bmatrix} 1 & 1 & 2 \\ 2 & 2 & 4 \end{bmatrix} = 1,$$

these equations are consistent.

If the equations $A\underline{x} = \underline{b}$ are consistent, then they have either one solution or an infinite number. The difference depends on A. If A is square and full rank, then $A^{-1}$ exists and there is only one solution, which is easily found by solving for $\underline{x}$:

$$A\underline{x} = \underline{b}$$

implies that

$$A^{-1}A\underline{x} = A^{-1}\underline{b}$$

and so

$$\underline{x} = A^{-1}\underline{b}. \tag{A.8}$$

For example, consider the three simultaneous equations described by equation A.2. Using A.8 produces the following unique solution to these equations:

$$\underline{x} = \begin{bmatrix} 1 & -1 & 2 \\ 3 & 1 & -1 \\ 5 & 2 & -1 \end{bmatrix}^{-1} \begin{bmatrix} 2 \\ 4 \\ 9 \end{bmatrix} = \begin{bmatrix} .2 & .6 & -.2 \\ -.4 & -2.2 & 1.4 \\ .2 & -1.4 & .8 \end{bmatrix} \begin{bmatrix} 2 \\ 4 \\ 9 \end{bmatrix} = \begin{bmatrix} 1 \\ 3 \\ 2 \end{bmatrix}.$$

We can verify that $x = 1$, $y = 3$, and $z = 2$ is the solution by substituting these values back into the original equations. MATLAB solves these equations via the commands

```
>> A = [1 −1 2;3 1 −1;5 2 −1];
>> b = [2; 4; 9];
>> x = inv(A)*b
```

The result is

```
        x =
1.0000
3.0000
2.0000
```

If the equations are consistent but A is not square and full rank, then there are an infinite number of solutions. In this case A has no inverse and may not even be a square matrix. The infinite number of solutions that exist can be found by using a generalization of the inverse called the generalized inverse, which is often denoted by A⁻. Every matrix has a generalized inverse, even matrices that are not square. For details on using the generalized inverse to solve linear equations, see for example, Searle (1966).

### Eigenvalues and Eigenvectors

One other useful topic in matrix algebra, which forms the basis of PCA (see chapter 10) for example, is eigenvalues and eigenvectors.

### Definitions

Consider an $n \times n$ matrix A. Suppose we are able to find an $n \times 1$ vector $\underline{v}$ and a scalar $d$ such that

$$A\underline{v} = d\underline{v}, \tag{A.9}$$

or in other words, when we post-multiply A by the vector $\underline{v}$, the result is still $\underline{v}$, except scaled by the constant $d$. In such a case, the vector $\underline{v}$ is called an *eigenvector* of A and the constant $d$ is called an *eigenvalue*. At least at the level of mathematics considered in this book, equation A.9 by itself does not offer any profound insights into the matrix A. So the definition of eigenvalues and eigenvectors is not particularly illuminating. Even so, eigenvectors and eigenvalues have many properties that are extremely useful, and it is for these properties, rather than for the definition, that eigenvectors and eigenvalues are so frequently used in statistics.

Next we consider methods for finding the eigenvectors and eigenvalues of a matrix. If equation A.9 holds, then

$$A\underline{v} - d\underline{v} = \underline{0},$$

where $\underline{0}$ is a vector of all zeroes. And therefore,

$$(A - dI)\underline{v} = \underline{0}. \tag{A.10}$$

Note that we needed to add the matrix I to make the difference inside the parentheses conformable.

An obvious solution to equation A.10 is that $\underline{v} = \underline{0}$, but this is not interesting because it is a solution no matter what the matrix A, and for this reason, it certainly cannot tell us anything useful about A. Thus, the only solutions of equation A.10 that could be of interest are when $\underline{v} \neq \underline{0}$. Now if $(A - dI)$ is nonsingular (i.e., full rank), then $\underline{v} = \underline{0}$ is the only solution. For this reason, we are interested in finding values of $d$ that make $(A - dI)$ singular. As we saw earlier, a square matrix is singular if and only if its determinant is zero. Therefore, our task is to find values of $d$ for which

$$|A - dI| = 0. \tag{A.11}$$

This is called the *characteristic equation* of the matrix A.

Note that unlike equation A.10, both sides of equation A.11 are scalars (rather than vectors). In fact, if A is $n \times n$, then its characteristic equation is an $n^{th}$ order polynomial. For example, in the case of the matrix

$$A = \begin{bmatrix} 3 & 1 \\ 1 & 3 \end{bmatrix},$$

the characteristic equation is

$$\begin{aligned}
0 &= \left\| \begin{bmatrix} 3 & 1 \\ 1 & 3 \end{bmatrix} - \begin{bmatrix} d & 0 \\ 0 & d \end{bmatrix} \right\|, \\
&= \begin{vmatrix} 3-d & 1 \\ 1 & 3-d \end{vmatrix} \\
&= (3-d)^2 - 1 \\
&= d^2 - 6d + 8 \\
&= (d-4)(d-2).
\end{aligned}$$

The two roots of this quadratic equation and, consequently, the two eigenvalues of A are $d = 4$ and $d = 2$. MATLAB will produce these eigenvalues in response to the command eig(A). For example, the commands

```
>> A = [3 1;1 3];
>> eig(A)
```

produce

```
        ans =
2
4
```

Once the eigenvalues are computed, the eigenvectors can be determined by solving equations A.10. In the current example

$$\begin{aligned}
\begin{bmatrix} 0 \\ 0 \end{bmatrix} &= \left( \begin{bmatrix} 3 & 1 \\ 1 & 3 \end{bmatrix} - \begin{bmatrix} d & 0 \\ 0 & d \end{bmatrix} \right) \begin{bmatrix} v_1 \\ v_2 \end{bmatrix} \\
&= \begin{bmatrix} 3-d & 1 \\ 1 & 3-d \end{bmatrix} \begin{bmatrix} v_1 \\ v_2 \end{bmatrix}.
\end{aligned}$$

We begin by substituting in the first eigenvalue $d = 4$:

$$\begin{bmatrix} -1 & 1 \\ 1 & -1 \end{bmatrix} \begin{bmatrix} v_1 \\ v_2 \end{bmatrix} = \begin{bmatrix} 0 \\ 0 \end{bmatrix},$$

which leads to two equations and two unknowns

$$-v_1 + v_2 = 0 \quad \text{and} \quad v_1 - v_2 = 0. \tag{A.12}$$

Note that these two equations have an infinite number of solutions. Of course, this was inevitable because we selected the eigenvalues $d = 4$ and $d = 2$ precisely because they are the only possible values of $d$ that lead to an infinite number of solutions of equations A.10.

Any set of $v_1$ and $v_2$ that satisfy equations A.12 define a legitimate eigenvector of the matrix A. Note that all such solutions fall on the line

$$v_2 = v_1.$$

Any vector can be considered as a directed line segment beginning at the origin (0,0) and ending at the vector coordinates. Thus, although there are an infinite number of solutions to equations A.12, they all point in the same direction. They differ only in length. The convention is to choose a solution so that the resulting eigenvector has a length of 1; that is, to choose $v_1$ and $v_2$ so that $\underline{v}'\underline{v} = 1$.

An easy way to do this is to choose any solution, compute $\underline{v}'\underline{v}$, and then divide both $v_1$ and $v_2$ by the square root of this value. In the example of equations A.12, we could choose $v_1 = 1$ and $v_2 = 1$.

Then

$$\underline{v}'\underline{v} = \begin{bmatrix} 1 & 1 \end{bmatrix} \begin{bmatrix} 1 \\ 1 \end{bmatrix} = 2,$$

and so the eigenvector associated with the eigenvalue $d = 4$ is

$$\underline{v}_1 = \begin{bmatrix} \frac{1}{\sqrt{2}} \\ \frac{1}{\sqrt{2}} \end{bmatrix}.$$

We use the subscript 1 to signify that this is the eigenvector associated with the first, or largest, eigenvalue. We can verify that the length of this eigenvector is 1 via

$$\begin{bmatrix} \frac{1}{\sqrt{2}} & \frac{1}{\sqrt{2}} \end{bmatrix} \begin{bmatrix} \frac{1}{\sqrt{2}} \\ \frac{1}{\sqrt{2}} \end{bmatrix} = \frac{1}{2} + \frac{1}{2} = 1.$$

By a similar process, we can determine that the eigenvector associated with the second eigenvalue $d = 2$ is

$$\underline{v}_2 = \begin{bmatrix} -\frac{1}{\sqrt{2}} \\ \frac{1}{\sqrt{2}} \end{bmatrix}.$$

## Properties

As previously mentioned, the definitions of eigenvalues and eigenvectors do not lead to any immediate insights into the matrix A. However, eigenvalues and eigenvectors have many properties that are extremely useful in a wide variety of applications, and it is for these properties that eigenvalues and eigenvectors are considered core topics in matrix or linear algebra. As we saw in chapter 10, several of these properties lie at the heart of PCA.

This section describes a few of the most important properties of eigenvalues and eigenvectors. Any text on linear algebra will include a variety of others.

*Property 1* *An n × n matrix has n eigenvalues, some of which may equal 0 and some of which may be repeated.* This follows because the characteristic equation of an $n \times n$ matrix is an $n^{th}$ order polynomial, which has $n$ roots. In our earlier numerical example, the $2 \times 2$ matrix

$$A = \begin{bmatrix} 3 & 1 \\ 1 & 3 \end{bmatrix}$$

has two eigenvalues; namely, 4 and 2.

*Property 2* *The number of nonzero eigenvalues of A equals the rank of A.* This property is extremely useful because it can be quite tedious to compute the rank of a matrix by determining the number of linearly independent rows or columns. Note that an important corollary to this property is that A is singular if and only if A has at least one eigenvalue equal to 0. In our earlier numerical example, A had two eigenvalues $d = 4$ and $d = 2$. These are both nonzero, so the rank of A is 2 and therefore A is nonsingular.

*Property 3* *The determinant of A equals the product of its eigenvalues.* So in our numerical example, the determinant of A must equal $4 \times 2 = 8$. Because A is $2 \times 2$, this is easily verified:

$$\begin{vmatrix} 3 & 1 \\ 1 & 3 \end{vmatrix} = (3 \times 3) - (1 \times 1) = 8.$$

With much larger matrices, however, computing the determinant directly is a time-consuming process. If the eigenvalues are known, property no. 3 makes this computation simple. Note also that if one of the eigenvalues of A is 0, then their product will be zero, and hence the determinant of A will be 0. In other words, if A has one or more eigenvalues equal to 0, then A must be singular—a result that also followed from property no. 2.

*Property 4* *The trace of A equals the sum of its eigenvalues.* The trace of a matrix is equal to the sum of all elements on the main diagonal. So

$$\text{trace}\left(\begin{bmatrix} 3 & 1 \\ 1 & 3 \end{bmatrix}\right) = 3 + 3 = 6,$$

and note that the sum of the eigenvalues of this matrix is also 6 (i.e., 4 + 2).

*Property 5    Diagonal Representation of a Symmetric Matrix. Suppose A is a symmetric $n \times n$ matrix. Construct the $n \times n$ diagonal matrix D that has the eigenvalues of A on its main diagonal (e.g., in descending order of magnitude). Construct the $n \times n$ square matrix V whose columns are the eigenvectors of A (so that the $i^{th}$ column of V is the eigenvector that corresponds with the eigenvalue in row i and column i of the matrix D). Then A = VDV'.*

In our numerical example, the diagonal representation of A is given by

$$A = \begin{bmatrix} \frac{1}{\sqrt{2}} & -\frac{1}{\sqrt{2}} \\ \frac{1}{\sqrt{2}} & \frac{1}{\sqrt{2}} \end{bmatrix} \begin{bmatrix} 4 & 0 \\ 0 & 2 \end{bmatrix} \begin{bmatrix} \frac{1}{\sqrt{2}} & \frac{1}{\sqrt{2}} \\ -\frac{1}{\sqrt{2}} & \frac{1}{\sqrt{2}} \end{bmatrix}$$

$$= \begin{bmatrix} 3 & 1 \\ 1 & 3 \end{bmatrix}.$$

A matrix in which all eigenvalues are positive is said to be *positive definite*, and a matrix in which all eigenvalues are non-negative (e.g., some may be zero) is said to be *positive semi-definite*. Note that, in this example, A is positive definite. PCA works on the eigenvalues and eigenvectors of the sample variance-covariance matrix. All variance-covariance matrices are symmetric and positive semidefinite.

MATLAB computes eigenvectors (and eigenvalues) using a similar form. Specifically, the command

[V,D] = eig(A)

returns a matrix V whose columns are the eigenvectors of A and a diagonal matrix D containing the eigenvalues of A. For example, the commands

```
>> A = [3 1;1 3];
>> [V,D] = eig(A)
```

produce the output

$$V =$$

$$\begin{matrix} -0.7071 & 0.7071 \\ 0.7071 & 0.7071 \end{matrix}$$

$$D =$$

$$\begin{matrix} 2 & 0 \\ 0 & 4 \end{matrix}$$

# Appendix B: Multivariate Probability Distributions

A *random vector* is a vector in which every entry is a random variable. For example, consider the vector

$$\underline{x} = \begin{bmatrix} x_1 \\ x_2 \\ \vdots \\ x_r \end{bmatrix}.$$

If $\underline{x}$ is a random vector, then each $x_i$ is a random variable. Let $f_i(x_i)$ denote the *probability density function* (pdf) of $x_i$. This function specifies the likelihood that a random sample drawn from the $x_i$ population exactly equals any specific numerical value.[1] If $x_i$ is normally distributed, then $f_i(x_i)$ is the familiar bell-shaped curve. With respect to the random vector $\underline{x}$, the pdfs $f_i(x_i)$ are known as the *marginal distributions*.

The marginal distributions of $\underline{x}$ provide much information about the sampling behavior of $\underline{x}$, but they do not tell us everything. In particular, they provide no information about any statistical relationships that might exist among the various $x_i$. Complete information about $\underline{x}$ is catalogued in the *joint probability density function* (or joint distribution)

$$f(x_1, x_2, \ldots, x_r) = f(\underline{x}).$$

This function specifies the likelihood that a random sample from the $\underline{x}$ population will produce any specific $r \times 1$ numerical vector.

If there is no statistical relationship among any of the $x_i$, then all information in the joint pdf is specified by the marginal pdfs. More specifically, the random variables $x_1, x_2, \ldots, x_r$ are *statistically independent* if and only if

---

1. This notation is sloppy because it does not discriminate between the name of the random variable or random vector and the specific numerical values that the random variable or vector can take. The current notation is simpler, and hopefully it is obvious from the context which interpretation is intended.

$$f(x_1, x_2, \ldots, x_r) = f_1(x_1) \times f_2(x_2) \times \cdots \times f_r(x_r), \tag{B.1}$$

for all possible values of $x_1, x_2, \ldots, x_r$. If equation B.1 fails for any combination of $x_1$, $x_2, \ldots, x_r$, then a statistical dependence exists among these random variables.

## Multivariate Normal Distributions

The *multivariate normal distribution* is, by far, the most widely used multivariate distribution in statistics. For example, it serves as the error model in the GLM and as the model that underlies PCA. A multivariate normal distribution has three assumptions: (1) the marginal distributions are all normal; (2) the only possible relationships among the $x_i$ are linear; and (3) all dependencies among the $x_i$ can be expressed as a function of the dependencies between all possible pairs of $x_i$ (i.e., there are no dependencies that depend on three-way or higher interactions). Thus, even if the $x_i$ are each normally distributed, the random vector $\underline{x}$ is not necessarily multivariate normally distributed. In addition, it must also be true that the only possible statistical dependencies that exist among the $x_i$ are pairwise linear relationships.

The well-known Pearson correlation coefficient (i.e., the Pearson's $r$) measures linear relationships between pairs of variables. This is the model of statistical dependence that underlies the multivariate normal distribution. Uncorrelated random variables have no linear relationship, but they could have a nonlinear relationship, in which case they would not be statistically independent (i.e., equation B.1 would not hold). Statistical independence implies zero correlation, but uncorrelated random variables are not necessarily independent. In a multivariate normal distribution, however, the only possible relationships are linear, so uncorrelated is equivalent to independent.

In the multivariate normal distribution, there is a mean and variance associated with each (random) variable and a correlation associated with each pair of variables. Let $\mu_i$ and $\sigma_i^2$ denote the mean and variance of $x_i$, respectively. The correlation between random variables $x_1$ and $x_2$ is defined as the standardized covariance:

$$\rho_{12} = \frac{\text{cov}_{12}}{\sigma_1 \sigma_2} = \frac{E[(x_1 - \mu_1)(x_2 - \mu_2)]}{\sigma_1 \sigma_2}. \tag{B.2}$$

If the means and variances are known, then note that it makes no difference whether we characterize the associations of a multivariate normal distribution in terms of correlations or covariances. From either one, equation B.2 allows us to solve for the other. The standard convention is to record the covariances.

The parameters of any multivariate normal distribution are catalogued in two structures: a mean vector $\underline{\mu}$ and a variance-covariance matrix $\Sigma$. The mean vector is a record of the mean of each marginal distribution,

$$\underline{\mu} = \begin{bmatrix} \mu_1 \\ \mu_2 \\ \vdots \\ \mu_r \end{bmatrix}, \tag{B.3}$$

and the variance-covariance matrix is a record of all variances and covariances,

$$\Sigma = \begin{bmatrix} \sigma_1^2 & \mathrm{cov}_{12} & \cdots & \mathrm{cov}_{1r} \\ \mathrm{cov}_{21} & \sigma_2^2 & \cdots & \mathrm{cov}_{2r} \\ \vdots & \vdots & \ddots & \vdots \\ \mathrm{cov}_{r1} & \mathrm{cov}_{r2} & \cdots & \sigma_r^2 \end{bmatrix}. \tag{B.4}$$

Because $\mathrm{cov}_{ij} = \mathrm{cov}_{ji}$, note that this is a symmetric matrix. It is also positive semidefinite (i.e., no eigenvalues can be negative; see appendix A).

Once numerical values are specified for the mean vector and the variance-covariance matrix, then the likelihood of any vector $\underline{x}$ can be computed from the multivariate normal pdf:

$$f(\underline{x}) = \frac{1}{(2\pi)^{r/2} |\Sigma|^{1/2}} \exp[-\tfrac{1}{2}(\underline{x} - \underline{\mu})' \Sigma^{-1} (\underline{x} - \underline{\mu})]. \tag{B.5}$$

Figure B.1 shows an example of this pdf for a bivariate normal distribution where the correlation between $x_1$ and $x_2$ is positive. The bottom panel shows some contours of equal likelihood from this distribution, which are created by slicing through the pdf shown in the top panel from different heights above the $(x_1, x_2)$ plane and looking down at the results from above. Note that these contours all have the same shape and differ only in size. A scatterplot of random samples from the distribution shown in the top panel would have the same overall shape as these contours. The positive correlation causes the major axis of the contours to have a positive slope. Note that random samples from the distribution that have a large $x_1$ value will also tend to have a large $x_2$ value.

A special case of the multivariate normal distribution that is widely used throughout this book assumes that all variables are independent and all variances are equal. In this case, note that

$$\Sigma = \begin{bmatrix} \sigma^2 & 0 & \cdots & 0 \\ 0 & \sigma^2 & \cdots & 0 \\ \vdots & \vdots & \ddots & \vdots \\ 0 & 0 & \cdots & \sigma^2 \end{bmatrix} = \sigma^2 \begin{bmatrix} 1 & 0 & \cdots & 0 \\ 0 & 1 & \cdots & 0 \\ \vdots & \vdots & \ddots & \vdots \\ 0 & 0 & \cdots & 1 \end{bmatrix} = \sigma^2 I.$$

The multivariate z-distribution is a special case of this in which the mean vector equals $\underline{0}$ and the variance-covariance matrix equals I.

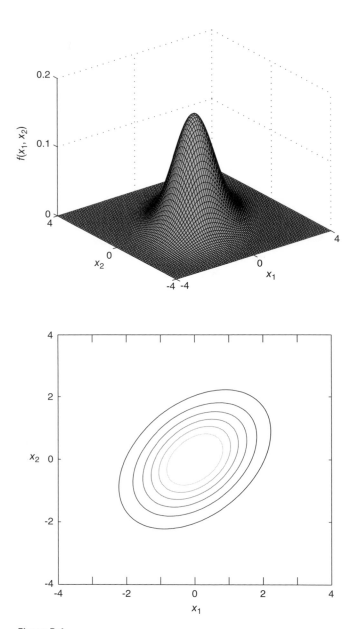

**Figure B.1**
(Top) The pdf of a bivariate normal distribution. (Bottom) Contours of equal likelihood from the pdf shown in the top panel. Note the positive correlation between $x_1$ and $x_2$.

Frequently in probability and statistics, and also in this book, we are interested in the distribution of a linear transformation of a random vector. More specifically, suppose $\underline{x}$ is an $r \times 1$ random vector, A is an $m \times r$ matrix of constants, and $\underline{b}$ is an $m \times 1$ vector of constants. Now consider the $m \times 1$ random vector

$$\underline{y} = A\underline{x} + \underline{b}.$$

Then regardless of the distribution of $\underline{x}$, the mean vector and variance-covariance matrix of $\underline{y}$ are equal to

$$\underline{\mu}_y = A\underline{\mu}_x + \underline{b}$$

and

$$\Sigma_{\underline{y}} = A\Sigma_{\underline{x}}A'.$$

Furthermore, if $\underline{x}$ has a multivariate normal distribution then $\underline{y}$ will also have a multivariate normal distribution (because linear transformations of normal random variables are normal).

# References

Adler, R. J. (1981). *The geometry of random fields*. New York: Wiley.

Aguirre, G., Zarahn, E., & D'Esposito, M. (1998). The variability of human, BOLD hemodynamic responses. *NeuroImage, 8,* 360–369.

Allen, R. L., & Mills, D. W. (2004). *Signal analysis: Time, frequency, scale, and structure*. New York: IEEE Press.

Amari, S., Cichocki, A., & Yang, H. (1996). A new learning algorithm for blind signal separation. *Advances in Neural Information Processing Systems, 8,* 757–763.

Andersson, J., Smith, S., & Jenkinson, M. (2008). FNIRT—FMRIB's nonlinear image registration tool. *Human Brain Mapping*, poster #496, Melbourne, Australia, June 15–19, 2008.

Ardekani, B. A., Guckemus, S., Bachman, A., Hoptman, M. J., Wojtaszek, M., & Nierenberg, J. (2005). Quantitative comparison of algorithms for inter-subject registration of 3D volumetric brain MRI scans. *Journal of Neuroscience Methods, 142,* 67–76.

Ashburner, J. (2007). A fast diffeomorphic image registration algorithm. *NeuroImage, 38,* 95–113.

Ashburner, J., & Friston, K. (2007a). Non-linear registration. In K. J. Friston, J. T. Ashburner, S. J. Kiebel, T. E. Nichols, & W. D. Penny (Eds.), *Statistical parametric mapping: The analysis of functional brain images* (pp. 63–80). London: Academic Press.

Ashburner, J., & Friston, K. (2007b). Rigid body registration. In K. J. Friston, J. T. Ashburner, S. J. Kiebel, T. E. Nichols, & W. D. Penny (Eds.), *Statistical parametric mapping: The analysis of functional brain images* (pp. 49–62). London: Academic Press.

Ashby, F. G. (1992). Multivariate probability distributions. In F. G. Ashby (Ed.), *Multidimensional models of perception and cognition* (pp. 1–34). Hillsdale, NJ: Lawrence Erlbaum Associates, Inc.

Ashby, F. G., & Townsend, J. T. (1986). Varieties of perceptual independence. *Psychological Review, 93,* 154–179.

Ashby, F. G., & Valentin, V. V. (2007). Computational cognitive neuroscience: Building and testing biologically plausible computational models of neuroscience, neuroimaging, and behavioral data. In M. J. Wenger & C. Schuster (Eds.), *Statistical and process models for cognitive neuroscience and aging* (pp. 15–58). Mahwah, NJ: Erlbaum.

Ashby, F. G., & Waldschmidt, J. G. (2008). Fitting computational models to fMRI data. *Behavior Research Methods, 40,* 713–721.

Attias, H. (1998). Independent factor analysis. *Neural Computation, 11,* 803–851.

Avants, B. B., Epstein, C. L., Grossman, M., & Gee, J. C. (2008). Symmetric diffeomorphic image registration with cross-correlation: Evaluating automated labeling of elderly and neurodegenerative brain. *Medical Image Analysis, 12,* 26–41.

Beckmann, C. F., & Smith, S. M. (2004). Probabilistic independent component analysis for functional magnetic resonance imaging. *IEEE Transactions on Medical Imaging, 23,* 137–152.

Beckmann, C. F., Jenkinson, M., & Smith, S. M. (2003). General multilevel linear modeling for group analysis in FMRI. *NeuroImage, 20,* 1052–1063.

Bell, A. J., & Sejnowski, T. J. (1995). An information-mazimization approach to blind separation and blind deconvolution. *Neural Computation, 7*, 1129–1159.

Benjamini, Y., & Hochberg, Y. (1995). Controlling the false discovery rate: A practical and powerful approach to multiple testing. *Journal of the Royal Statistical Society. Series B (Methodological), 57*, 289–300.

Bishop, C. (1995). *Neural networks for pattern recognition*. Oxford, UK: Clarendon.

Bishop, C. M. (2006). *Pattern recognition and machine learning*. New York: Springer.

Biswal, B. B., & Ulmer, J. L. (1999). Blind source separation of multiple signal sources of fMRI data sets using independent component analysis. *Journal of Computer Assisted Tomography, 23*, 265–271.

Bower, J. M., & Beeman, D. (1998). *The book of GENESIS: Exploring realistic neural models with the GEneral NEural SImulation System* (2nd Ed.). New York: Springer-Verlag.

Boynton, G. M., Engel, S. A., Glover, G. H., & Heeger, D. J. (1996). Linear systems analysis of functional magnetic resonance imaging in human V1. *Journal of Neuroscience, 16*, 4207–4221.

Bracewell, R. N. (1965). *The Fourier transform and its applications*. New York: McGraw-Hill.

Brillinger, D. R. (1975). *Time series—Data analysis and theory*. New York: Holt, Rinehart & Winston.

Buckner, R. L., Andrews-Hanna, J. R., & Schacter, D. L. (2008). The brain's default network: Anatomy, function, and relevance to disease. *Annals of the New York Academy of Sciences, 1124*, 1–38.

Buhmann, M. D. (2003). *Radial basis functions: Theory and implementations*. New York: Cambridge University Press.

Bullmore, E., Brammer, M., Williams, S. C. R., Rabe-Hesketh, S., Janot, N., David, A., Mellers, J., Howard, R., & Sham, P. (1996). Statistical methods of estimation and inference for functional MR image analysis. *Magnetic Resonance in Medicine, 35*, 261–277.

Buxton, R. B. (2002). *Introduction to functional magnetic resonance imaging: Principles and techniques*. New York: Cambridge University Press.

Buxton, R. B., & Frank, L. R. (1998). A model for coupling between cerebral blood flow and oxygen metabolism during neural stimulation. *Journal of Cerebral Blood Flow and Metabolism, 17*, 64–72.

Buxton, R. B., Wong, E. C., & Frank, L. R. (1998). Dynamics of blood flow and oxygenation changes during brain activation: The balloon model. *Magnetic Resonance in Medicine, 39*, 855–864.

Cahn, B. R., & Polich, J. (2006). Meditation states and traits: EEG, ERP, and neuroimaging studies. *Psychological Bulletin, 132*, 180–211.

Calhoun, V. D., Adali, T., Pearlson, G. D., & Pekar, J. J. (2001). Spatial and temporal independent component analysis of functional MRI data containing a pair of task-related waveforms. *Human Brain Mapping, 13*, 43–53.

Calvo-Merino, B., Glaser, D. E., Grèzes, J., Passingham, R. E., & Haggard, P. (2005). Action observation and acquired motor skills: An fMRI study with expert dancers. *Cerebral Cortex, 15*, 1243–1249.

Cao, J. (1999). The size of the connected components of excursion sets of $\chi^2$, $t$ and $F$ fields. *Advances in Applied Probability, 31*, 577–593.

Cardoso, J.-F. (1997). Infomax and maximum likelihood for blind source separation. *IEEE Letters on Signal Processing, 4*, 112–114.

Chen, C. T. (1970). *Introduction to linear systems theory*. New York: Holt, Rinehart and Winston.

Chen, Y., Bressler, S. L., & Ding, M. (2006). Frequency decomposition of conditional Granger causality and application to multivariate neural field potential data. *Journal of Neuroscience Methods, 150*, 228–237.

Churchill, R. V., Brown, J. W., & Verhey, R. F. (1974). *Complex variables and applications* (Third Ed.). New York: McGraw-Hill.

Clark, V. P., Maisog, J. M., & Haxby, J. V. (1998). FMRI studies of face memory using random stimulus sequences. *Journal of Neurophysiology, 79*, 3257–3265.

Cohen, J. (1992). A power primer. *Psychological Bulletin, 112*, 155–159.

Cohen, J., Cohen, P., West, S. G., & Aiken, L. S. (2003). *Applied multiple regression/correlation analysis for the behavioral sciences* (Third Ed.). Mahwah, NJ: Erlbaum.

Cohen, M. S. (1997). Parametric analysis of fMRI data using linear systems methods. *NeuroImage, 6*, 93–103.

Comon, P. (1994). Independent component analysis: A new concept? *Signal Processing, 36*, 11–20.

Cox, R. W. (1996). AFNI: Software for analysis and visualization of functional magnetic resonance neuroimages. *Computers and Biomedical Research, 29*, 162–173.

Cox, R. W., & Hyde, J. S. (1997). Software tools for analysis and visualization of fMRI data. *NMR in Biomedicine, 10*, 171–178.

Dale, A. M. (1999). Optimal experimental design for event-related fMRI. *Human Brain Mapping, 8*, 109–114.

Dale, A. M., & Buckner, R. L. (1997). Selective averaging of rapidly presented individual trials using fMRI. *Human Brain Mapping, 5*, 329–340.

Davies, M. (2004). Identifiability issues in noisy ICA. *IEEE Signal Processing Letters, 11*, 470–473.

Dempster, A. P., Laird, N. M., & Rubin, D. B. (1977). Maximum likelihood from incomplete data via the EM algorithm. *Journal of the Royal Statistical Society, Series B, 39*, 1–38.

Desmond, J. E., & Glover, G. H. (2002). Estimating sample size in functional MRI (fMRI) neuroimaging studies: Statistical power analyses. *Journal of Neuroscience Methods, 118*, 115–128.

Disbrow, E. A., Slutsky, D. A., Roberts, T. P., & Krubitzer, L. A. (2000). Functional MRI at 1.5 Tesla: A comparison of the blood oxygenation level-dependent signal and electrophysiology. *Proceedings of the National Academy of Sciences, USA, 97*, 9718–9723.

Dum, R. P., & Strick, P. L. (2005). The origin of corticospinal projections from the premotor areas in the frontal lobe. *Journal of Neuroscience, 11*, 667–689.

Evans, A. C., Marrett, S., Torrescorzo, J., Ku, S., & Collins, L. (1991). MRI-PET correlative analysis using a volume of interest (VOI) atlas. *Journal of Cerebral Blood Flow and Metabolism, 11*, A69–A78.

Firbank, M. J., Harrison, R. M., Williams, E. D., & Coulthard, A. (2000). Quality assurance for MRI: Practical experience. *The British Journal of Radiology, 73*, 376–383.

Fisher, R. A. (1935). *The design of experiments*. Edinburgh: Oliver & Boyd.

Fransson, P., Kruger, G., Merboldt, K.-D., & Frahm, J. (1999). MRI of functional deactivation: Temporal and spatial characteristics of oxygenation-sensitive responses in human visual cortex. *NeuroImage, 9*, 611–618.

Fransson, P., Merbolt, K.-D., Petersson, K. M., Ingvar, M., & Frahm, J. (2002). On the effects of spatial filtering—A comparative fMRI study of episodic memory encoding at high and low resolution. *NeuroImage, 16*, 977–984.

Friston, K. J., Ashburner, J. T., Kiebel, S. J., Nichols, T. E., & Penny, W. D. (Eds.) (2007). *Statistical parametric mapping: The analysis of functional brain images*. London: Academic Press.

Friston, K. J., Frith, C. D., Liddle, P. F., & Frackowiak, R. S. (1991). Comparing functional (PET) images: The assessment of significant change. *Journal of Cerebral Blood Flow Metabolism, 11*, 690–699.

Friston, K. J., Harrison, L., & Penny, W. (2003). Dynamic causal modeling. *NeuroImage, 19*, 1273–1302.

Friston, K. J., Holmes, A. P., & Ashburner, J. (1999). *Statistical Parametric Mapping (SPM)*. http://www.fil.ion.ucl.ac.uk/spm/.

Friston, K. J., Holmes, A., Poline, J.-B., Grasby, P., Williams, S., Frackowiak, R., & Turner, R. (1995a). Analysis of time-series revisited. *NeuroImage, 2*, 45–53.

Friston, K., Holmes, A., Worsley, K., Poline, J., Frith, C., & Frackowiak, R. (1995b). Statistical parametric maps in functional imaging: A general linear approach. *Human Brain Mapping, 2*, 189–210.

Friston, K. J., Josephs, O., Ress, G., & Turner, R. (1998). Nonlinear event-related responses in fMRI. *Magnetic Resonance in Medicine, 39*, 41–52.

Friston, K. J., & Penny, W. (2003). Posterior probability maps and SPMs. *NeuroImage, 19*, 1240–1249.

Friston, K. J., Penny, W., Phillips, C., Kiebel, S., Hinton, G., & Ashburner, J. (2002). Classical and Bayesian inference in neuroimaging: Theory. *NeuroImage, 16*, 465–483.

Friston, K. J., Worsley, K. J., Frackowiak, R. S. J., Mazziotta, J. C., & Evans, A. C. (1994). Assessing the significance of focal activations using their spatial extent. *Human Brain Mapping, 1*, 210–220.

Gaeta, M., & Lacoume, J.-L. (1990). Source separation without prior knowledge: The maximum likelihood solution. In E. Masgrau, L. Torres, & M. A. Lagunas (Eds.), *Proceedings of EUSIPCO 1990* (pp. 621–624). Amsterdam: Elsevier.

Gavrilescu, M., Shaw, M. E., Stuart, G. W., Eckersley, P., Svalbe, I. D., & Egan, G. F. (2002). Simulation of the effects of global normalization procedures in functional MRI. *NeuroImage, 17*, 532–542.

Genovese, C. R. (2000). A Bayesian time-course model for functional magnetic resonance imaging data. *Journal of the American Statistical Association, 95*, 691–703.

Geweke, J. (1982). Measurement of linear dependence and feedback between multiple time series. *Journal of the American Statistical Association, 77*, 304–313.

Geweke, J. (1984). Measures of conditional linear dependence and feedback between time series. *Journal of the American Statistical Association, 79*, 907–915.

Glover, G. H. (1999). Deconvolution of impulse response in event-related BOLD fMRI. *NeuroImage, 9*, 416–429.

Goebel, R., Esposito, F., & Formisano, E. (2006). Analysis of functional image analysis contest (FIAC) data with brainvoyager QX: From single-subject to cortically aligned group general linear model analysis and self-organizing group independent component analysis. *Human Brain Mapping, 27*, 392–401.

Granger, C. W. J. (1969). Investigating causal relations by econometric models and cross-spectral methods. *Econometrica, 37*, 424–438.

Graybill, F. A. (1976). *Theory and application of the general linear model*. North Scituate, MA: Duxbury.

Green, C. G., Nandy, R. R., & Cordes, D. (2002). PCA-preprocessing of fMRI data adversely affects the results of ICA. *Proceedings of the International Society of Magnetic Resonance in Medicine*, 10th Scientific Meeting and Exhibition, Honolulu, Hawaii, May 18–24.

Greene, J. D., Sommerville, R. B., Nystrom, L. E., Darley, J. M., & Cohen, J. D. (2001). An fMRI investigation of emotional engagement in moral judgment. *Science, 293*, 2105–2108.

Haacke, E. M., Brown, R. W., Thompson, M. R., & Venkatesan, R. (1999). *Magnetic resonance imaging: Physical principles and sequence design*. New York: Wiley.

Hashemi, R. H., Bradley, Jr., W. G., & Lisanti, C. J. (2004). *MRI: The basics* (2nd Ed.). Philadelphia, PA: Lippincott Williams & Wilkins.

Haynes, J., & Rees, G. (2006). Decoding mental states from brain activity in humans. *Nature Reviews Neuroscience, 7*, 523–534.

Haxby, J. V., Gobbini, M. I., Furey, M. L., Ishai, A., Schouten, J. L., & Pietrini, P. (2001). Distributed and overlapping representations of faces and objects in ventral temporal cortex. *Science, 293*, 2425–2430.

Herrington, J. D., Sutton, B. P., & Miller, G. A. (2007). Data-storage formats in neuroimaging: Background and tutorial. In J. T. Cacioppo, L. G. Tassinary, & G. G. Berntson (Eds.), *Handbook of psychophysiology, third edition* (pp. 859–866). New York: Cambridge University Press.

Hill, D. L. G., Batchelor, P. G., Holden, M., & Hawkes, D. J. (2001). Medical image registration. *Physics in Medicine and Biology, 46*, R1–R45.

Hinrichs, H., Scholz, M., Tempelmann, C., Woldorff, M. G., Dale, A. M., & Heinze, H. J. (2000). Deconvolution of event-related fMRI responses in fast-rate experimental designs: Tracking amplitude variations. *Journal of Cognitive Neuroscience, 12*, 76–89.

Höskuldsson, A. (1988). PLS regression methods. *Journal of Chemometrics, 2*, 211–228.

Hu, D., Yan, L., Liu, Y., Zhou, Z., Friston, K. J., Tan, C., & Wu, D. (2005). Unified SPM–ICA for fMRI analysis. *NeuroImage, 3*, 746–755.

Huettel, S. A., & McCarthy, G. (2000). Evidence for a refractory period in the hemodynamic response to visual stimuli as measured by MRI. *Neuroimage, 11*, 547–553.

Huettel, S. A., Singerman, J. D., & McCarthy, G. (2001). The effects of aging upon the hemodynamic response measured by functional MRI. *NeuroImage, 13*, 161–175.

Huettel, S. A., Song, A. W., & McCarthy, G. (2004). *Functional magnetic resonance imaging*. Sunderland, MA: Sinauer.

Hyvärinen, A. (1999). Fast and robust fixed-point algorithms for independent component analysis. *IEEE Transactions on Neural Networks, 10*, 626–634.

Hyvärinen, A., Karhunen, J., & Oja, E. (2001). *Independent component analysis*. New York: Wiley.

Hyvärinen, A., & Oja, E. (1997). A fast fixed-point algorithm for independent component analysis. *Neural Computation, 9,* 1483–1492.

Jezzard, P., & Balaban, R. S. (1995). Correction for geometric distortions in echoplanar images from B0 field variations. *Magnetic Resonance in Medicine, 34,* 65–73.

Johnston, D., & Wu, S. M.-S. (1995). *Foundations of cellular neurophysiology.* Cambridge, MA: MIT Press.

Kayser, A. S., Sun, F. T., & D'Esposito, M. (2009). A comparison of Granger causality and coherency in fMRI-based analysis of the motor system. *Human Brain Mapping, 30,* 3475–3494.

Kiebel, S. J., & Holmes, A. P. (2007). The general linear model. In K. J. Friston, J. T. Ashburner, S. J. Kiebel, T. E. Nichols, & W. D. Penny (Eds.), *Statistical parametric mapping: The analysis of functional brain images* (pp. 101–125). London: Academic Press.

Klein, A., Andersson, J., Ardekani, B. A., Ashburner, J., Avants, B., Chiang, M.-C., Christensen, G. E., Collins, D. L., Gee, J., Hellier, P., Song, J. H., Jenkinson, M., Lepage, C., Rueckert, D., Thompson, P., Vercauteren, T., Woods, R. P., Mann, J. J., & Parsey, R. V. (2009). Evaluation of 14 nonlinear deformation algorithms applied to human brain MRI registration. *Neuroimage, 46,* 786–802.

Koch, C. (1999). *Biophysics of computation.* New York: Oxford.

Le Bihan, D., Mangin, J. F., Poupon, C., Clark, C. A., Pappata, S., Molko, N., & Chabriat, H. (2001). Diffusion tensor imaging: Concepts and applications. *Journal of Magnetic Resonance Imaging, 13,* 534–546.

Lee, L., Friston, K., & Horwitz, B. (2006). Large-scale neural models and dynamic causal modeling. *NeuroImage, 30,* 1243–1254.

Lieberman, M. D., Berkman, E. T., & Wager, T. D. (2009). Correlations in social neuroscience aren't voodoo: Commentary on Vul et al. (2009). *Perspectives on Psychological Science, 4,* 299–307.

Lloyd, D. (2002). Functional MRI and the study of human consciousness. *Journal of Cognitive Neuroscience, 14,* 818–831.

Logothetis, N. K. (2003). The underpinnings of the BOLD functional magnetic resonance imaging signal. *The Journal of Neuroscience, 23,* 3963–3971.

Logothetis, N. K., Pauls, J., Augath, M., Trinath, T., & Oeltermann, A. (2001). Neurophysiological investigation of the basis of the fMRI signal. *Nature, 412,* 150–157.

Luce, R. D. (1986). *Response times: Their role in inferring elementary mental organization.* New York: Oxford.

Lund, T. E., Madsen, K. H., Sidaros, K., Luo, W. L., & Nichols, T. E. (2006). Non-white noise in fMRI: Does modelling have an impact? *NeuroImage, 29,* 54–66.

Marreiros, A. C., Kiebel, S. J., & Friston, K. J. (2008). Dynamic causal modelling for fMRI: A two-state model. *NeuroImage, 39,* 269–278.

McIntosh, A. R., Bookstein, F. L., Haxby, J. V., & Grady, C. L. (1996). Spatial pattern analysis of functional brain images using partial least squares. *NeuroImage, 3,* 143–157.

McIntosh, A. R., Chau, W. K., & Protzner, A. B. (2004). Spatiotemporal analysis of event-related fMRI data using partial least squares. *NeuroImage, 23,* 764–775.

McIntosh, A. R., & Lobaugh, N. J. (2004). Partial least squares analysis of neuroimaging data: Applications and advances. *NeuroImage, 23,* S250–S263.

McKeown, M. J., Hansen, L. K., & Sejnowski, T. J. (2003). Independent component analysis of functional MRI: What is signal and what is noise? *Current Opinion in Neurobiology, 13,* 620–629.

McKeown, M. J., Makeig, S., Brown, G. G., Jung, T.-P., Kindermann, S. S., Bell, A. J., & Sejnowski, T. J. (1998). Analysis of fMRI data by blind separation into independent spatial components. *Human Brain Mapping, 6,* 160–188.

Mechelli, A., Price, C. J., & Friston, K. J., (2001). Nonlinear coupling between evoked rCBF and BOLD signals: A simulation study of hemodynamic responses. *NeuroImage, 14,* 862–872.

Miller, K. L., Luh, W. M., Liu, T. T., Martinez, A., Obata, T., Wong, E. C., Frank, L. R., & Buxton, R. B. (2001). Nonlinear temporal dynamics of the cerebral blood flow response. *Human Brain Mapping, 13,* 1–12.

Miller, M. M., Donovan, C.-L., Van Horn, J. D., German, E., Sokol-Hessner, P., & Wolford, G. L. (2009). Unique and persistent individual patterns of brain activity across different memory retrieval tasks. *NeuroImage, 48,* 625–635.

Mori, S. (2007). *Introduction to diffusion tensor imaging*. Amsterdam, The Netherlands: Elsevier, B. V.

Mumford, J. A., & Nichols, T. E. (2008). Power calculation for group fMRI studies accounting for arbitrary design and temporal autocorrelation. *NeuroImage, 39*, 261–268.

Murphy, K., Birn, R. M., Handwerker, D. A., Jones, T. B., & Bandettini, P. A. (2009). The impact of global signal regression on resting state correlations: Are anti-correlated networks introduced? *NeuroImage, 44*, 893–905.

Nichols, T. E., & Holmes, A. P. (2001). Nonparametric permutation tests for functional neuroimaging: A primer with examples. *Human Brain Mapping, 15*, 1–25.

Nichols, T. E., & Poline, J.-B. (2009). Commentary on Vul et al.'s (2009). "Puzzlingly High Correlations in fMRI Studies of Emotion, Personality, and Social Cognition." *Perspectives on Psychological Science, 4*, 291–293.

Norman, K., Polyn, S. M., Detre, G., & Haxby, J. V. (2006). Beyond mind-reading: Multi-voxel pattern analysis of fMRI data. *Trends in Cognitive Sciences, 10*, 424–430.

Nosko, V. P. (1969). Local structure of Gaussian random fields in the vicinity of high level shines. *Soviet Mathematics Doklady, 10*, 1481–1484.

Ogawa, S., Lee, T. M., Kay, A. R., & Tank, D. W. (1990). Brain magnetic resonance imaging with contrast dependent on blood oxygenation. *Proceedings of the National Academy of Sciences, USA, 87*, 9868–9872.

Ogawa, S., Lee, T. M., Nayak, A. S., & Glynn, P. (1990). Oxygenation-sensitive contrast in magnetic resonance imaging of rodent brain at high magnetic fields. *Magnetic Resonance in Medicine, 16*, 9–18.

Ogawa, S., Lee, T. M., Stepnoski, R., Chen, W., Zhu, X. H., & Ugurbil, K. (2000). An approach to probe some neural systems interaction by functional MRI at neural time scale down to milliseconds. *Proceeding of the National Academy of Sciences, USA, 97*, 11026–11031.

Ollinger, J. M., Corbetta, M., & Shulman, G. L. (2001a). Separating processes within a trial in event-related functional MRI. II. Analysis. *NeuroImage, 13*, 218–229.

Ollinger, J. M., Shulman, G. L., & Corbetta, M. (2001b). Separating processes within a trial in event-related functional MRI. I. The method. *NeuroImage, 13*, 210–217.

Papoulis, A. (1965). *Probability, random variables, and stochastic processes*. New York: McGraw-Hill.

Papoulis, A., & Pillai, S. U. (1991). *Probability, random variables and stochastic processes* (Fourth Ed.). New York: McGraw-Hill.

Pauling, L., & Coryell, C. D. (1936). The magnetic properties and structure of hemoglobin, oxygenated hemoglobin, and carbonmonoxygenated hemoglobin. *Proceedings of the National Academy of Sciences USA, 22*, 210–236.

Pearlmutter, B. A., & Parra, L. C. (1997). Maximum likelihood blind source separation: A context-sensitive generalization of ICA. *Advances in Neural Information Processing Systems, 9*, 613–619.

Pereira, F., Mitchell, T., & Botvinick, M. (2009). Machine learning classifiers and fMRI: A tutorial overview. *Neuroimage, 45*(1 Suppl), S199–209.

Petersson, K. M., Nichols, T. E., Poline, J. B., & Holmes, A. P. (1999). Statistical limitations in functional neuroimaging. I. Non-inferential methods and statistical models. *Philosophical Transactions of the Royal Society of London B, 354*, 1239–1260.

Pfeuffer, J., McCullough, J. C., Van de Moortele, P.-F., Ugurbil, K., & Hu, X. (2003). Spatial dependence of the nonlinear BOLD response at short stimulus duration. *NeuroImage, 18*, 990–1000.

Pham, D.-T., & Garrat, P. (1997). Blind separation of a mixture of independent sources through a quasi-maximum likelihood approach. *IEEE Transactions on Signal Processing, 45*, 1712–1725.

Poldrack, R. A., & Mumford, J. A. (2009). Independence in ROI analysis: Where is the voodoo? *Social Cognitive and Affective Neuroscience, 4*, 208–213.

Poline, B., Worsley, K. J., Evans, A. C., & Friston, K. J. (1997). Combining spatial extent and peak intensity to test for activations in functional imaging. *NeuroImage, 5*, 83–96.

Poole, D. (2006). *Linear algebra: A modern introduction* (Second Ed.). Belmont, CA: Thomson.

Ratcliff, R. (1979). Group reaction time distributions and an analysis of distribution statistics. *Psychological Bulletin, 86*, 446–461.

Rayens, W. S., & Andersen, A. H. (2006). Multivariate analysis of fMRI data by oriented partial least squares. *Magnetic Resonance Imaging, 24*, 953–958.

Richter, W., & Richter, M. (2003). The shape of the fMRI BOLD response in children and adults changes systematically with age. *NeuroImage, 20*, 1122–1131.

Rosenberg, J. R., Amjad, A. M., Breeze, P., Brillinger, D. R., & Halliday, D. M. (1989). The Fourier approach to the identification of functional coupling between neuronal spike trains. *Progress in Biophysics and Molecular Biology, 53*, 1–31.

Rueckert, D., Sonoda, L. I., Hayes, C., Hill, D. L. G., Leach, M. O., & Hawkes, D. J. (1999). Nonrigid registration using free-form deformations: Application to breast MR Images. *IEEE Transactions on Medical Imaging, 18*, 712–721.

Schacter, D. L., Buckner, R. L., Koutstaal, W., Dale, A. M., & Rosen, B. R. (1997). Late onset of anterior prefrontal activity during true and false recognition: An event-related fMRI study. *NeuroImage, 6*, 259–269.

Schetzen, M. (1980). *The Volterra & Wiener theories of nonlinear systems*. New York: Wiley.

Schwarz, G. (1978). Estimating the dimension of a model. *The Annals of Statistics, 6*, 461–464.

Searle, S. R. (1966). *Matrix algebra for the biological sciences*. New York: Wiley.

Serences, J. (2004). A comparison of methods for characterizing the event-related BOLD timeseries in rapid fMRI. *NeuroImage, 21*, 1690–1700.

Shannon, C. E., & Weaver, W. (1949). *The mathematical theory of communication*. Urbana, IL: University of Illinois Press.

Smith, A. M., Lewis, B. K., Ruttimann, U. E., Ye, F. Q., Sinnwell, T. M., Yang, Y., Duyn, J. H., & Frank, J. A. (1999). Investigation of low frequency drift in fMRI signal. *NeuroImage, 9*, 526–533.

Smith, S. M., Jenkinson, M., Woolrich, M. W., Beckmann, C. F., Behrens, T. E. J., Johansen-Berg, H., Bannister, P. R., De Luca, M., Drobnjak, I., Flitney, D. E., Niazy, R., Saunders, J., Vickers, J., Zhang, Y., De Stefano, N., Brady, J. M., & Matthews, P. M. (2004). Advances in functional and structural MR image analysis and implementation as FSL. *NeuroImage, 23*, 208–219.

Stephan, K. E., Harrison, L. M., Kiebel, S. J., David, O., Penny, W. D., & Friston, K. J. (2007). Dynamic causal models of neural system dynamics: Current state and future extensions. *Journal of Biosciences, 32*, 129–144.

Stephan, K. E., Penny, W. D., Moran, R., Den Ouden, H. E., Daunizeau, J., & Friston, K. J. (2010). Ten simple rules for dynamic causal modelling. *NeuroImage, 49*, 3099–3109.

Sternberg, S. (1966). High-speed scanning in human memory. *Science, 153*, 652–654.

Stone, J. V. (2004). *Independent component analysis*. Cambridge, MA: MIT Press.

Sun, F. T., Miller, L. M., & D'Esposito, M. (2004). Measuring interregional functional connectivity using coherence and partial coherence analyses of fMRI data. *NeuroImage, 21*, 647–658.

Sun, F. T., Miller, L. M., & D'Esposito, M. (2005). Measuring temporal dynamics of functional networks using phase spectrum of fMRI data. *NeuroImage, 28*, 227–237.

Talairach, J., & Tournoux, P. (1988). *Co-planar stereotaxic atlas of the human brain: 3-dimensional proportional system—an approach to cerebral imaging*. New York: Thieme Medical Publishers.

Vazquez, A. L., & Noll, D. C. (1998). Non-linear aspects of the blood oxygenation response in functional MRI. *NeuroImage, 8*, 108–118.

Vul, E., Harris, C., Winkielman, P., & Pashler, H. (2009). Puzzlingly high correlations in fMRI studies of emotion, personality, and social cognition. *Perspectives on Psychological Science, 4*, 274–290.

Wager, T. D., Vazquez, A., Hernandez, L., & Noll, D. C. (2005). Accounting for nonlinear BOLD effects in fMRI: parameter estimates and a model for prediction in rapid event-related studies. *NeuroImage, 25*, 206–218.

Winer, B. J., Brown, D. R., & Michels, K. M. (1991). *Statistical principles in experimental design* (3rd Ed.). New York: McGraw-Hill.

Woods, R. P., Mazziotta, J. C., & Cherry, S. R. (1993). MRI-PET registration with automated algorithm. *Computer Assisted Tomography, 17*, 536–546.

Woolrich, M. W., Behrens, T. E. J., Beckmann, C. F., Jenkinson, M., & Smith, S. M. (2004). Multilevel linear modelling for FMRI group analysis using Bayesian inference. *NeuroImage, 21*, 1732–1747.

Woolrich, M. W., Jbabdi, S., Patenaude, B., Chappell, M., Makni, S., Behrens, T., Beckmann, C., Jenkinson, M., & Smith, S. M. (2009). Bayesian analysis of neuroimaging data in FSL. *NeuroImage, 45*, 173–186.

Worsley, K. J. (1995). Estimating the number of peaks in a random field using the Hadwiger characteristic of excursion sets with applications to medical images. *Annals of Statistics*, *23*, 640–669.

Worsley, K. J., Evans, A. C., Marrett, S., & Neelin, P. (1992). A three-dimensional statistical analysis for rCBF activation studies in human brain. *Journal of Cerebral Blood Flow Metabolism*, *12*, 900–918.

Worsley, K. J., & Friston, K. J. (1995). Analysis of time-series revisited—Again. *NeuroImage*, *2*, 173–181.

Worsley, K. J., Marrett, S., Neelin, P., Vandal, A. C., Friston, K. J., & Evans, A. C. (1996). A unified statistical approach for determining significant signals in images of cerebral activation. *Human Brain Mapping*, *4*, 58–73.

Zarahn, E., Aquirre, G., & D'Esposito, M. (1997). A trial-based experimental design for fMRI. *NeuroImage, 6*, 122–138.

Zheng, Y., Martindale, J., Johnston, D., Jones, M., Berwick, J., & Mayhew, J. (2002). A model of the hemodynamic response and oxygen delivery to brain. *NeuroImage*, *16*, 617–637.

# Index

Affine transformation, 65
AFNI, 9, 14
Amplitude of a complex number, 193–194
Analysis of variance, 101–102, 167, 176–177, 289
Analyze data format, 13
ANOVA. *See* Analysis of variance
ART, 68
Atlas, brain, 64
Autocorrelation function, 188–190
Autoregressive model, 221
 order of, 221, 233

Balloon model, 25, 35, 293
Bayesian information criterion, 233
Bayesian statistics, 294–295
Between-subject variance, 164, 175–178
Bilinear models of neural activation, 293–294
Bit of information, 267
Block design, 6, 97–99, 113–114
 percent signal change, 119–120
 power analysis, 180–183
 preprocessing considerations, 42, 75–76
BOLD signal, 3, 17–42
Bonferroni correction, 129–130, 145–146
Boxcar model, 23, 26, 92–93
Brain Voyager, 8–9

Canonical correlation, 292
Causality, 211–219, 226–231, 242–243
Central limit theorem, 69, 263
Characteristic equation, 311
Chi-square map, 116–117, 137, 153
Cholesky factorization, 265
Cluster, 147
Cluster height, 153–156
Cluster-based approaches to the multiple comparisons
 problem, 147–156
Cocktail-party problem, 257–258
Coherence analysis, 185–219, 242–243
Coherency, 210
Commutative property, 298–299
Complex number, 193–194

Computational neuroscience, 22–23, 294
Confirmatory data analysis, 219, 293
Conformable matrices, 298
Connectivity analysis, 185
Consistent linear equations, 306–310
Contour of equal likelihood, 246, 317–318
Convolution integral, 20–21
Coordinate system, MRI 4–5, 52–53
Coregistration, 58–63
Correlation coefficient, 60, 188, 197, 262, 316
Correlation model, 81, 91–99, 123–125, 163,
 287–289
Covariance, 188
Cross-correlation function, 190–192
Cross-power spectrum, 197, 214
Cross-spectral density, 196–197
CT scanning, 2

Deconvolution, 22–24
Degrees of freedom
 chi-square map, 116–118
 GLM, 105, 112–113, 124
 group analysis, 166, 168–171, 173, 176
 power analysis, 179, 183
Delta function, 18–20, 32–33, 82
Design matrix, 88, 99–100, 102
Determinant, 303
Diagonal matrix, 297
DICOM data format, 11–13
DICOM to MINC conversion, 15
DICOM to NIfTI conversion, 14
Diffusion tensor imaging, 5
Distortion correction, 78–79
Dynamic causal modeling, 293–294

Eigenvalue, 104–105, 246–248, 310–314
Eigenvector, 104, 246–248, 310–314
Empirical Bayesian methods, 294–295
Entropy. *See* Information
Error variance, 41, 89–90, 103, 105, 226–230
Euler characteristic, 134–138, 149
Euler's formula, 193

Even function, 194
Event-related design, 6–7, 42, 75, 81–97, 120–123
  rapid, 6–7
  slow, 6, 33, 292
Excel, 30
Excursion set, 134
Expectation-maximization algorithm, 295
Exploratory data analysis, 219, 289, 293

False discovery rate, 141–146
False positive rate, 127
  experiment-wise, 128, 141
  single test, 128
FastICA, 270, 285–287
FBR model, 81–91, 123–125, 287–289
Field map, 5, 79
Finite BOLD response model. *See* FBR model
FIR model. *See* Hrf
Fixed effects model, 164–170, 175–176
Fixed factor, 162–170
F-map, 137, 153
Fourier transform, 24, 26, 45–46, 193, 215
FSL, 8, 11, 13–14, 16, 75, 79, 106, 117, 283–286, 295
  FNIRT, 68
  FSLUTILS, 14–15
  MELODIC, 283
Full width at half maximum. *See* FWHM
FWHM, 70–71, 132

Gaussian kernel. *See* Kernel
Gaussian random field, 130–141, 147–156
Gauss-Markov theorem, 103, 105
Generalized inverse, 310
General linear model, 87–90, 100–118, 231–232
Geometric distribution, truncated, 85–86
Global normalization, 79
Grand mean scaling, 79–80
Granger causality, 222–243
  conditional, 235–242
Group map, 160–161, 175
Group variance. *See* Between-subject variance

Hanning window, 46–48
Header component, 12–13
Head motion correction, 51–58
Hemodynamic response function. *See* Hrf
Homogeneity of variance, 103, 106, 166
Hemoglobin, 3
Hrf, 20–33, 47–51, 92–93, 125
  basis function model, 30–33, 96, 113–117
  difference of gamma functions, 30, 47–51
  FIR model, 32–33, 81–82, 87, 125
  gamma function, 25–26, 28–29
  parameter estimation, 29–30
  temporal derivative, 47–51
Hypothesis testing
  in coherence analysis, 207
  in Granger causality, 234–235

in ICA, 283–285
in the GLM, 107–118

Identity matrix, 301
Image component, 12–13
Impulse response function, 20–21
Inconsistent linear equations, 306–310
Independence, statistical, 106–107, 261–263, 268,
  273–274, 315–316
Infomax, 272–277
Infomax learning algorithm, 274–277
Information, 60, 266–271
Interpolation, 43–47, 66
  linear, 43–44
  sinc, 45–47
  spline, 44
IRTK, 68

Jittering, 7, 84–86, 104–105
Joint information, 267, 271, 273
Joint probability density function, 315

Kernel, 69–73, 77, 132–134
Knot, 44
Kurtosis, 262, 269

Laplace distribution, 263–264
Landmark identification, 59, 63–64
Least squares parameter estimation, 103
Leptokurtic distributions, 263, 269
Linear interpolation. *See* Interpolation
Linear system, 17–21
Linearly independent, 304
Local field potential, 3, 17
Localizer, 4
Logistic distribution, 272–275
Low-pass filter, 205

Machine learning, 291–292
Macrolinearity, 86–87, 95, 123
Magnetic field inhomogeneities, 5
Marginal distribution, 315
Matched filter theorem, 71
MATLAB, 15–16, 20–21, 24, 56, 103, 198, 207, 216,
  297–314
  conv, 21
  fft, 24
  ifft, 24
  optimization toolbox, 30, 56
  signal processing toolbox, 198, 216
Matrix, 297
  addition, 298
  diagonal form, 104
  ill-conditioned, 105
  inverse, 302–304
  multiplication, 298–299
  nonsingular, 303–304
  orthogonal, 253, 265–266, 271

rank, 304–306
  singular, 303
  transpose, 299–300
Maximum likelihood parameter estimation, 105
Maximum likelihood ICA, 271–277
Mean-centered data, 188, 249, 263–264
Mean vector, 316–317
Microlinearity, 86–87, 92, 95, 124, 198, 201
MINC data format, 14
Minimum variance unbiased estimator, 103
Mixed effects model, 171
Mixing matrix, 261
Mixture of normal distributions, 284–285
Modulus of a complex number, 193–194
Moments, 262–263, 269
MNI atlas, 64
MNI software, 14
Multi-level group analysis, 175–178
Multiple factor experiments, 176–178
Multivariate normal distribution, 316–319
  Gaussian random fields, 130–131
  GLM, 88, 101
  ICA, 257, 281–283
  PCA, 246–248, 251
Multivariate statistics, 81, 245, 287, 289, 292–293
Mutual information, 60, 268, 270–271, 273

Naïve Bayes classifier, 292
Negentropy, 269–271, 285
NIfTI data format, 13–14
Noise, 7–8, 41, 263
  coherence, effects on, 198
  GLM model of, 87, 106, 124
  Granger causality, effects on, 230
  PCA to reduce, 251–255
  preprocessing steps to reduce, 69, 71–77
Noise reduction with PCA, 251–255
Noise, effects on correlation, 186–187
Noisy ICA model, 281–285
Noninformative prior, 294
Nonlinear BOLD response, 33–39
Nonlinear registration, 66–68
Nonlinear transformation, 65
Non-normality in ICA, 263, 269–271
Nonparametric methods, 118–119, 156–157
Normal equations, 32, 103, 231–232
Normalization, 63–68
Nyquist-Shannon sampling theorem, 46, 73, 75, 218

Order of a matrix, 297
Order of a statistic, 262

Parameter estimation, 103–107, 231–233
Partial coherence, 209–211
Partial correlation, 210
Partial least squares, 292–293
Partial trials design, 91
Pattern classifiers, 291–292

Percent signal change, 119–123, 180
Permutation methods, 118–119, 156–157
PET scanning, 2, 79
Phantoms, 78
Phase of a complex number, 194
Phase spectrum, 211–219
Platykurtic distributions, 269
Positive definite, 314
Positive semi-definite, 247, 314
Postprocessing, 8
Power analysis, 178–183
Power spectrum, 193–196
Preprocessing, 8, 41–80
Preprocessing pipeline, 80
Prewhitening, 106
Principle components analysis, 246–257, 265,
  285–287, 292–293, 314
Prior distribution, 294
Probability density function, 315
Probabilistic ICA. See Noisy ICA
Proportional scaling, 79

Quality assurance, 78

Radial basis function, 66
Random effects model, 163–165, 170–176
Random factor, 162–165
Random field, 130. See also Gaussian random field
Random vector, 315
Region of interest, 113, 119, 136, 138, 205
Regression model, 102, 231
Resel, 132, 138–141

Satterthwaite approximation, 118
Scalar, 298
Scalar multiplication, 299
Scanner drift, 75–79, 88–89
Seed region, 205–207
Shimming, 5, 78
Sidak correction, 128–130
Signal-to-noise ratio, 69, 71–72, 106
Sinc function, 45
Sinc interpolation. See Interpolation
Singular-value decomposition, 293
Skewness, 262
Slice-timing correction, 42–51, 57–58
Smoothing, spatial, 68–73
Spatial extent, 147, 150–156
Spatial ICA, 258–261
Spline interpolation. See Interpolation
SPM, 8, 11, 13–14, 16, 45–46, 75, 79, 99–100, 106,
  113, 295
  DARTEL, 68
Square matrix, 297
Stationarity, 289
Statistical parametric map, 107–118, 127, 131, 147,
  159
Structural equation modeling, 292, 294

Structural scan, 4
Super-Gaussian distributions, 263, 269, 274, 284
Superposition principle, 18, 20, 33–34, 82, 86, 198, 201
Support vector machine, 292
SyN, 68

Talairach atlas, 64
Temporal correlation, 106–107, 117–118
Temporal derivative. *See* Hrf
Temporal filtering, 73–77
Temporal ICA, 258–260
Testable hypothesis, 110–111
Testing set, 292
Time-invariant linear system, 20–21
T-map, 112–115, 136–137, 153, 180
TR, 4
Tractography, 5
Training set, 292
Type I error, 113, 118, 127, 178
Type II error, 178

Uncertainty. *See* Information
Uniform distribution, 273
Univariate statistics, 81, 245, 287
Unmixing matrix, 261

Variance-covariance matrix, 246, 316–317
  diagonal representation, 246–247, 314
Vector, 298
Voodoo correlations, 157–158
Volterra series model, 35–39
Voxel, 4–5
Voxel size, 5, 58–59

Whitening, 263–266, 270
Within-subject variance, 163–167, 170–171, 175–178

Z-map, 131, 136